Comprehensive Computer Studies

Peter Bishop

Edward Arnold

First published 1981
by Edward Arnold (Publishers) Ltd
41 Bedford Square, London WC1B 3DQ

British Library Cataloguing in Publication Data

Bishop, Peter
Comprehensive computer studies.
1. Electronic data processing
I. Title
001.6′4 QA76

ISBN 0-7131-0371-X

Phototypesetting and illustrations by Parkway Group, London and Abingdon.
Printed in Great Britain by
Butler and Tanner Limited, London and Frome

Preface

The purpose and scope of this book

The purpose of this book is to provide a comprehensive introduction to electronic computers and computing. It is intended for use by school pupils taking an O Level, C.S.E. or equivalent course in Computer Studies, though it is also suitable for the general reader.

The book covers most of the topics common to O Level and C.S.E. Computer Studies syllabuses currently in use. A large number of questions from past examination papers are included in the exercises. To overcome the problem of the differences in the depth of treatment required by different syllabuses, several chapters have more than one section. The first section deals with the topic in broad outline, while further sections cover some aspects in slightly more detail. These further sections may be omitted without loss of continuity.

The small amount of mathematics that is used, is introduced very gradually. Special background mathematics sections are included for reference if necessary. Computer programming, using CESIL and BASIC languages, is discussed in several places, but this book does not aim to teach computer programming.

The structure of the book

The material of the book naturally divides itself into several parts:

The first three chapters introduce the basic ideas of information storage and processing, and describe the structure of a computer in broad outline. Chapters 4 to 8 describe the devices that make up a computer, in slightly more detail. Chapters 9 to 15 introduce and develop the logical processes used in computers. Chapters 16 to 20 describe how computers are put to work, and introduce analogue computers. Chapters 21 and 22 describe the history and social effects of computers.

The final chapter provides some material for projects on computers, as required by most examination boards. A wide variety of topics is introduced. Each includes a brief summary of the topic, followed by questions and suggestions for further study.

Terminology

An attempt is made to give a painless introduction to the more common technical terms used in connection with computers. A glossary is to be found at the end of the book to assist with this. All the terms used conform to the British Computer Society's Glossary of Computing Terms for Introductory Courses and to the ICL Glossary of Basic Computer Terms.

A model computer – the IMC-1

Computers are far too complicated for an introductory course to be able to describe any part of their internal working in detail. In order to give a 'feel' for some of the step-by-step processes carried out by computers, a much simplified model computer, the IMC-1 (Introductory Model Computer, Mark 1) is introduced. It contains the essential features of a digital computer, without any of the details.

At certain stages of the book, examples and exercises use the IMC-1 as a basis. These are, however, confined to chapters concerned with the detailed workings of computers. Most chapters refer to actual computers.

The world of computing

The world of computing is one of rapid progress. Every effort has been made to make this book an introduction to the current state of computers and computing, but as it works its way through the publication process, new developments will pass it by. The line has been drawn for inclusion of information at the time of completion of the manuscript – 18th March, 1979. Further developments will have to wait for further editions.

Acknowledgements

This book has been written from teaching notes developed and revised during several years of teaching Computer Studies at a comprehensive school. My colleagues Mr Peter Walker and Mrs Susan Stevens have given valuable help, both in reviewing material and in trying out sections of the book in the classroom.

The Publishers would like to thank Mr Paul McGee for reviewing early drafts of this book.

The CESIL language is used in this book by kind permission of the ICL Computer Education in Schools Project.

My thanks go to the following Examinations Boards who have given permission for questions from past examinations in Computer Studies to be included in the book:

AEB	Associated Examining Board
EAEB	East Anglian Examinations Board
JMB	Joint Matriculation Board
MREB	Metropolitan Regional Examinations Board
OLE	Oxford Delegacy of Local Examinations
UCLES	University of Cambridge Local Examinations Syndicate
WJEC	Welsh Joint Education Committee
WMEB	West Midlands Examinations Board
YREB	Yorkshire Regional Examinations Board

In addition to the examination board abbreviations, the year and paper number (where appropriate) are indicated after each question. For example:

(EAEB 78 I) means East Anglian Examinations Board, 1978, Paper I.

The Publisher's thanks are also due to the following for permission to reproduce photographs: pp 13, 141 & 143 left and right, Crown Copyright and the Science Museum; pp 129 & 130, Crown Copyright and the C.O.I.; p 147, Crown Copyright, The Science Museum and the United States Army; pp 1, 32 & 35 bottom, I.C.L.; p 2 top, Ford Motor Co. Ltd; p 2 bottom, Keystone Press and N.A.S.A.; p 3 top, Alfa-Laval; p 3 bottom & 16, the National Computing Centre Ltd; pp 4 top & 5 top, Merilyn Thorold; p 4 bottom, B.B.C.; pp 10, 27, 34, 36, 37, 38, 40, 41, 42 top & bottom, 57, 102, 146 bottom, 153 & 159, I.B.M. UK Ltd; pp 26 & 31, Honeywell and Geoffrey Sturdy; p 28, Ferranti Electronics Ltd; p 33, 92, 134, Data General; p 80, Intel Corporation; pp 100 & 160, Novosti Press; p 101, Burroughs Machines Ltd; p 111, British Airways; pp 117, 158, 164, Commodore Personal Computer Centre; p 127 top, Lloyds Bank Ltd; p 127 bottom, Williams & Glyn's Bank Ltd; p 131, British Aerospace and G.E.C.–Marconi Electronics; p 132, Keystone Press; p 139 top and bottom, Electronic Assoc. Ltd; p 144, 157 right, The Science Museum; p 146 top, The Public Records Office; p 148 left, The Dept. of Computer Science, University of Manchester; p 148, The Science Museum; p 152, Fiat Motor Co. Ltd; p 156, Associated Newspapers Ltd; p 161, The Anglo Chinese Educational Institute and Hsinhua News Agency; p 163 top left, Canon; p 163 top right, Seiko Time Ltd; p 163 centre left, Hewlett-Packard Ltd; p 163 centre right, and bottom, Aston Martin Lagonda; p 165, Julia Howlett, St. Margarets Software Ltd; p 167, The Tate Gallery and Arthur Tooth and Sons Ltd.

Note to the reader

In all the exercises, questions of above average difficulty are marked *. Some sections of the text are also marked in this way. These may be omitted without loss of continuity.

The Publishers would like to thank Microsense Computers Ltd and Lion Micro Computers for their help in producing the photograph on the front cover, showing a Beckman microchip image produced on the Apple II microcomputer.

Contents

1

Introduction

Electronic computers are an essential tool of modern society. In the thirty years since their beginnings in back rooms of universities and military research establishments, they have become the centre of an enormous industry. They have found a place in offices and factories, have landed on the moon, and will perhaps soon be as common in homes as television sets. A constant flow of new ideas, new devices, and new applications has kept up the rapid pace of development, a pace which shows no signs of slackening.

This chapter lays the foundations for a study of computers. It describes their capabilities and limitations, and introduces two ideas essential to computers – data and programs. It also introduces a very useful tool for working with computers – flow diagrams.

At first, computers had the image of mysterious electronic brains, with enormous power, and a will of their own. With computers becoming increasingly common, and more and more people working with them, much of this mystery has disappeared. They are seen to be reliable, fast and efficient, and, in common with all machines, capable of occasional breakdowns. Most important, it is being realised that computers can do no more than carry out their instructions.

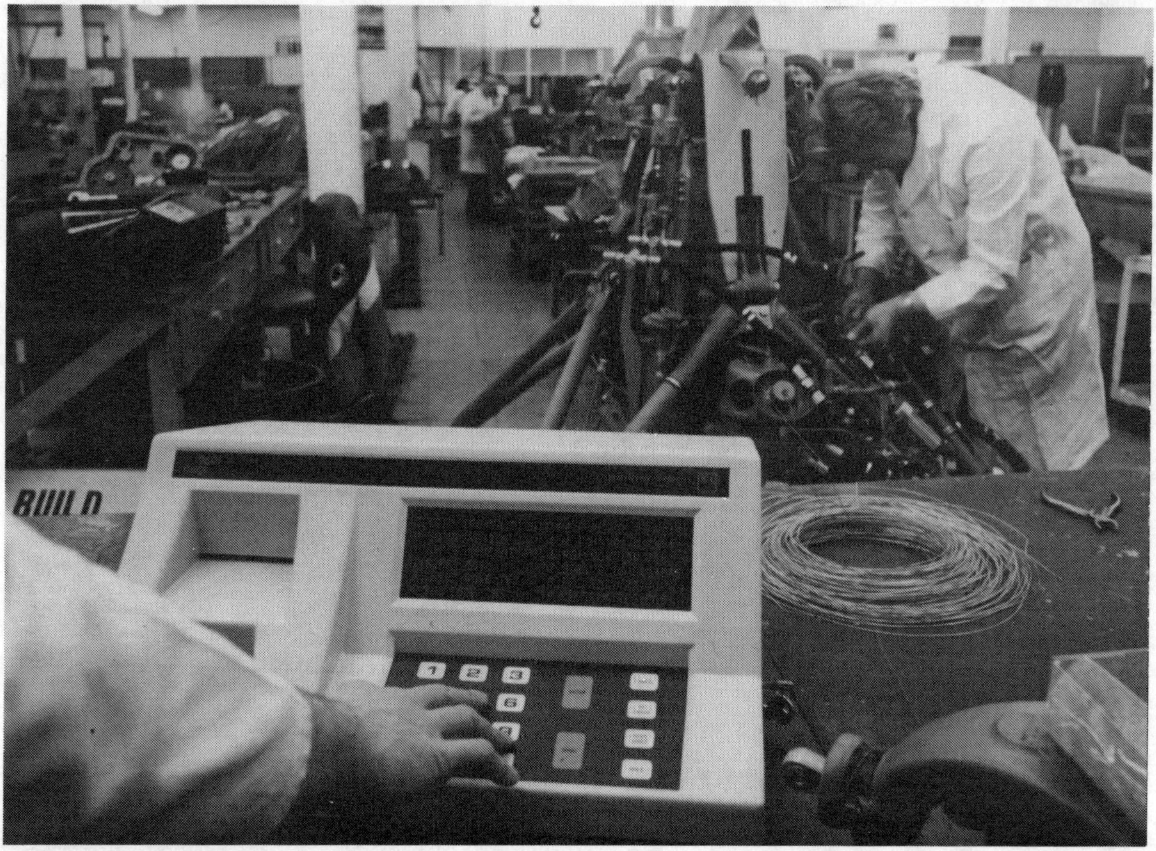

A computer terminal in a factory

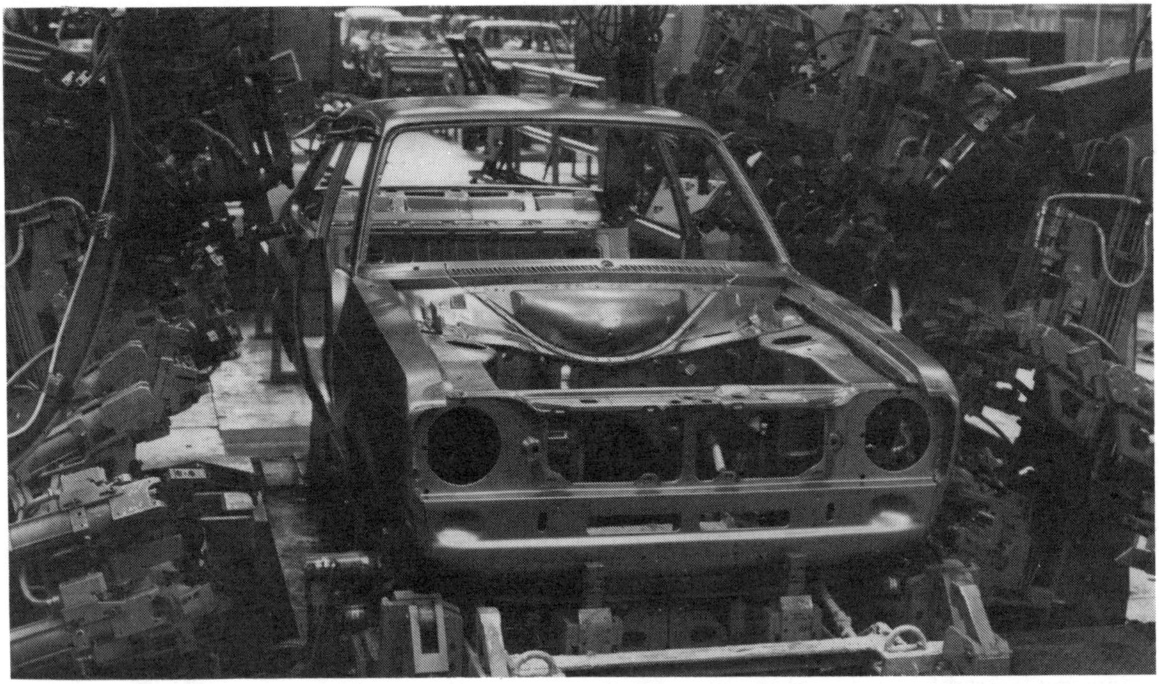

Computer-controlled welding equipment in a car factory

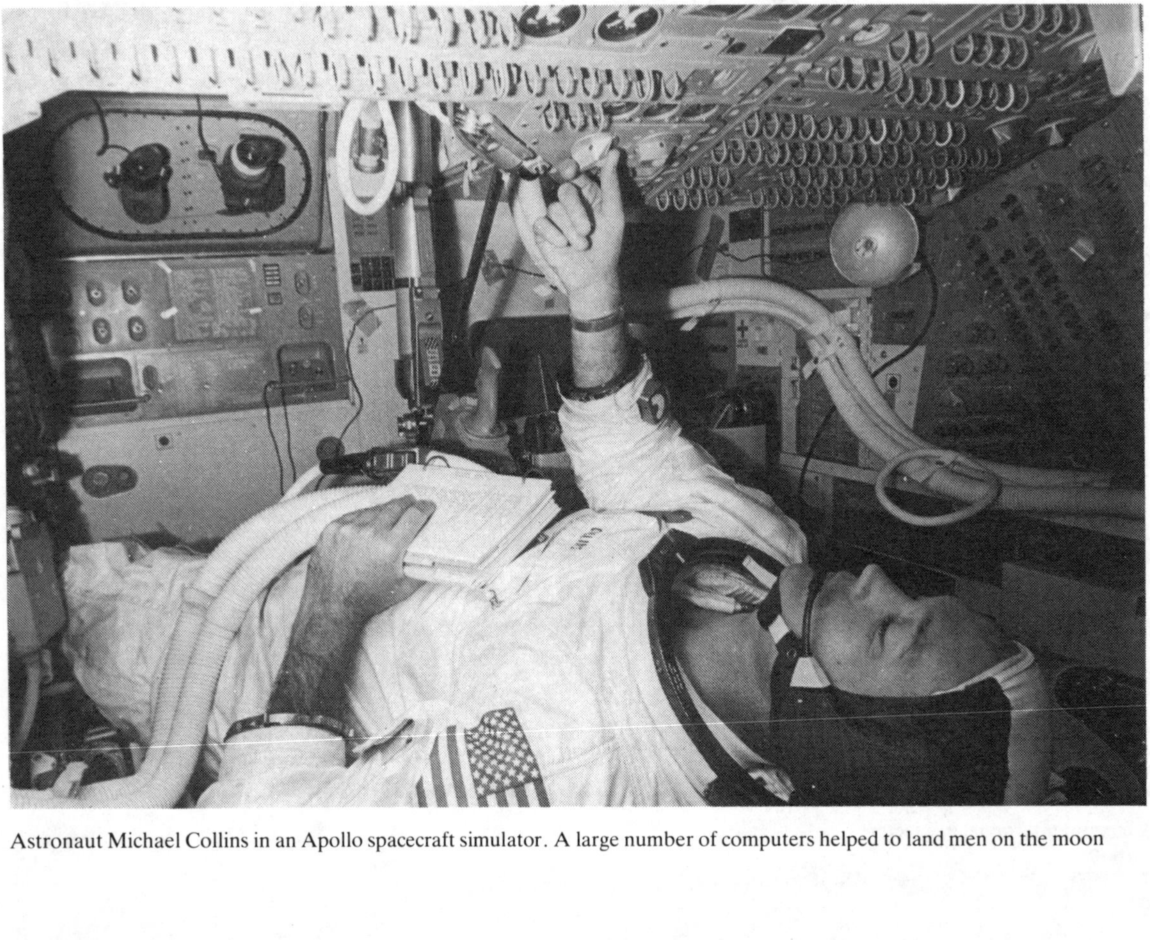

Astronaut Michael Collins in an Apollo spacecraft simulator. A large number of computers helped to land men on the moon

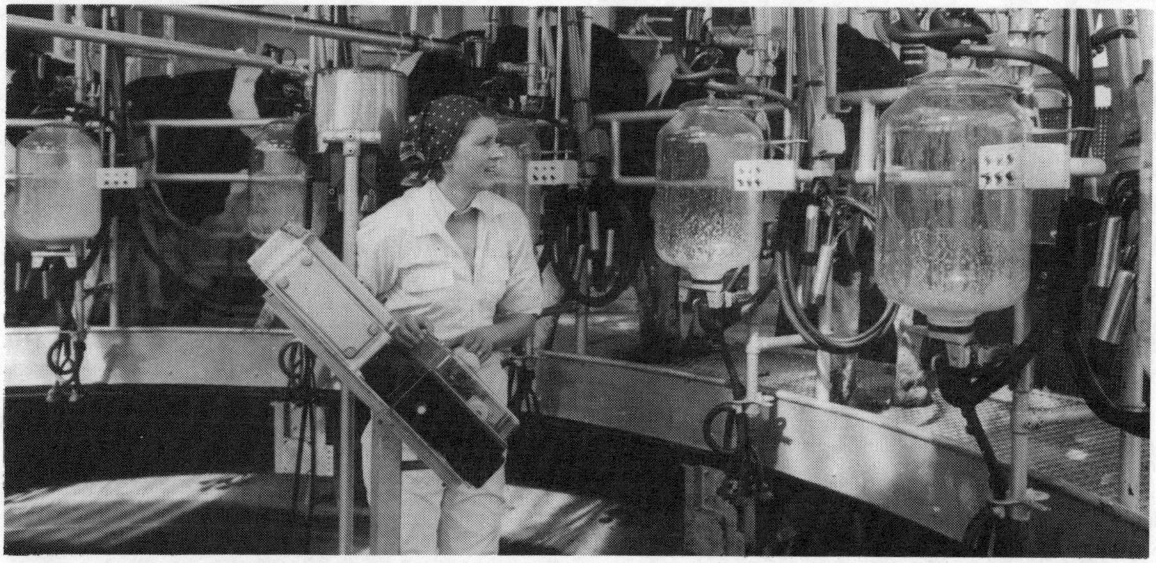

A microprocessor-controlled milking machine

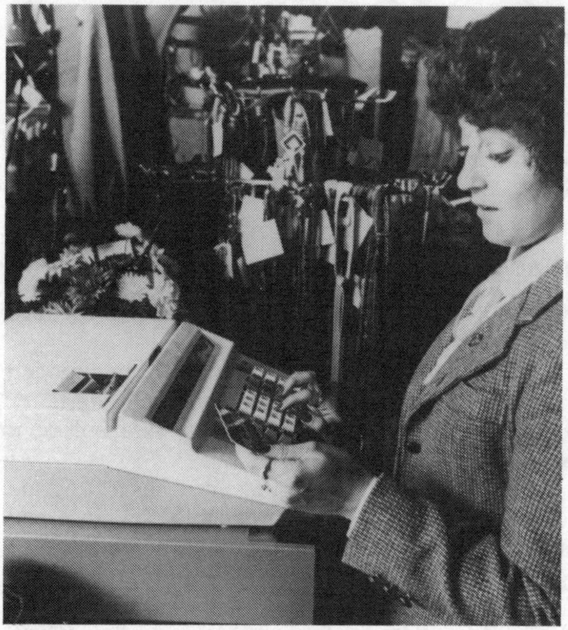

A computer terminal in a clothes shop

What can computers do?

Many people have very strange ideas about what computers can and cannot do. At the start of a study of computers, it is essential to be quite clear what their capabilities and limitations are.

Computers can calculate. They can also store information, and find it when needed. Computers can sort information and combine it in different ways. This information is not always numbers. It can be words or codes.

Computers can be instructed to make certain decisions, but a computer cannot think for itself, or understand anything.

Therefore a brief answer to the question, 'what can computers do?' is:

computers can process information

Information for a computer: Data

Computers process many different kinds of information:

prices, bank balances, names and addresses, wages, taxes, temperatures and a host of others.

However, while it is being used by a computer, information must be in a special form, often in a code.

Data
Information in a form which can be processed by a computer is called **data.**
Large stores of information are very common:

telephone directories, dictionaries, catalogues, bank statements, election registers and many others.

Similar large stores of information are often kept on computers.

Hopefully, when a person uses some information, that person understands what the information means. But this is not so with computers. Although a computer processes data, it does not understand it. Data means nothing to a computer. For

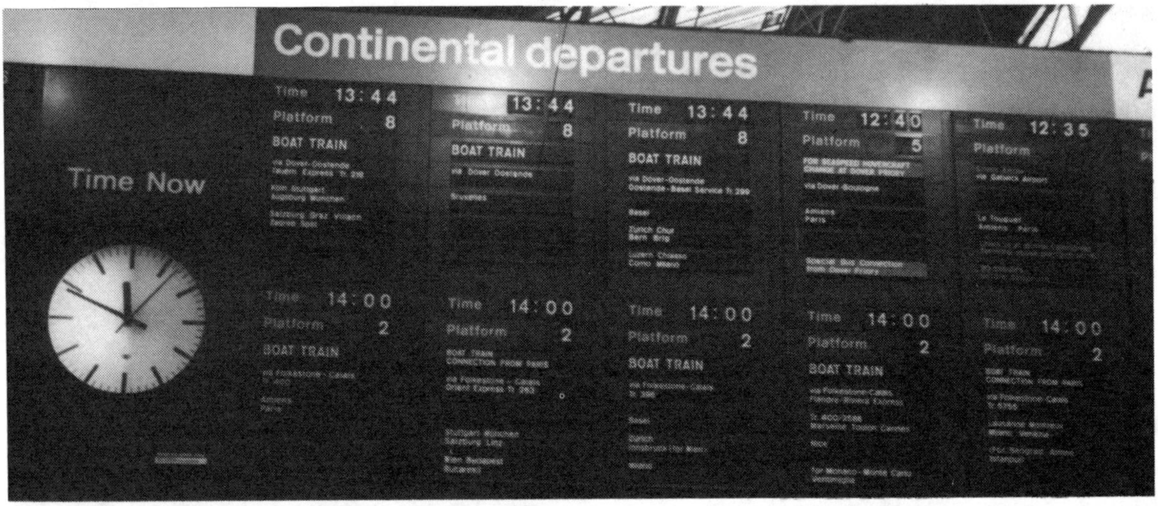

Information for the rail traveller

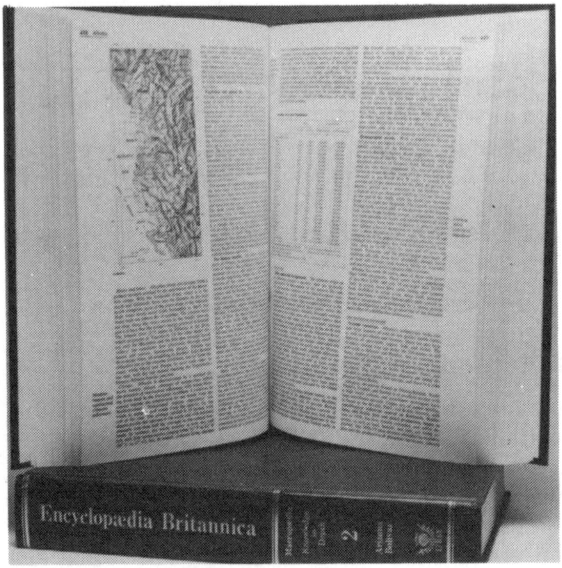

A rich source of information – an encyclopaedia

example, if a person's name is spelled wrongly, a computer will not usually notice. Most important, if the data used by a computer is wrong, the results it produces will be wrong. In the computer world, there is a saying about this: **Garbage in, garbage out,** sometimes shortened to GIGO.

Instructions to a computer

Everything a computer does is in response to instructions. A computer cannot do anything without being instructed.

One might argue that a number of other devices only work in response to instructions. What makes computers different from pocket calculators, lifts, stoves, taps and windscreen wipers?

Programs

The answer is that computers can store a large number of instructions, and then work through them one at a time. A set of instructions to a computer is called a **program.**

It's rather like an automatic washing machine

Computers and automatic washing machines have much in common.

An automatic washing machine must be supplied with clothes, soap and water before it starts. A computer must be supplied with data before it starts.

An automatic washing machine has a program which tells it how many times to wash, rinse and spin the clothes. It works through the entire program by itself. A computer has a program which tells it how to process the data – what calculations to do, what data to store, etc. It works through all the steps of the program by itself.

At the end of the process, the washing is taken out of the washing machine. Similarly, a computer prints out its results when it has finished processing.

However, this analogy must not be taken too far. A computer can do a much wider range of tasks than a washing machine.

Input, process and output

All data processing, whether it is done by a com-

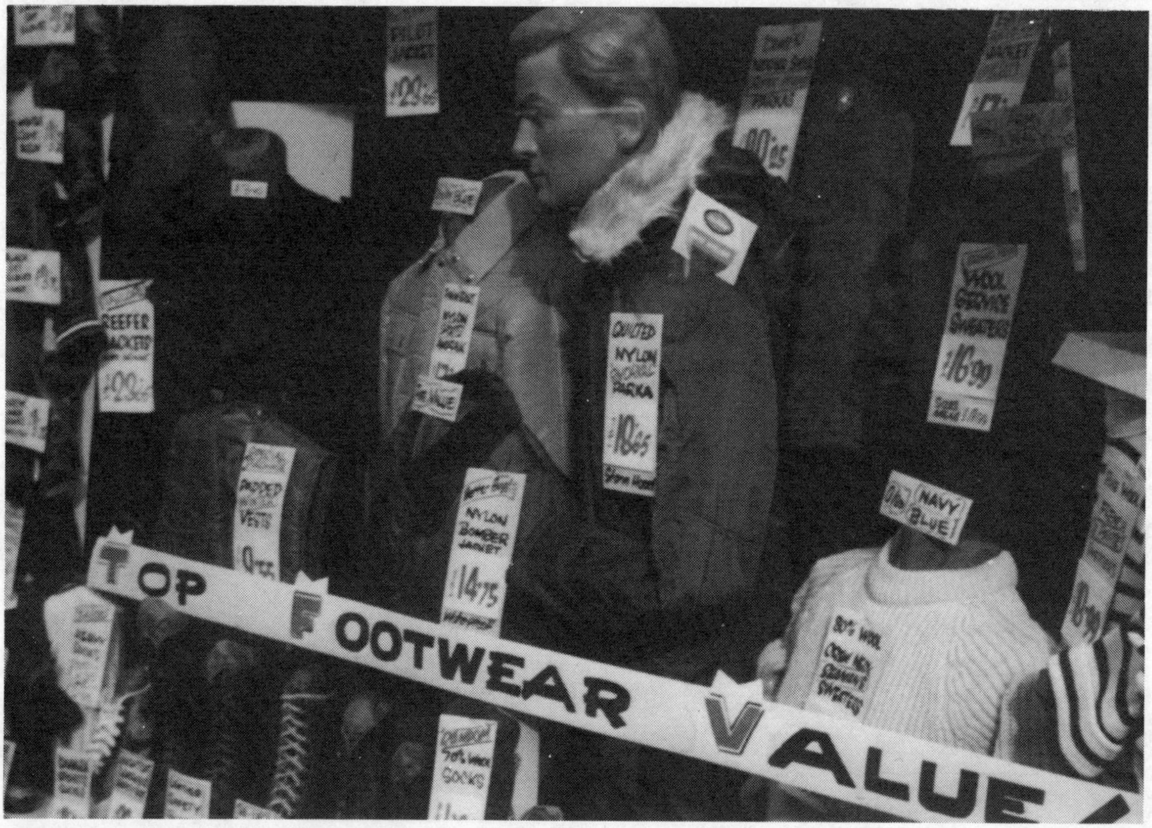

Information on display

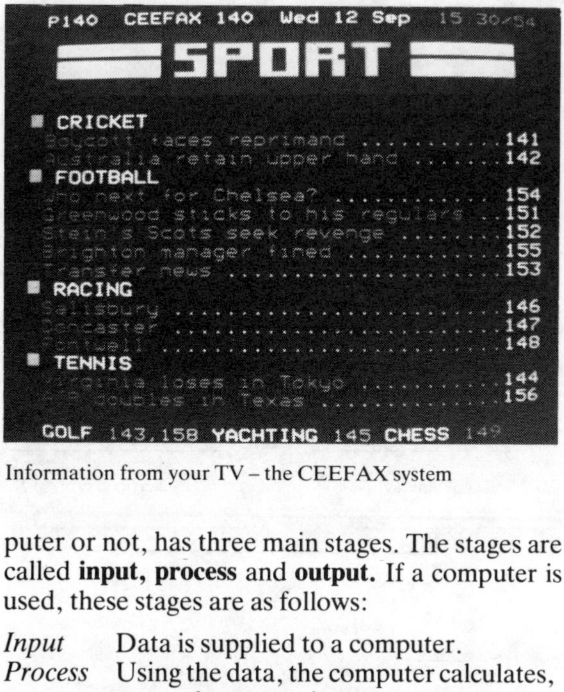

Information from your TV – the CEEFAX system

puter or not, has three main stages. The stages are called **input, process** and **output.** If a computer is used, these stages are as follows:

Input Data is supplied to a computer.
Process Using the data, the computer calculates, stores data, sorts it, etc.
Output The results are printed out by the computer.

The data processing questions

Unlike some people, a computer cannot work in a haphazard way. Data processing must be done in an orderly fashion. One way of ensuring this is to ask three questions about any data processing task:

1 What input is required?
2 What processing is done?
3 What is the output?

These questions can be asked about many everyday tasks. They make the task easier to understand, and also easier to do.

For example, asking the questions about the task of replying to a letter from a friend:

1 *What input is required?* Read the friend's letter.
2 *What processing is done?* Decide what to write.
3 *What is the output?* Write a letter in reply.

Another example is producing a gas bill:

1 *What input is required?* The old and new meter

readings, the account number, name and address, and the price of the gas.
2 *What processing is done?* The amount of gas used and the cost are calculated.
3 *What is the output?* A gas bill, showing an account number, name, address, meter readings and amount to pay.

Replying to a letter is not usually done on a computer, but working out a gas bill usually is. Both tasks have input, process and output stages.

Flow diagrams

Another systematic way to describe the various steps of a task is to use a **flow diagram.** Each step is written in a box, and arrows are used to join the boxes. Different types of step have different shapes of box. The ones most frequently used are shown in Figure 1.1.

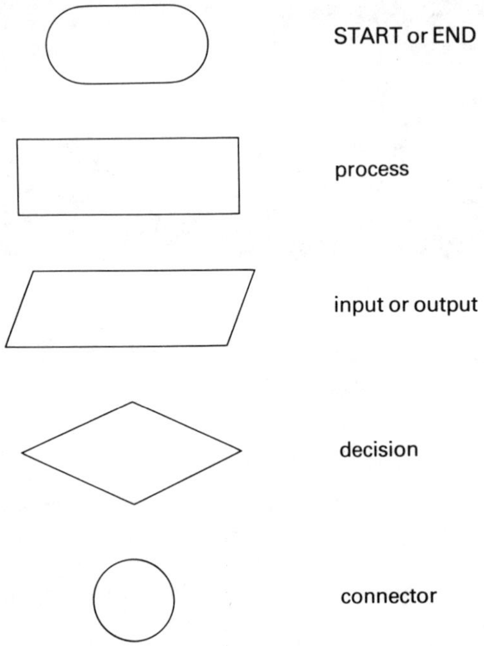

Fig. 1.1. Flow diagram symbols

A flow diagram is sometimes called a **flowchart.** Flow diagrams can be used to describe many everyday situations, as well as tasks which are done on computers.

Example 1 Replying to a letter from a friend. See Figure 1.2.

Example 2 A person has collected a number of leaflets about holidays from travel agents. He will select a holiday if (a) it is in July, (b) it costs less than £400, (c) he has not been there before.

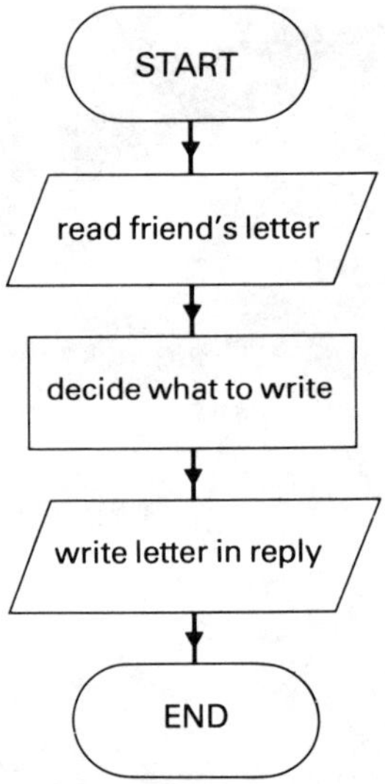

Fig. 1.2. Flowchart of replying to a letter from a friend

Draw a flowchart of the process of accepting or rejecting a holiday. (Figure 1.3)

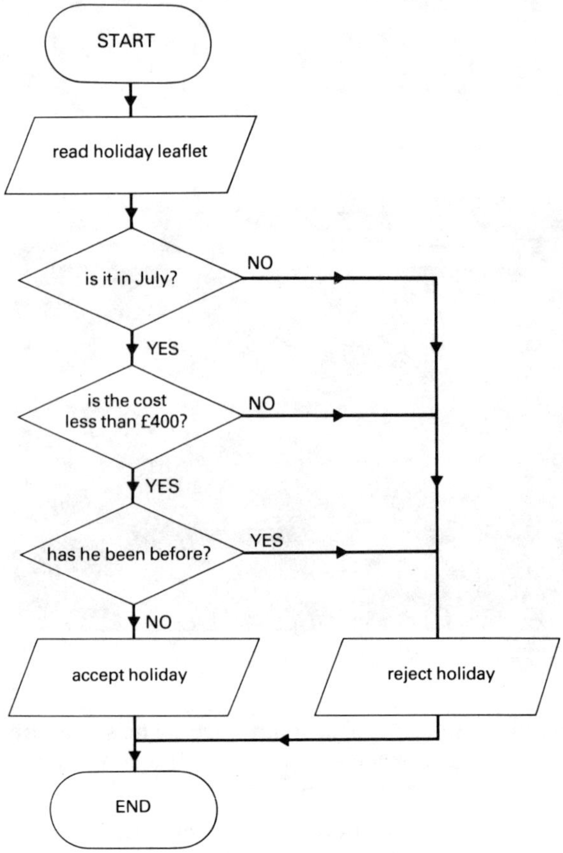

Fig. 1.3. Flowchart of accepting or rejecting a holiday

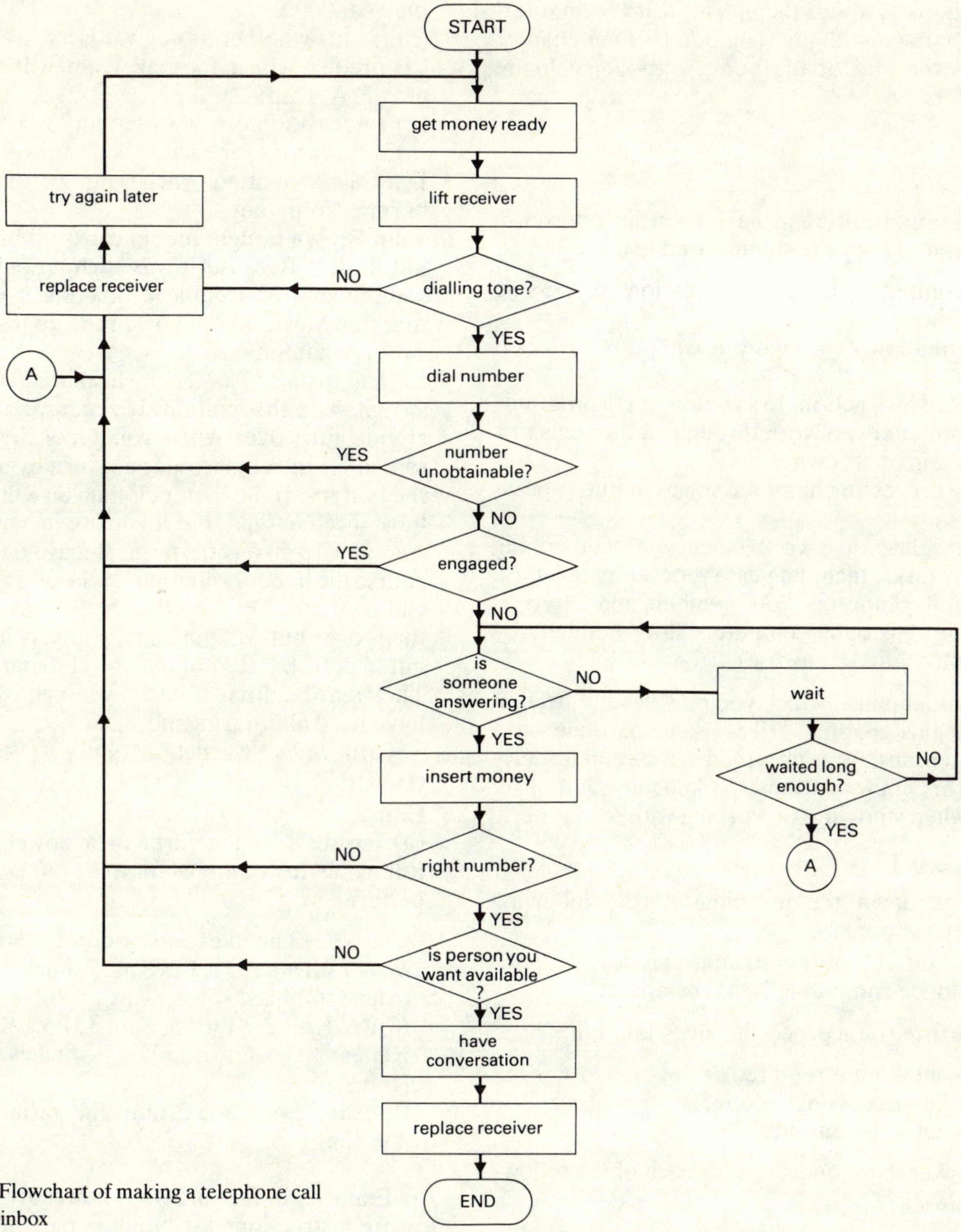

Fig. 1.4. Flowchart of making a telephone call from a coinbox

Example 3 Draw a flow diagram to show all the steps involved in using a public (coin operated) telephone. Assume that you have the right money, know the number you want, and can dial it directly. (Figure 1.4)

Analogue and digital computers

Electronic computers can be divided into two types, depending on the way they represent information. In the first type, called **digital computers,** numbers and letters are represented as digits, in some code.

In the second type, called **analogue computers,** numbers are represented by the strengths of electric currents. The stronger the current, the larger the number.

Another example of analogue and digital devices is clocks. Ordinary clocks are analogue devices – they show the time by the position of their hands. Digital clocks represent the time as digits.

Most computers are digital computers, and most

of this book is about them. The word 'computer' normally means 'digital computer'. One chapter towards the end of the book is about analogue computers.

Summary

Several important ideas have been introduced in this chapter. They are summarized here:

- ☐ A computer is an information processing machine.
- ☐ Information as used by a computer is called data.
- ☐ A set of instructions to a computer is a program.
- ☐ A computer can work through all the steps of a program on its own.
- ☐ Data processing has three stages: input, process and output.
- ☐ A flow diagram is a convenient way of describing many tasks, including data processing tasks.
- ☐ Digital computers store numbers and letters as digits. Analogue computers store numbers by the strengths of electric currents.

One final point, which you may have noticed in reading this chapter. All work to be done on a computer must be approached in a careful, orderly way. This approach must be kept in mind at all times when studying, or working with, computers.

Exercise 1

1 Write down the meanings of the following words or phrases:
data; GIGO; program; input; process; output; analogue computer; digital computer.

2 The three data processing questions are:

1 What input is required?
2 What processing is done?
3 What is the output?

Answer these questions for each of the following tasks:

(a) Baking a cake.
(b) Making a model aeroplane.
(c) Producing a telephone bill.
(d) Growing vegetables.
(e) Repairing a motor car.

3 Draw flow diagrams for the tasks in question **2.**

4 Do you think that computers can be programmed to

(a) calculate the positions of the planets in the year 2000.
(b) estimate the number of people on earth in the year 2000.
(c) decide whether or not war is a bad thing.
(d) predict which football team will win the next F.A. Cup.
(e) forecast tomorrow's weather?
Give reasons for each of your answers.

***5** Data is information which is not worth remembering. Comment.

6 John Brown bought an old car from his friend Sid Smart. Because it was such an old car he sometimes had trouble in making it go. The first time it would not go he rang up his friend. This is what Sid said.

'Will it start? No! Then check that you have switched on the ignition. If you have, does the engine turn over when you press the starter switch? If the engine does not turn over, check the battery. If the battery is flat you will have to have it re-charged, but if you are in a hurry get someone to give you a push. It may go then. Of course the battery wires may be loose or broken. Check them. On the other hand if the engine turns over but will not start, you may have run out of petrol. If it's not that, try the spark plugs. They may be dirty. If it still won't go when you have tried all this ring me again.'

Turn Sid's instructions into a flowchart. (EAEB 76 II)

7 Either

(a) Express, in the form of a flowchart, the following instructions for part of a knitting pattern:

Use No. 12 needles and cast on 121 stitches.
Row 1 *Knit 1, Purl 1, Knit 5, Purl 1. Repeat from * until last stitch. Knit 1.
Row 2 Knit 2, *Purl 5, Knit 1, Purl 1, Knit 1. Repeat from * to the last 7 stitches. Purl 5, Knit 2.
Repeat rows 1 and 2 until the garment is 10 inches long.

Or

(b) Express, in the form of a flowchart, the following instructions for building part of a brick wall.

Row 1 Lay 30 red bricks.
Row 2 Lay $\frac{1}{2}$ a red brick, 1 red brick, *5 white bricks, 2 red bricks. Repeat from * until the last $\frac{1}{2}$ brick. Lay $\frac{1}{2}$ a red brick.
Row 3 *Lay 1 red brick, $\frac{1}{2}$ a red brick, $\frac{1}{2}$ a white brick, 4 white bricks, $\frac{1}{2}$ a white brick, $\frac{1}{2}$ a red brick. Repeat from * until the last 2 bricks. Lay 2 red bricks.
Repeat rows 2 and 3 until the wall is over 80 cm high. (WMEB 74 II)

2

The overall structure of a computer

The previous chapter introduced some general ideas of information processing. This chapter shows how the design of a computer puts these ideas into practice.

Computers come in many shapes and sizes. The smallest computers are no larger than a typewriter, the biggest fill several large rooms. Prices range from a few hundred to several million pounds.

A typical medium sized computer

This chapter is concerned with the overall structure of a typical medium sized computer. It would be housed in a room about 8 metres square, and cost between £20000 and £200000. This chapter describes the purpose of each part of the computer, and the way the parts are linked together.

At first sight, most computers appear to be a collection of grey boxes, of various shapes and sizes. Here and there a few lights flash, and every now and then reels of magnetic tape, and a long roll of paper, are seen to move. But on the whole it is not at all obvious what is happening.

Units

Each of the grey boxes is called a **device,** or a **unit.** Each does part of the whole information processing operation. The units are connected by a large number of wires underneath the floor of the computer room.

A typical medium sized computer consists of the following units: a central processing unit (called a **CPU** for short), input devices, output devices, backing store, terminals and an operator's console. The photograph and Figure 2.1 show what they look like, and how they are linked together. Notice the flow of data between the various units, and how they are controlled.

The central processing unit

The actual processing of data takes place in the **central processing unit.** It has no moving parts. It consists entirely of solid state electronic components such as transistors and integrated circuits. In older computers there are small rings of a magnetic substance for storing data. All the work of the CPU is done by means of small pulses of electricity.

The CPU has three parts, as shown in Figure 2.2.

The **control unit** co-ordinates the step-by-step running of the whole computer. It shares control of all the units of the computer with the operator's console. The **arithmetic and logic unit** (ALU) does the calculations and makes the decisions. The **memory** stores the data and programs that are in use at the time.

The other devices connected to the CPU are called **peripherals.** They communicate data to and from the CPU, and provide additional storage.

Input devices

The **input devices** receive data from sources outside the computer. The data may be typed in directly, or read from punched cards, paper tape or other storage **media.** The input devices convert the data to the patterns of electrical pulses used by the CPU.

Output devices

The **output devices** change the electrical pulses from the CPU into printed or displayed characters.

Backing store

Backing store gives the computer rapid access to very large quantities of data, far more than can be stored in the CPU memory. The most common backing store media are magnetic tapes and magnetic discs.

Terminals

Terminals provide direct communication between the computer and a person using it. Terminals can be connected to the computer from a long distance, via telephone lines. Terminals can be used to program the computer, or for input and output of data.

Operator's console

Of course a computer cannot work entirely on its

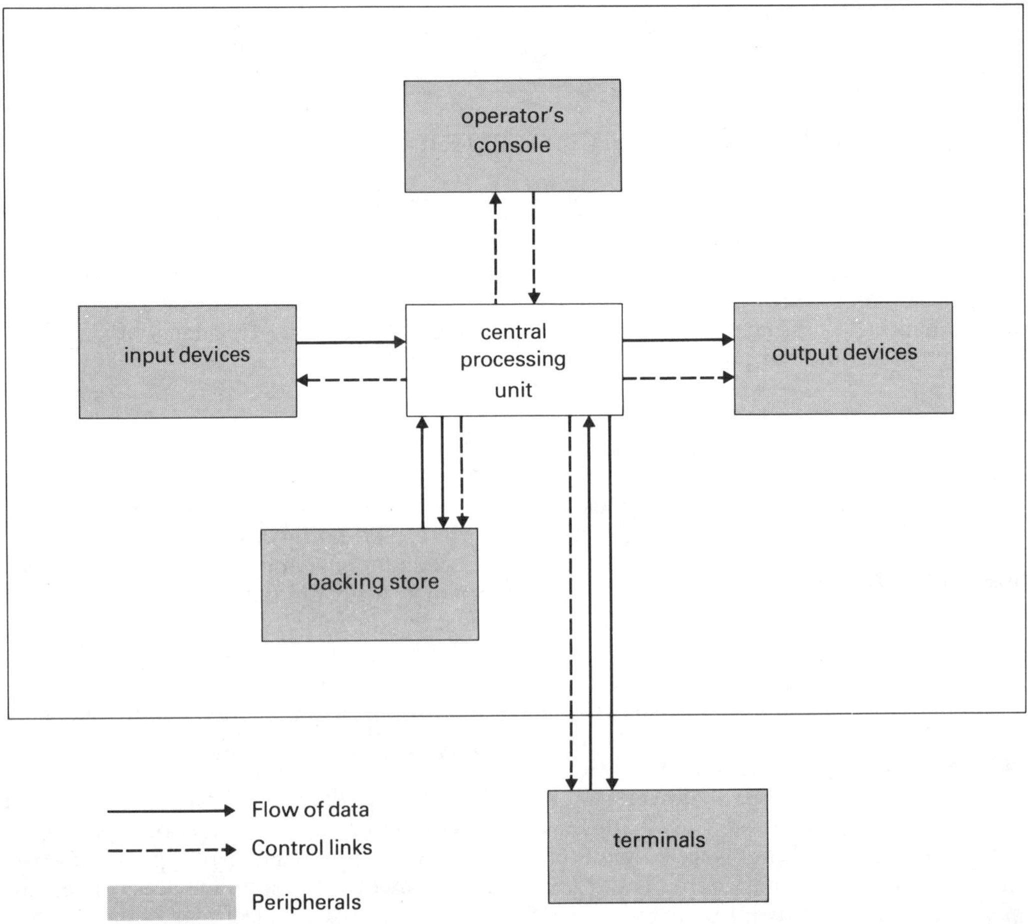

Fig. 2.1. The units of a typical medium sized computer

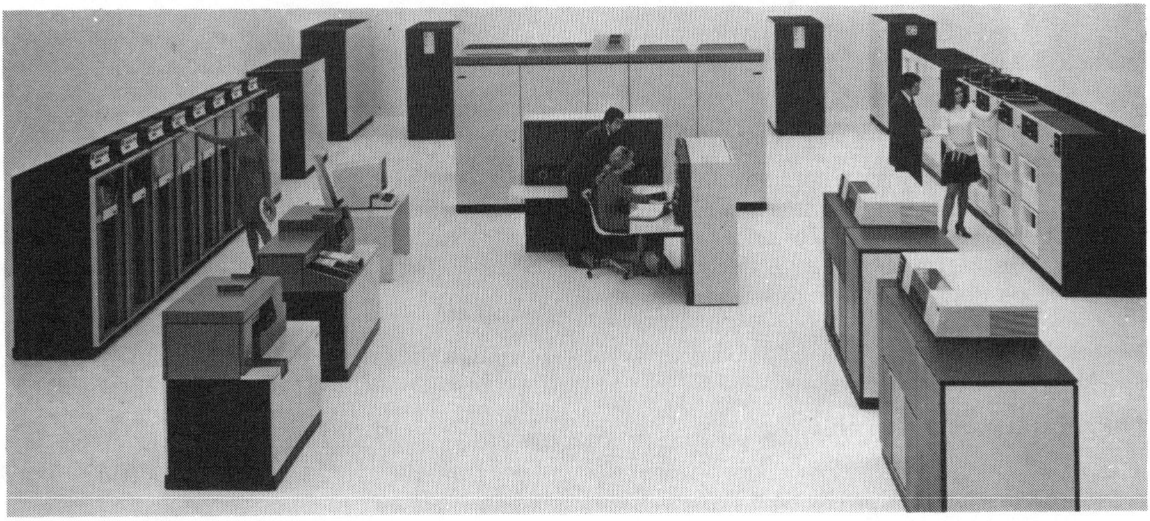

A computer of the sort described in the text. In the centre is the operator's console, behind which is the CPU. On the far left and right are backing store units, magnetic tape units and magnetic disc drives respectively. In the foreground, on the left are two card readers and on the right are two line printers

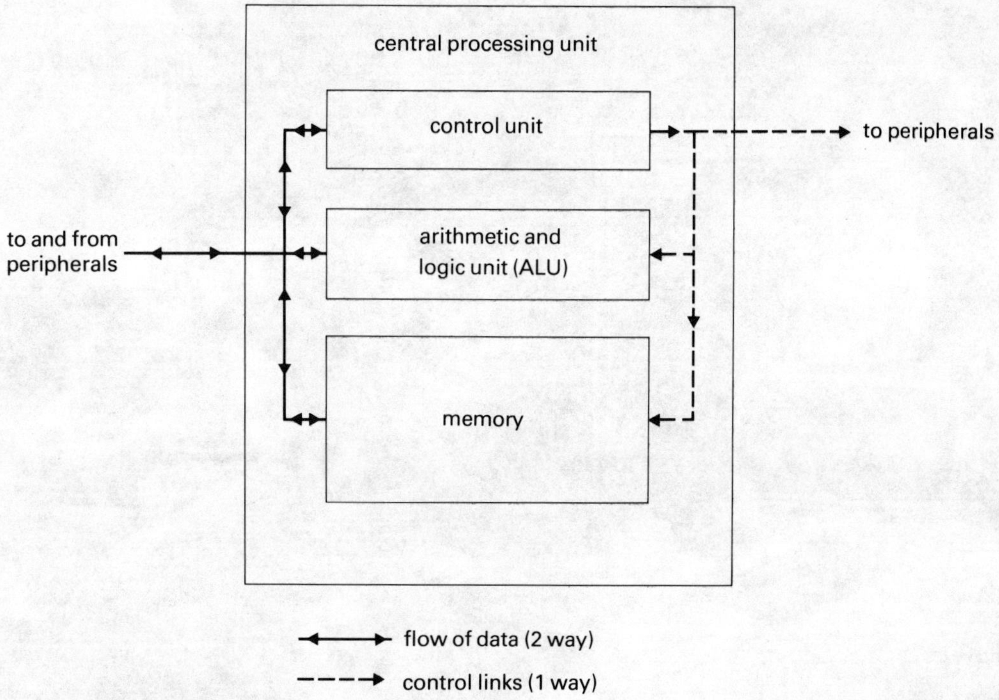

Fig. 2.2. The parts of a central processing unit

own. There is an **operator's console,** which connects with the control unit of the CPU. It has a keyboard similar to that on a typewriter. Instructions are typed by the computer operator, and messages are sent by the computer to the operator. In this way, control of the computer is shared between the person operating it, and the control unit of the CPU.

Large and small computers

Computers vary considerably in size. Large computers may have more than one CPU, and many peripheral units. Small computers are called **minicomputers.** The smallest computers, called **microcomputers,** are often enclosed in a single unit. The unit contains input, output and processing devices, and sometimes backing store. The input device is also used for operating instructions.

Some popular computers

Several computer manufacturers make computers which closely resemble the description in this chapter. Some popular models are:
ICL 1900 and **ICL 2900** series, made by International Computers Limited, a British company.
IBM 360 and **IBM 370** series, made by International Business Machines, based in the U.S.A.
PDP8 and **PDP11** series of minicomputers, made by Digital Equipment Corporation, also based in the U.S.A.

Popular microcomputers include the Commodore PET, the Research Machines 380Z, the Tandy TRS-80, the Sinclair ZX80 and the Apple 2.

Hardware and software

This chapter has provided a very brief introduction to the **hardware** of a computer – the components which make up a computer. The programs which enable the hardware to be put to work are called **software.**

Each hardware device mentioned in this chapter is described in more detail later in the book. When each device is discussed separately, it is important to bear in mind how it fits in to the overall structure of a computer.

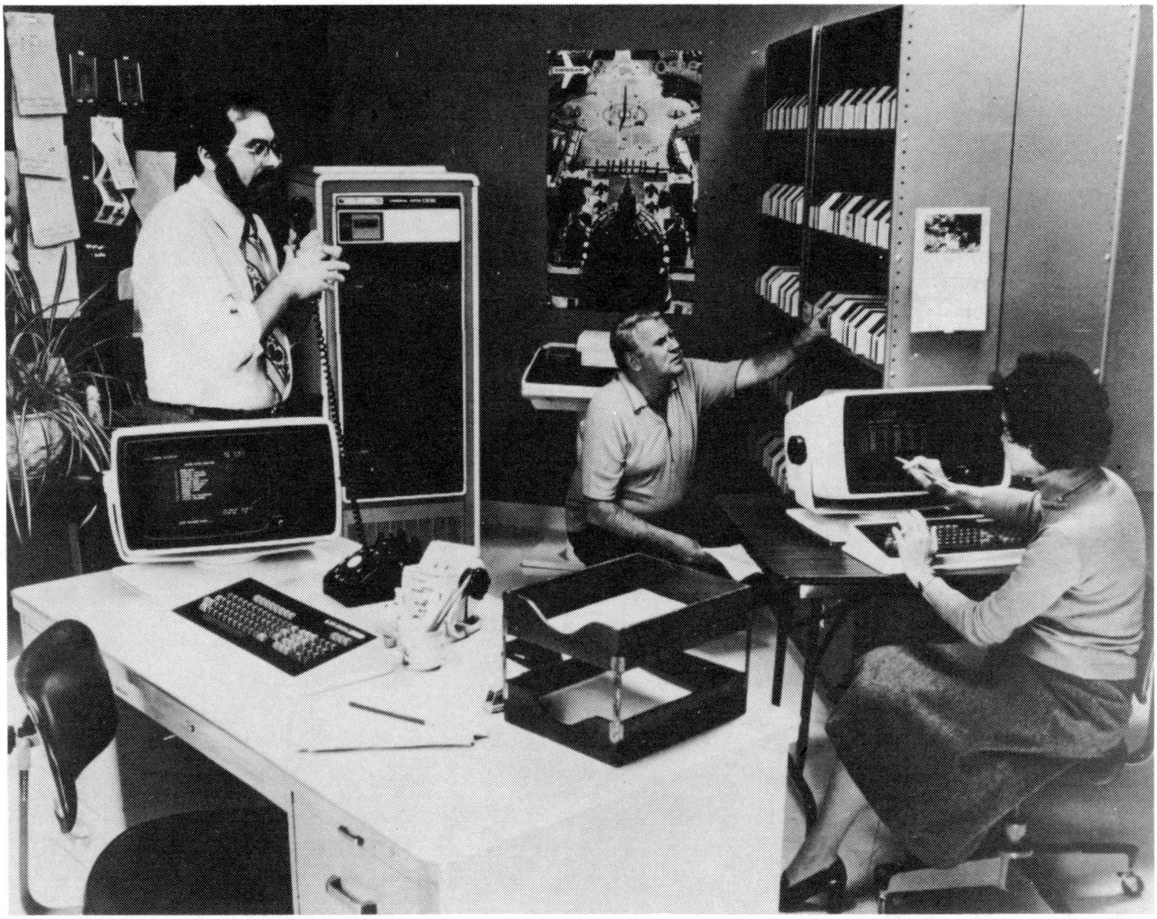

A Data General small business computer

Exercise 2

1 Write down the meanings of the following words or phrases:
device; CPU; control unit; ALU; memory; peripheral; input devices; output devices; backing store; terminal; operator's console; hardware; software.

2 Which of the following are parts of the CPU? ALU, backing store, memory, control unit, operator's console

3 Which unit of a computer has no moving parts?

4 List some types of peripheral devices.

5 Which unit co-ordinates the step-by-step running of the whole computer?

6 Find some photographs of computers. Try to identify the different units.

7 Figure 2.3 shows a clerk at work calculating and making out bills. If a computer was used for the same task what devices or units of the computer would correspond to

(a) the filing cabinet,
(b) the calculating machine, (c) the IN tray,
(d) the clerk? (EAEB 78 I)

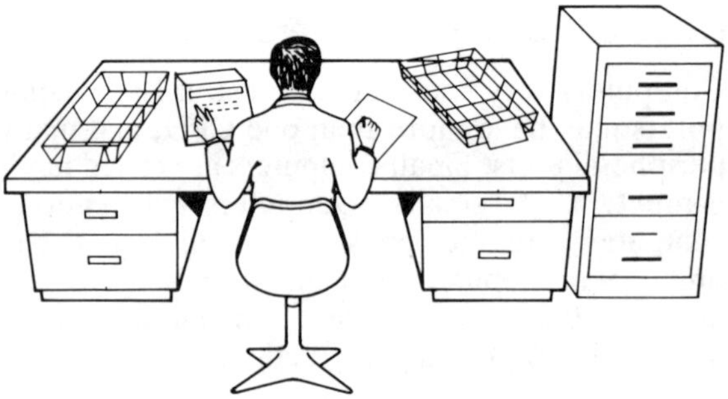

Fig. 2.3.

3

Coding and storing data

Section A

You will remember from a previous chapter that data is information in a form which can be used by a computer. In other words, data is a representation of information. This chapter explains some of the ways in which data is coded and stored on computers.

Unfortunately, different computers use different ways of representing data. Very often the same item of data is coded differently during input, processing, storage and output on one computer. The way in which data is represented depends on the physical medium storing it, or the device processing it, and the nature and purpose of the data.

Bits and bistable devices

Coding and storing of data is made simpler by the fact that all the storage media and processing devices in a computer have one feature in common – they have two **states** only. For example, a switch has two states – on and off. Figure 3.1 shows some more examples. Devices with only two stable states are called **bistable devices.**

The codes most suited to these storage media and processing devices use only two characters. For this reason, all the codes which represent data on a computer use only two characters, the digits 0 and 1.

There is a number system which only uses the digits 0 and 1, namely the base two or **binary** system. Binary forms the basis of most number codes on computers. The binary digits 0 and 1 are called **bits.**

Different data codes

As mentioned previously, there are a number of different codes for representing data on computers. The most widely used ones, which are discussed in the chapter, are **character codes, sign-and-magnitude, 2's complement** and **1's complement** codes for numbers. **Fixed point** and **floating point** numbers are introduced in the second section of the chapter, as well as the use of base eight and base sixteen numbers to describe data coded in binary.

The next few sections depend on some knowledge of binary numbers, and of negative numbers. If you are not familiar with either of these, you are advised to read the section on binary numbers and negative numbers at the end of the chapter.

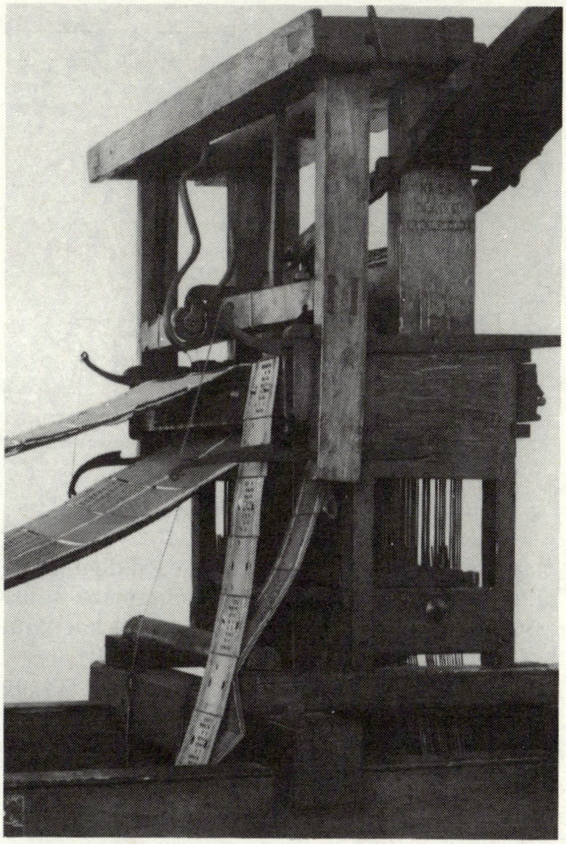

Information in a binary code on punched cards controlling a weaving loom

Place value

In these sections the idea of **place value** is also important. Here is a brief reminder of what it means:

A number in any base is written as a set of digits. In base ten, the digits are 0, 1, . . . 9, and in base two

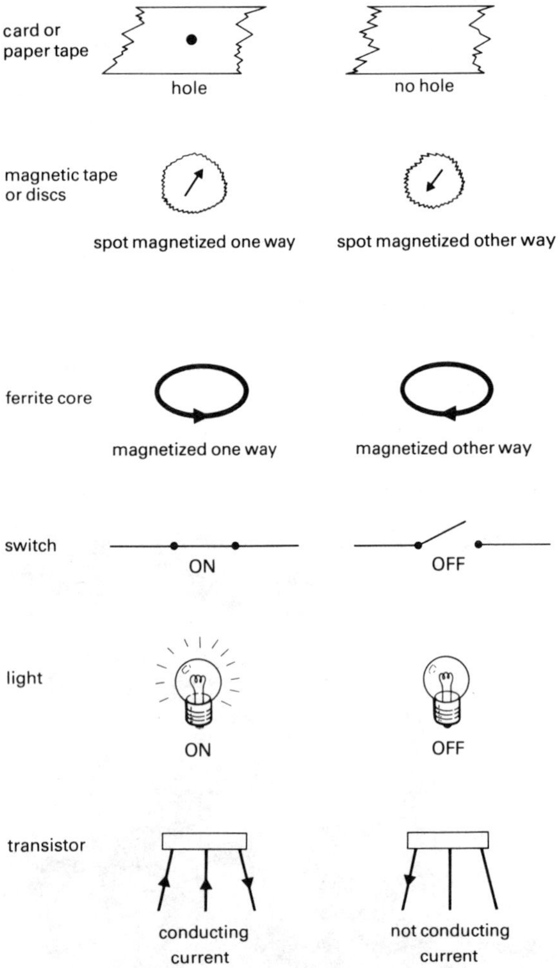

Fig. 3.1. Bistable devices and two state storage media

they are 0 and 1. The position of each digit in the number is important. There is a place value associated with each position. In a base ten number, the place values are (from right to left), units, tens, hundreds etc., and in a base two number they are units, twos, fours, eights, etc.

The digit with the highest place value is called the **most significant** digit, and the one with the lowest place value the **least significant** digit. For example:

In base two 1 0 0 1 0 1 0

most significant digit — least significant digit

In base ten 361 497

most significant bit — least significant bit

Character codes

Data for use by digital computers is generally expressed as characters. Characters include the digits 0 to 9, letters and punctuation marks. They are called **numeric, alphabetic** (together known as **alphanumeric**) and **special** characters respectively.

The characters which a computer can store and process form the **character set** of that computer. Different types of computer have different character sets.

Character code is a type of code where a group of binary digits (usually six or eight) is used to represent each character. Figure 3.2 shows the character set and character code for ICL 1900 series computers.

On almost all computers, input and output data, and data stored on backing store is in character code. Numbers are sometimes kept in character code during calculations, and at other times changed to one of the codes mentioned later, depending on the type of computer, and the purpose of the calculations.

character	code	character	code
0	0 0 0 0 0 0	@	1 0 0 0 0 0
1	0 0 0 0 0 1	A	1 0 0 0 0 0
2	0 0 0 0 1 0	B	1 0 0 0 1 0
3	0 0 0 0 1 1	C	1 0 0 0 1 1
4	0 0 0 1 0 0	D	1 0 0 1 0 0
5	0 0 0 1 0 1	E	1 0 0 1 0 1
6	0 0 0 1 1 0	F	1 0 0 1 1 0
7	0 0 0 1 1 1	G	1 0 0 1 1 1
8	0 0 1 0 0 0	H	1 0 1 0 0 0
9	0 0 1 0 0 1	I	1 0 1 0 0 1
:	0 0 1 0 1 0	J	1 0 1 0 1 0
;	0 0 1 0 1 1	K	1 0 1 0 1 1
<	0 0 1 1 0 0	L	1 0 1 1 0 0
=	0 0 1 1 0 1	M	1 0 1 1 0 1
>	0 0 1 1 1 0	N	1 0 1 1 1 0
?	0 0 1 1 1 1	O	1 0 1 1 1 1
space	0 1 0 0 0 0	P	1 1 0 0 0 0
!	0 1 0 0 0 1	Q	1 1 0 0 0 1
"	0 1 0 0 1 0	R	1 1 0 0 1 0
#	0 1 0 0 1 1	S	1 1 0 0 1 1
£	0 1 0 1 0 0	T	1 1 0 1 0 0
%	0 1 0 1 0 1	U	1 1 0 1 0 1
&	0 1 0 1 1 0	V	1 1 0 1 1 0
'	0 1 0 1 1 1	W	1 1 0 1 1 1
(	0 1 1 0 0 0	X	1 1 1 0 0 0
)	0 1 1 0 0 1	Y	1 1 1 0 0 1
*	0 1 1 0 1 0	Z	1 1 1 0 1 0
+	0 1 1 0 1 1	[	1 1 1 0 1 1
,	0 1 1 1 0 0	$	1 1 1 1 0 0
–	0 1 1 1 0 1	]	1 1 1 1 0 1
.	0 1 1 1 1 0	↑	1 1 1 1 1 0
/	0 1 1 1 1 1	new line	1 1 1 1 1 1

Fig. 3.2. The ICL 1900 series character code

Binary coded decimal

You will notice that the character code for the digits 0 to 9 in Figure 3.2 is the binary equivalent of these numbers.

For example

$$9 = \frac{8\ \ 4\ \ 2\ \ 1}{1\ \ 0\ \ 0\ \ 1} = 8 + 1$$

If this method of coding is used on each digit of a decimal number separately, the binary code produced is called **binary coded decimal** (BCD). For example, using four bits for each decimal digit:

$$73 = 0111\ \ 0011 \quad \text{(BCD)}$$
and
$$594 = 0101\ \ 1001\ \ 0100 \quad \text{(BCD)}$$

BCD is a very convenient code for converting to and from base ten, though more bits are needed than if the whole decimal number is converted to a single binary number.

Negative numbers

The three commonest ways of coding negative numbers on computers are now introduced: sign-and-magnitude, twos complement and ones complement. The main reason for using the last two rather complicated codes for negative numbers is that they enable subtraction to be performed by a modified form of addition.

In these sections, all the numbers used as examples are integers (whole numbers). These codes may, however, be used to represent fractions.

Sign-and-magnitude coding

In this code, one bit represents the sign of the number, and the other bits represent the size (or magnitude) of the number. The convention for the sign bit is that 1 represents negative, and 0 positive. The sign bit may be at either end of the binary number.

Here are some examples (the sign bit is underlined):

$$\underline{1}01001 = -9$$
$$1100\underline{0} = +12$$
$$\underline{0}1011001 = +89$$
$$\underline{1}1000 = -8$$

Notice the difference between the second and fourth examples.

Twos complements

In twos complement coding, the bits have the same place values as binary numbers, except that the most significant bit represents a negative quantity.

The place values for a six bit, twos complement number are:

−32	16	8	4	2	1

For example

$$1\ 0\ 0\ 1\ 1\ 0 = -32 + 4 + 2 = -32 + 6 = -26$$

There is a fairly simple relationship between the code for a positive number and the corresponding negative number (its **twos complement**).

	−32	16	8	4	2	1
11 =	0	0	1	0	1	1
−11 = −32 + 21 =	1	1	0	1	0	1
23 =	0	1	0	1	1	1
−23 = −32 + 9 =	1	0	1	0	0	1
8 =	0	0	1	0	0	0
−8 = −32 + 24 =	1	1	1	0	0	0

In the first two examples, it can be seen that, apart from the units column, the bits for the negative number are the opposite of those for the positive number. One method of changing from a positive to a negative number in twos complement form is as follows:

Change the 0's to 1's and the 1's to 0's, and then add 1. This method also works for the third example (8 and −8). Try it for yourself.

Subtraction using twos complement

You will know that subtraction can be done by adding a negative number. For example 16 + (−7) gives the same result as 16 − 7. Computers which use twos complement coding do subtraction by making the second number negative as described above, and adding it to the first number.

For example, the stages of calculating 24 − 17 using twos complements are:

		−32	16	8	4	2	1
store 17		0	1	0	0	0	1
reverse bits		1	0	1	1	1	0
add 1, gives −17		1	0	1	1	1	1
store 24		0	1	1	0	0	0
add −17 and 24	(1)	0	0	0	1	1	1

↑ overflow bit

The extra bit, carried from the −32 column, is called the **overflow bit.** In this case, it is ignored.

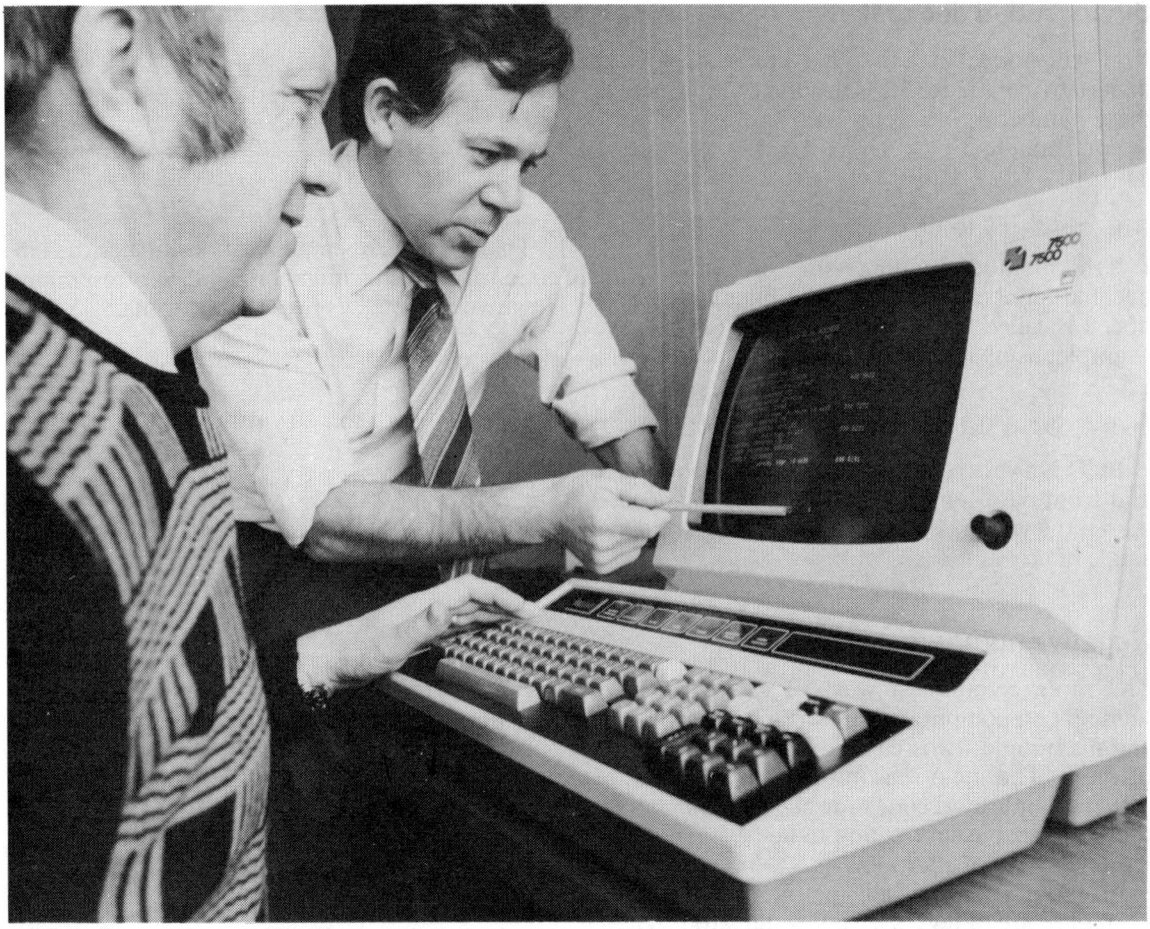

An ICL visual display terminal being used for information retrieval

The six bit answer is 0 0 0 1 1 1 (= 7) as required.

The steps of calculating 19 − 16 are:

		−32	16	8	4	2	1
store 16		0	1	0	0	0	0
reverse bits		1	0	1	1	1	1
add 1, gives − 16		1	1	0	0	0	0
store 19		0	1	0	0	1	1
add − 16 and 19	(1)	0	0	0	0	1	1

In this example, the overflow bit is again ignored, giving the required answer, 3. The question of overflow is discussed in more detail in Chapter 10.

Ones complements

You will recall that the twos complement of a binary number is found by reversing the bits and adding 1. A simpler type of complement is found by merely reversing the bits. This is called the **ones complement.** For example, using six bits:

	−31	16	8	4	2	1
5 =	0	0	0	1	0	1
−5 =	1	1	1	0	1	0

Notice that the most significant bit now represents −31, rather than −32 in twos complement numbers.

Subtraction using ones complements

This is similar to the method using twos complements, except that the overflow must be added to the units column of the sum to give the correct answer.

For example, the stages of calculating 24 − 17 using ones complements are:

		−31	16	8	4	2	1	
store 17		0	1	0	0	0	1	
reverse bits, gives − 17		1	0	1	1	1	0	
store 24		0	1	1	0	0	0	
add − 17 and 24	1	0	0	0	1	1	0	
add overflow bit	└	→	→	→	→	→	1	
		0	0	0	1	1	1	= 7

The stages of calculating 19 − 16 are:

		−31	16	8	4	2	1	
store 16		0	1	0	0	0	0	
reverse bits, gives − 16		1	0	1	1	1	1	
store 19		0	1	0	0	1	1	
add − 16 and 19	1	0	0	0	0	1	0	
add overflow bit	└	→	→	→	→	→	1	
		0	0	0	0	1	1	= 3

Adding the overflow bit from one end of the number to another is called **wrap-around carry.**

Storing data: bits, bytes and words

An advantage of coding data in terms of bits is that each bit can only have the value 0 or 1. A disadvantage is that a large number of bits are needed to store most data items.

To avoid the complexity of handling bits individually, all computers deal with bits in groups. The size of the group depends on the type of computer, the type of data and the storage medium. Bits may be grouped differently by the same computer for different purposes. The most common groups of bits are called **bytes** and **words.**

Bytes

A byte is usually regarded as a group of bits storing the code for one character. Most computer memories use eight bits for this purpose. Data on punched cards, paper tape, magnetic tape and magnetic discs is almost always coded in bytes.

Words

A word is a larger grouping of bits, ranging from sixteen to sixty-four bits on different types of computers. On some computers, a word is the smallest unit of memory. On most computers, a word is the number of bits which can be processed in one operation. A word can store several characters, or a complete number in one of the numeric codes mentioned in this chapter, or an instruction to the computer, as described in chapter 11.

Parity

One bit in a byte or a word is sometimes used for checking purposes. It is called a **parity bit.** The parity bit contains a 0 or a 1 so that there is an even number of 1's in the whole byte or word (even parity). For odd parity, there must be an odd number of 1's. For example, using even parity on an eight bit byte:

parity bit

1 1 0 0 1 0 0 1

The parity bit contains a 1 to make up an even number of 1's.

Here is another example, using even parity on a sixteen bit word:

parity bit

0 1 1 0 1 1 1 1 0 1 1 0 1 1 0 0

Parity bits are used in **parity checks** as follows: When an even parity word or byte is copied from one part of a computer to another, the number of 1's in the word or byte is checked. If there is no longer an even number, then a bit has been copied wrongly. The check is similar for odd parity.

The main use of parity checks is during input, as this is where errors are most likely to occur.

Exercise 3a

1 Write down the meanings of the following words or phrases:
bistable device;
numeric, alphabetic and special characters;
place value; most significant digit;
alphanumeric character; character set;
character code; bit; byte; word; BCD;
overflow bit; wrap-around carry; parity bit;
parity check; sign-and-magnitude code.

2 Increasing use is being made of codes for everyday information. Post codes, income tax codes and vehicle licence codes are obvious examples. Make a list of other common information which is written in code.

3 Using the character code on page 14:
(a) Decode the message (four letters) in this 24 bit word:

1 0 0 0 1 0 1 1 1 0 0 1 1 1 0 1 0 0
1 0 0 1 0 1

(b) Encode the word ABLE in a 24 bit word.

4 Convert these base ten numbers to binary coded decimal, using four bits per decimal digit:
(a) 91 (b) 56 (c) 493
Convert these BCD numbers to base ten:
(d) 1 0 0 1 0 1 1 0 (e) 1 0 0 0 0 1 1 1
(f) 0 1 1 0 0 1 0 0 0 1 1 1

5 The place values for eight bit sign-and-magnitude coding are as follows:

sign bit	64	32	16	8	4	2	1	
For example								
1	1	0	0	1	0	0	1	= −73

Encode the following decimal numbers in this code:
(a) 39 (b) −61 (c) 117
Decode the following sign-and-magnitude binary numbers:
(d) 0 0 1 1 0 1 1 0 (e) 1 0 1 0 0 1 1 0
(f) 1 1 0 1 1 1 0 1
(g) What are the largest and smallest (decimal) numbers which can be coded in this manner?

6 Write the following decimal numbers as six bit, twos complement binary numbers:
(a) 27 (b) − 13 (c) 31
Change the following six bit, twos complement binary numbers to decimal numbers:
(d) 0 1 0 0 1 0 (e) 1 1 1 0 1 1 (f) 1 1 1 1 1 0
Carry out the following subtractions using six bit, twos complement binary numbers:
(g) 15 − 7 (h) 28 − 18 *(i) 19 − 22
(j) What are the largest and smallest (decimal) numbers which can be coded as six bit, twos complement binary numbers.

7 Do parts (a) to (j) of question **6** using six bit, ones complement binary numbers.

8 How many different numbers can be written as:
(a) one bit (b) two bits (c) three bits
(d) six bits (e) eight bits (f) *n* bits?

9 Fill in the missing parity bits (even parity);
(a) _ 1 0 0 1 0 1 1 (b) _ 1 0 1 0 0
(c) One of the following numbers, which include a parity bit, has been coded wrongly. Use a parity check to determine which one it is.

1 0 1 1 0 1 1 1 0 1 1 1 1 0 0 1 0 1

10 A certain computer application requires dates of birth to be written as follows: 27/03/62.
Using four bit BCD for the numbers, and the code 1 1 1 1 for the /, encode the following dates of birth in 32 bit words:
(a) 31/01/54 (b) 29/02/64
(c) Decode the following date of birth:

0 0 0 0 0 0 0 1 1 1 1 1 0 0 0 0 0 1 0 0
1 1 1 1 0 1 1 0 0 0 0 1

11 The IMC-1 model computer uses eight bit, twos complement storage for integers. The place values are:

−128	64	32	16	8	4	2	1	
For example								
1	0	0	0	1	1	0	0	= −116

Write the following decimal numbers in this form:
(a) 29 (b) −48 (c) − 103
Change the following eight bit, twos complement binary numbers to decimal:
(d) 0 0 1 0 1 1 1 1 (e) 1 0 1 0 0 1 1 0
(f) 1 1 0 1 0 0 0 1
Carry out the following subtractions using eight bit, twos complement numbers:
(g) 68 − 13 (h) 53 − 27 (i) 79 − 58
(j) What is the range of decimal numbers that can be stored as eight bit twos complement numbers?

***12** ICL 2900 series computers store decimal integers as follows:
Each eight bit byte stores two decimal digits in four bit BCD. The sign is stored in the least significant four bits, coded as follows:

positive: 1 0 1 0, 1 1 0 0, 1 1 1 0 or 1 1 1 1
negative: 1 0 1 1 or 1 1 0 1

As many bytes are used as are needed to store the whole decimal number. For example, using two bytes:

1 0 0 0	0 1 0 1	0 0 1 1	1 0 1 1	= −853
digit	digit	digit	sign	

Encode the following decimal numbers, using one or two bytes as required:
(a) 5 (b) −9 (c) 421 (d) −219 (e) −57
Change the following binary numbers, coded as above, to decimal:
(f) 0 0 1 1 0 0 0 0 0 0 0 1 1 1 1 1
(g) 0 0 1 0 1 1 0 1
(h) 1 0 0 0 1 0 0 1 0 0 1 0 1 1 1 0

This method of storing two decimal digits per byte is called **packed decimal.** It is used on many popular types of computers.

13 Car registration numbers are made up in any of the following formats:

(1) 1 to 3 letters followed by 1 to 3 digits followed by a single letter (e.g. ABC 123R).
(2) 1 to 3 letters followed by 1 to 3 digits (e.g. ABC 123).
(3) 1 to 3 digits followed by 1 to 3 letters (e.g. 123 ABC).
(4) 1 or 2 letters followed by 4 digits (e.g. AB 1234).
(5) 4 digits followed by 1 or 2 letters (e.g. 1234 AB).

(a) What is the least number of bits needed to represent an alphabetic character?
(b) What is the least number of bits needed to represent a 3-digit number?
(c) What is the least number of bits needed to represent a 4-digit number?
(d) Suggest a way of encoding registration numbers of the above types in an economical manner (i.e. using as few bits as possible). State the code which you have used.
(e) Fully encode, in binary, the following registration number: WNO 205F.
(AEB 78 II)

14 State, with reasons for your answer, the number of characters you would expect to store in a 24 bit word, assuming that the character set contains not more than 60 members, but more than 50 members. (UCLES 76 I)

15 The twos complement method of representing number in 4 bit cells is as follows:

The first bit is the number of −8's.
The second bit is the number of 4's.
The third bit is the number of 2's.
The fourth bit is the number of 1's.

Thus 0 1 1 0 represents $(0 \times -8) + (1 \times 4) + (1 \times 2) + (0 \times 1) = 0 + 4 + 2 + 0 = 6$ and 1 1 0 1 represents $(1 \times -8) + (1 \times 4) + (0 \times 2) + (1 \times 1) = -8 + 4 + 0 + 1 = -3$

(a) In this system what would be the representations of the numbers 5 and −6?
(b) List all the negative numbers which can be represented in this system.
(c) If cell A contains 0 0 1 0, cell B contains 1 0 1 1, and the contents of cell B are subtracted from cell A and the result stored in cell C, what would be the bit pattern in cell C? (WMEB 74 I)

In the following questions, choose the correct answer from the ones given:

16 The **ones complement** of a six-digit binary number is found by replacing each 0 by 1 and each 1 by 0, e.g. the ones complement of 0 1 1 0 0 0 is 1 0 0 1 1 1.

In a special system positive numbers are represented by their actual binary representation, e.g. 13 would be 0 0 1 1 0 1 and negative numbers, e.g. −13 can be represented by the ones complement of 13 which is 1 1 0 0 1 0. In this system
(a) The ones complement of 1 0 1 1 0 0 is
(i) 0 0 1 1 0 1, (ii) 0 1 0 1 0 0,
(iii) 1 1 0 0 1 0, (iv) 0 1 0 0 1 1,
(v) none of these.
(b) How would −3 be represented?
(i) 0 0 0 0 1 1, (ii) 1 1 1 1 0 0,
(iii) 1 1 0 0 0 0, (iv) 0 0 0 1 1 1,
(v) 1 1 1 0 0 0.
(c) What negative number would 1 0 0 0 0 0 represent?
(i) −31, (ii) −64, (iii) −32, (iv) −16,
(v) −1 0 0 0 0 0. (WMEB 75 I)

17 In a binary-coded-decimal system of representing numbers in a computer the following code is used:

0 = 0 0 0 0	5 = 1 0 0 0
1 = 0 0 0 1	6 = 1 0 0 1
2 = 0 0 1 0	7 = 1 0 1 0
3 = 0 0 1 1	8 = 1 0 1 1
4 = 0 1 0 0	9 = 1 1 0 0

No other representations are allowed. For example, in this system the number 21 is represented by 0 0 1 0 0 0 0 1, and the number 54 is represented by 1 0 0 0 0 1 0 0.
(a) In this system the number 68 is represented by
(i) 0 1 0 0 0 0 1 0, (ii) 0 1 1 0 0 1 0 0,
(iii) 0 1 1 0 1 0 1 1, (iv) 1 0 0 1 1 0 1 1,
(v) 1 0 0 1 0 1 0 0.
(b) In this system 0 0 1 1 + 0 1 0 0 is equal to
(i) 1 1 1, (ii) 1 0 1 0, (iii) 0 1 1 1,
(iv) 0 0 1 1 0 1 0 0, (v) 0 0 0 0 0 1 1 1.
(c) In this system 1 0 1 1 0 0 1 0 − 1 0 0 1 0 1 0 0 is equal to
(i) 0 0 0 1 1 1 1 0, (ii) 0 0 0 1 0 0 1 0,
(iii) 0 0 1 0 1 1 1 0, (iv) 1 1 0 0 1 1 0 0,
(v) 0 0 0 1 1 0 1 1. (WMEB 77 I)

Section B

The rest of the chapter concerns some further aspects of information storage. It introduces some other number bases that are frequently used, in addition to base two. Methods of storing fractions, and very large and very small numbers are also described.

* Other number bases

In working with computers, it is sometimes necessary to write down numbers in the way in which they are stored on the computer. As you will have noticed from the previous section, using base two is very slow and cumbersome. However, writing numbers in base ten means that it takes a long time to convert them to base two.

What is needed are number bases that make numbers easy to convert to base two, but also short. There are in fact two such number bases, base eight (**octal**) and base sixteen (**hexadecimal**), in common use.

Octal numbers

The place values in base eight are as follows:

	512	64	8	1	
For example	1	2	5	3	= 683 in base ten

To show how to convert from base two to base eight, compare these numbers:

base ten	**base two**	**base eight**
1	1	1
8	1 000	1 0
64	1 000 000	1 0 0
512	1 000 000 000	1 0 0 0

Notice that three place values in base two correspond to one place value in base eight. The method of conversion is as follows:

To change from base two to base eight, group the base two digits in threes, starting with the least significant bit, and convert each set of three to one base eight digit. For example:

base two	1 1 0	0 1 0	1 1 1	(= 423 in base ten)
base eight	6	2	7	

To change from base eight to base two, convert each base eight digit to three binary digits, putting 0's on the front where necessary. For example:

base eight	2	1	4	(= 140 in base ten)
base two	0 1 0	0 0 1	1 0 0	

Hexadecimal numbers

The place values in base sixteen are as follows:

	256	16	1	
For example	3	9	2	= 914 in base ten

Base sixteen needs extra digits for numbers from ten to fifteen. The letters A to F are used:

base ten	0	1	2 . . .	9	10	11	12	13	14	15	16
base sixteen	0	1	2 . . .	9	A	B	C	D	E	F	10

The method of converting base two to base sixteen is similar to the one for base eight, except that groups of four bits are used. That is:

To change from base two to base sixteen, group the base two digits in fours, starting with the least significant bit, and convert each set of four to one base sixteen digit. For example:

base two	1 0 0 1	0 1 0 1	(= 149 in base ten)
base sixteen	9	5	

Changing from base sixteen to base two is done by converting each base sixteen digit into four binary digits, filling in 0's in front if necessary. For example:

base sixteen	3	6	(= 54 in base ten)
base two	0 0 1 1	0 1 1 0	

and

base sixteen	B	9	(= 185 in base ten)
base two	1 0 1 1	1 0 0 1	

For these reasons, numbers stored on computers are sometimes written down, not in binary, but as octal or hexadecimal numbers. This is usually done when a computer program is being checked. Normal input and output numbers are almost always in base ten.

* Fractions

All of the numeric codes mentioned in the first part of this chapter can, with suitable modifications, be used to store fractions. Most codes for fractions are based on the place values for binary fractions, which are as follows:

	$\frac{1}{2}$	$\frac{1}{4}$	$\frac{1}{8}$	$\frac{1}{16}$	$\frac{1}{32}$	etc.
For example	1	0	1	0	0	$= \frac{5}{8}$ or 0.625

Sign-and-magnitude fractions have the most significant bit as the sign bit, as before.

sign	$\frac{1}{2}$	$\frac{1}{4}$	$\frac{1}{8}$	$\frac{1}{16}$	$\frac{1}{32}$	
For example						
1	0	1	1	0	0	$= -\frac{3}{8}$ or -0.375

Twos complement fractions have the most significant bit representing -1.

-1	$\frac{1}{2}$	$\frac{1}{4}$	$\frac{1}{8}$	$\frac{1}{16}$	$\frac{1}{32}$	
For example						
1	0	1	1	0	0	$= -1 + \frac{3}{8} = -\frac{5}{8}$ or -0.625

Converting base ten fractions to binary is generally rather difficult. However, if the base ten fraction can obviously be expressed as a sum of halves, quarters, eights, etc., then conversion is fairly simple. For example:

	$\frac{1}{2}$	$\frac{1}{4}$	$\frac{1}{8}$	$\frac{1}{16}$	$\frac{1}{32}$
$\frac{7}{16} = \frac{1}{4} + \frac{1}{8} + \frac{1}{16} =$	0	1	1	1	0
$0.75 = \frac{3}{4} = \frac{1}{2} + \frac{1}{4} =$	1	1	0	0	0

One way of dealing with fractions which cannot be converted by the above method, is as follows:

Change the numerator and denominator of the fraction to binary, and then divide the binary denominator into the binary numerator. For example:

$\frac{4}{5} = \frac{100}{101}$

```
          .110011
101 ) 100.000000
       10 1
       01 10
          1 01
            1000
             101
              110
              101
                1 etc.
```

Thus, correct to six binary places,

	$\frac{1}{2}$	$\frac{1}{4}$	$\frac{1}{8}$	$\frac{1}{16}$	$\frac{1}{32}$	$\frac{1}{64}$
$\frac{4}{5} =$	1	1	0	0	1	1

Notice that the binary fraction is not exact. The errors which arise in storing binary fractions are discussed in Chapter 10.

* Fixed point numbers

Integers or fractions in sign-and-magnitude, complementary or BCD coding are called **fixed point** numbers. This is because the binary point is in a fixed position (although the point itself is not coded). For integers, the point is assumed to be to the right of the least significant bit. For fractions it is to the left of the $\frac{1}{2}$'s bit. For example, using six bit, twos complement numbers:

integer

−32	16	8	4	2	1	
1	0	1	1	0	1	.

fraction

−1	$\frac{1}{2}$	$\frac{1}{4}$	$\frac{1}{8}$	$\frac{1}{16}$	$\frac{1}{32}$
0 .	1	1	0	0	1

assumed position of binary point

However, the main use of the term 'fixed point' is to distinguish these numbers from **floating point numbers,** which are now introduced.

* Floating point numbers

A way of storing very large or very small numbers on a computer is to code them as **floating point numbers.** The name floating point means that the binary point always 'floats' to the front of the number.

Floating point storage is similar to the method of writing large or small numbers in base ten, called **standard form.** For example:

		standard form
3600000 =	3.6 × 1000000 =	3.6×10^{6}
0.00003 =	3.0 × 0.00001 =	3.0×10^{-5}

Standard form numbers are written in terms of powers of ten. In place of powers of ten, floating point numbers use powers of two. A floating point number is stored as a fraction (called the **mantissa**) multiplied by a power of two (called the **exponent**). For example:

mantissa				**exponent**				
±	$\frac{1}{2}$	$\frac{1}{4}$	$\frac{1}{8}$	±	4	2	1	
0	1	0	0	0	0	1	1	$= \frac{1}{2} \times 2^{3} = \frac{1}{2} \times 8 = 4$

Notice that the above example uses sign-and-magnitude coding for the mantissa and exponent. Complementary form may also be used. Some further examples of numbers coded this way are shown in table 3.1.

Table 3.1

mantissa				**exponent**						
±	$\frac{1}{2}$	$\frac{1}{4}$	$\frac{1}{8}$	±	4	2	1			
0	1	0	0	0	0	0	1	$= \frac{1}{2} \times 2^{1}$	$= \frac{1}{2} \times 2$	$= 1$
0	1	1	1	0	0	1	1	$= \frac{7}{8} \times 2^{3}$	$= \frac{7}{8} \times 8$	$= 7$
0	1	0	1	1	0	1	0	$= \frac{5}{8} \times 2^{-2}$	$= \frac{5}{8} \times \frac{1}{4}$	$= \frac{5}{32}$
1	1	0	0	0	1	1	1	$= -\frac{1}{2} \times 2^{7}$	$= -\frac{1}{2} \times 128$	$= -64$

To convert a decimal number to binary floating point form, first change it to a fraction multiplied by a power of 2, and then convert these to binary. Always use the next power of 2 larger than the number. For some examples see table 3.2.

Storage of floating point numbers

In most computers, the storage space for a floating point number is large. One, two or four complete words are commonly used. Many computers allow a choice of size of storage space for floating point numbers.

The number of significant figures in a number that can be stored is proportional to the number of bits allocated to the mantissa. To ensure maximum utilisation of the available space, the fraction is always adjusted so that there is a 1 in the $\frac{1}{2}$'s bit, unless the number stored is 0. This is called **normalization.** (If the mantissa is in twos complement form, the first two bits must be 0 1 or 1 0 unless the whole number is zero.)

The range of numbers that can be stored is related to the number of bits allocated to the exponent. A compromise must always be reached when dividing the available storage space between mantissa and exponent. In most computers, the mantissa has approximately four times the number of bits allocated to the exponent.

Exercise 3b

1 Write down the meanings of the following words or phrases:
octal; hexadecimal; standard form; mantissa; exponent; fixed point number;
floating point number; normalization;

2 Convert these binary numbers to octal:
(a) 1 0 1 0 1 0 (b) 1 1 0 1 1 1 0 0 0
(c) 1 1 1 1 1 1 1 1 1 (d) 1 0 0 0 1
(e) 1 0 0 1 1 1 0 0 1 1 1

3 Convert these octal numbers to binary:
(a) 74 (b) 61 (c) 132 (d) 153 (e) 472

4 Convert these binary numbers to hexadecimal:
(a) 0 1 1 0 0 1 0 1 (b) 1 1 0 0 0 1 0 1
(c) 1 0 0 1 0 1 1 1 1 1 1 0 1 0

5 Convert these hexadecimal numbers to binary:
(a) 71 (b) 7E (c) 132 (d) 103 (e) 35B

6 How many octal digits can be stored in a 24 bit word?

7 How many hexadecimal digits can be stored in a 24 bit word?

8 Convert these twos complement binary fractions to base ten fractions:

	-1	$\frac{1}{2}$	$\frac{1}{4}$	$\frac{1}{8}$	$\frac{1}{16}$	$\frac{1}{32}$
(a)	0	1	1	1	0	0
(b)	0	1	0	0	0	1
(c)	0	0	1	1	0	0
(d)	1	1	1	1	0	0
(e)	1	1	0	0	1	0

9 Convert these base ten fractions into six bit, twos complement fractions:
(a) $\frac{3}{16}$ (b) $\frac{5}{16}$ (c) $\frac{17}{32}$ (d) $-\frac{1}{4}$ (e) $-\frac{7}{32}$

10 What is the largest fraction that can be written as a six bit, twos complement fraction?

11 Convert these floating point numbers to base ten numbers or fractions:

	mantissa				**characteristic**			
	$\pm$	$\frac{1}{2}$	$\frac{1}{4}$	$\frac{1}{8}$	$\pm$	4	2	1
(a)	0	1	0	1	0	0	1	1
(b)	0	1	1	0	0	1	0	1
(c)	0	1	1	1	0	1	0	1
(d)	1	1	1	0	0	1	1	0
(e)	0	1	1	0	1	0	1	0
(f)	0	1	1	1	1	0	1	0
(g)	1	1	1	0	1	1	0	0
(h)	0	1	0	1	0	0	0	0

12 Convert these base ten numbers and fractions to floating point numbers, with place values as in question **11**.
(a) 3 (b) 6 (c) 10 (d) -14 (e) $\frac{1}{4}$ (f) $\frac{5}{16}$ (g) $\frac{3}{32}$ (h) $-\frac{5}{64}$

Table 3.2

	mantissa				**exponent**			
	$\pm$	$\frac{1}{2}$	$\frac{1}{4}$	$\frac{1}{8}$	$\pm$	4	2	1
$5 = \frac{5}{8} \times 8 = \frac{5}{8} \times 2^3 =$	0	1	0	1	0	0	1	1
$40 = \frac{5}{8} \times 64 = \frac{5}{8} \times 2^6 =$	0	1	0	1	0	1	1	0
$\frac{3}{8} = \frac{3}{4} \times \frac{1}{2} = \frac{3}{4} \times 2^{-1} =$	0	1	1	0	1	0	0	1
$-\frac{7}{8} = -\frac{7}{8} \times 1 = -\frac{7}{8} \times 2^0 =$	1	1	1	1	0	0	0	0

13 (a) What is the largest positive decimal number that can be written as a floating point number, with place values as in question **11**?
(b) What is the smallest positive decimal number that can be coded in this way?

*__14__ Change the binary number 1 0 0 1 0 1 0 1 to a decimal number or fraction, using each of the following codes:
(a) BCD, four bits per binary digit,
(b) twos complement integer,
(c) ones complement integer,
(d) sign-and-magnitude fraction,
(e) twos complement fraction,
(f) floating point (place values as in question **11**).
Comment on your answers.

*__15__ Find out, for as many different kinds of computers as possible:
(a) Which codes are used to store data.
(b) Whether bytes, words (or both) are used in the memory, and how many bits there are in each.
(c) If floating point coding is used, the number of bits allocated to the mantissa and to the exponent.
Comment on your findings.

16 The binary equivalent of 0.2 (base 10) is 0.0 0 1 1 0 0 1 1 0 0 1 1 . . . recurring.
If $A = 0.2$ (base ten) and $S = A + A + A + A + A$,
(a) Write the value of A in base 2 using 4 bits in the binary fraction.
(b) Find the value of S in base 2 using binary arithmetic to evaluate the formula.
(c) Express answer (b) in base 10.
(d) Why does answer (c) differ from the value of S that would be obtained if you had worked in denary? (EAEB 77 II)

17 (a) Convert the binary number 1 1.0 1 into its denary equivalent.
(b) Floating point numbers are held in a computer store having 16-bit storage locations as follows:

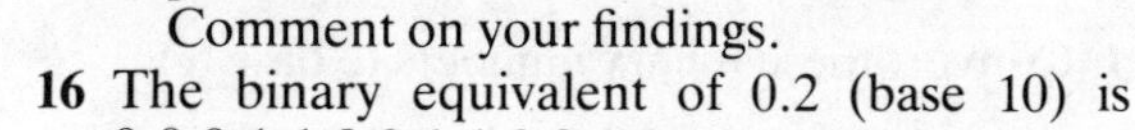

S_1 and S_2 are sign bits such that 0 indicates a positive number and 1 a negative number. Copy the diagrams below and indicate how the binary numbers 1 1 0 1 1.1 and 0.1 0 1 might be represented in floating point form. (UCLES 78 I)

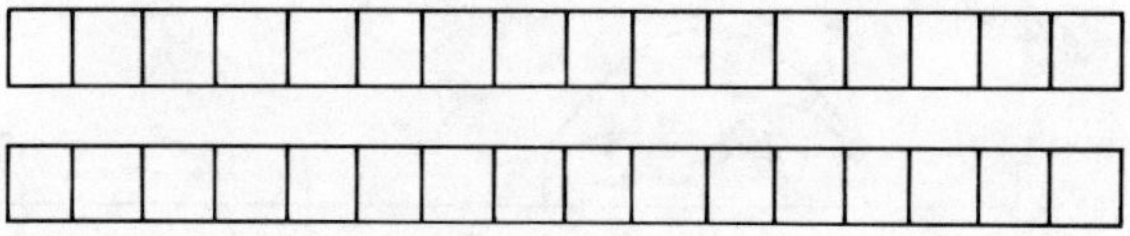

18 (a) Why are binary numbers suitable for computers but not very convenient for people, whereas the decimal number system is convenient for people but less so for computers?
(b) Explain with examples both the sign-and-magnitude (or sign-and-modulus) and twos complement representations of negative binary numbers.
(c) Why is complement form frequently used in computers?
(d) In a location of 12 bits, using twos complement form for negative numbers what is (i) the largest positive number, and (ii) the largest negative number that can be stored, and what are their decimal equivalents? (OLE 78 II)

Section C: Background mathematics

This section gives a very brief introduction to negative numbers, and to binary numbers. It is intended only for anyone who is not familiar with these topics.

Negative numbers

Numbers may be written along a line, with 0 not at the end, but in the middle. Positive numbers are on the right of 0, negative numbers on the left.

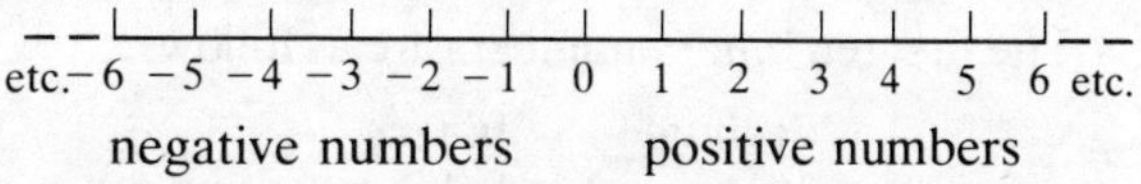

When adding positive numbers, one moves forwards along the line. When adding negative numbers, one moves backwards. Always start at 0. For example:

4 + 2:

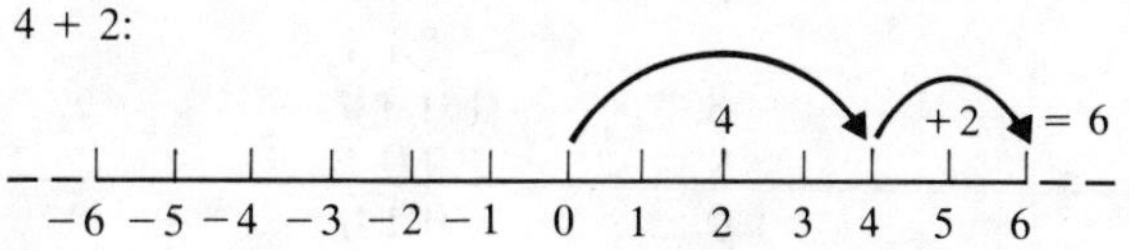

4 + (−2):

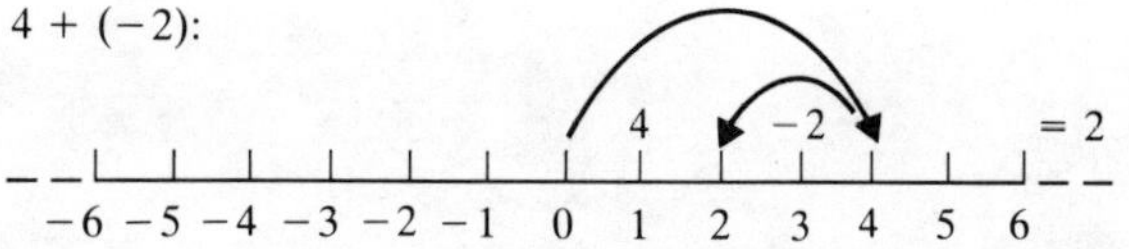

$-4 + 2$:

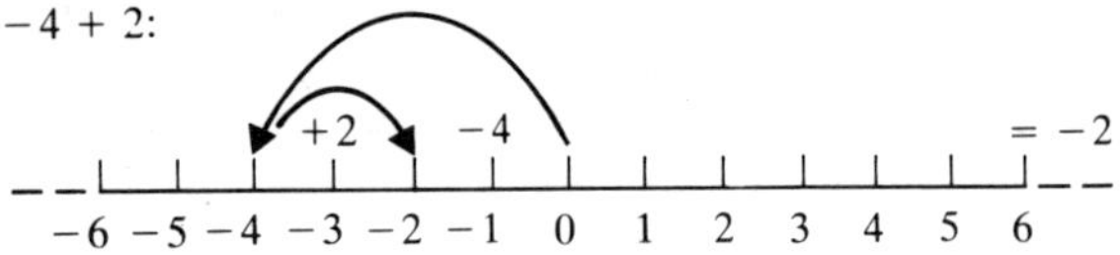

$-4 + (-2)$;

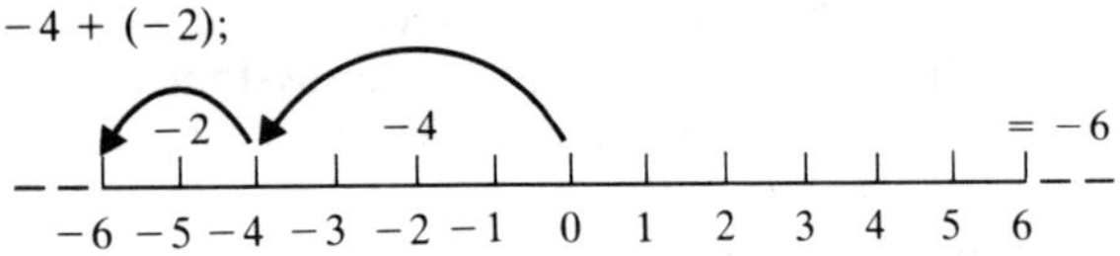

Exercise 3c

Try the following questions yourself. You should soon be able to do them without drawing lines and arrows.

1 $2 + 3$
2 $2 + (-3)$
3 $-2 + 3$
4 $-2 + (-3)$
5 $4 + (-7)$
6 $5 + (-3)$
7 $-1 + (-5)$
8 $4 + (-9)$
9 $-11 + 8$
10 $7 + (-13)$
11 $-3 + 2 + (-5)$
12 $3 + 4 + (-7)$

Binary numbers

Ordinary base ten numbers have place values of units, tens, hundreds etc. Base two, or binary, numbers have place values of units, twos, fours, eights, sixteens etc. The only digits needed are 0 and 1.

The first ten binary numbers are as follows:

decimal 10 1	**binary** 8 4 2 1
1	1
2	1 0
3	1 1
4	1 0 0
5	1 0 1
6	1 1 0
7	1 1 1
8	1 0 0 0
9	1 0 0 1
1 0	1 0 1 0

The rules for adding binary numbers are as follows:

$0 + 0 = 0$
$0 + 1 = 1$
$1 + 0 = 1$
$1 + 1 = 1\,0$ (i.e. 0 carry 1)
$1 + 1 + 1 = 1\,1$ (i.e. 1 carry 1)

Here are some complete binary numbers added together:

```
     1 0 1 1 0
  +    1 0 1 1
  ------------
   1 0 0 0 0 1
  ------------
     1 1 1 1      ← carried numbers
```

and

```
     1 1 0 1 1
  +  1 0 1 1 1
  ------------
   1 1 0 0 1 0
  ------------
   1 1 1 1 1
```

Exercise 3d

1 Convert these binary numbers to base ten:

1 1 0 0   1 1 1 1   1 0 0 1 0

2 Convert these decimal numbers to binary:

13   19   27

3 Add the following binary numbers. Check the answers by converting all the numbers to base ten.

```
   1 0 1 1 1      1 0 0 1 1      1 1 0 1 1
 +   1 0 1 0    + 1 1 0 0 1    +   1 1 1 1
 ----------     ----------     ----------

 ----------     ----------     ----------

     1 1 1 1      1 0 1 1 0
   + 1 1 1 1    + 1 1 1 0 1
 ----------     ----------

 ----------     ----------
```

Although this section is very brief, it contains just enough information to enable your to do the work in the first part of the chapter.

4

The computer memory

The memory is the part of the central processing unit of a computer which is used for storing the data and instructions that the computer is processing at the time. It is sometimes called the **main store.**

The memory consists of a large number of storage spaces called cells. Depending on the type of computer, each cell stores a byte or a word, using one of the codes explained in the previous chapter. The memory is an **immediate access** store. Data can be fetched from any cell, or stored in any cell, extremely rapidly. Memory cells do not have to be used in order. Access to the memory is very fast – about one millionth of a second in many computers.

Addresses

Each cell in the memory is located by means of a number called its address. In this respect, a computer memory is arranged rather like a row of houses. (See Figure 4.1.) It is worth emphasizing that the address of a memory cell is different from the data stored in that cell. (In a similar way, the address of a house is different from the name of its occupants.) However, in a computer both data and addresses are in binary.

An example of a computer memory

The memory of the IMC-1 model computer is a simple example of a computer memory. It has 32 cells, each capable of storing an eight bit word. The addresses are from 0 to 31 (0 0 0 0 0 to 1 1 1 1 1 in binary). Notice that five bits are needed for a memory address. Figure 4.2 shows the complete IMC-1 memory. Notice that the memory cell with address 1 0 0 1 1 contains the word 1 0 1 1 0 1 1 0.

Ferrite cores

Looking inside the memory of many older computers one will find a large number of small metal rings, all threaded by thin wires. The rings are called **ferrite cores.** They are small rings of soft iron, which can be magnetized in one direction or the other. The two directions of magnetization store the two binary digits 0 and 1. The wires which pass through the cores are used to change their magnetization. A pulse of current in a wire, in the required direction, will achieve this. See Figure 4.3. The pulse must be bigger than a certain **threshold size** or it has no effect on the core.

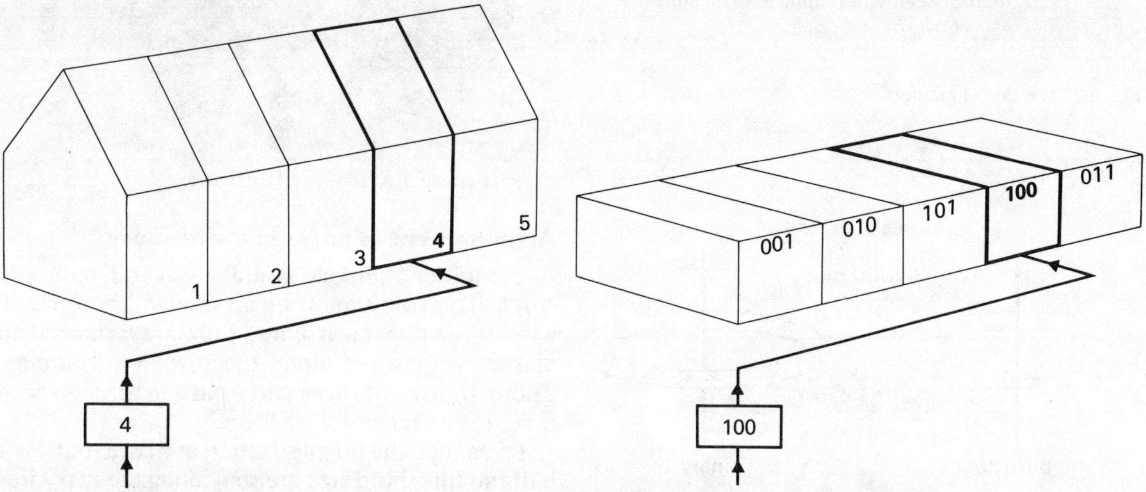

Address locates house

Address (in binary) locates computer memory cell

Fig. 4.1. Addressing

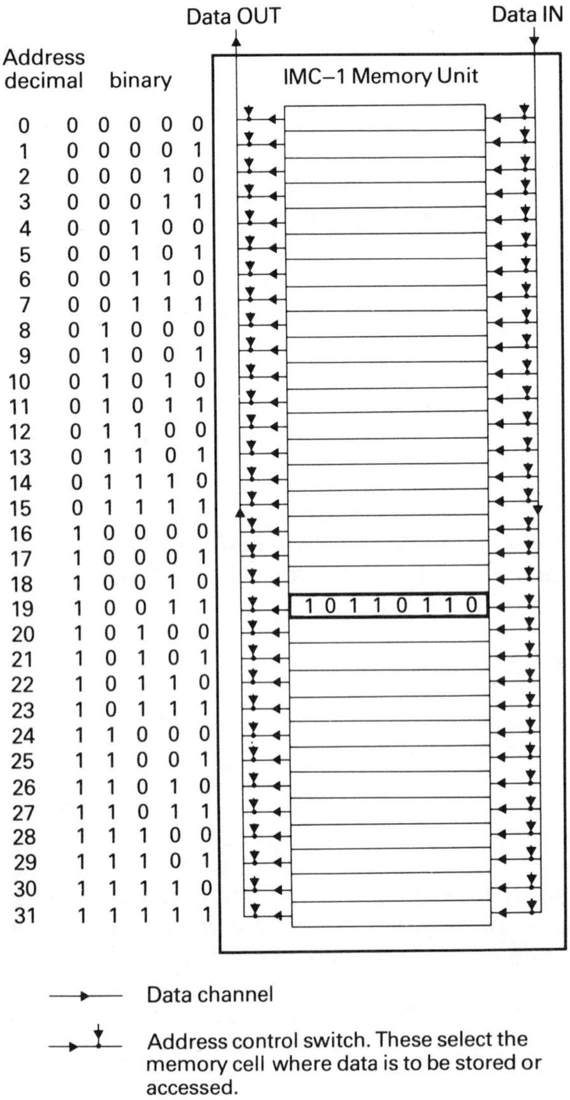

Fig. 4.2. The IMC-1 memory

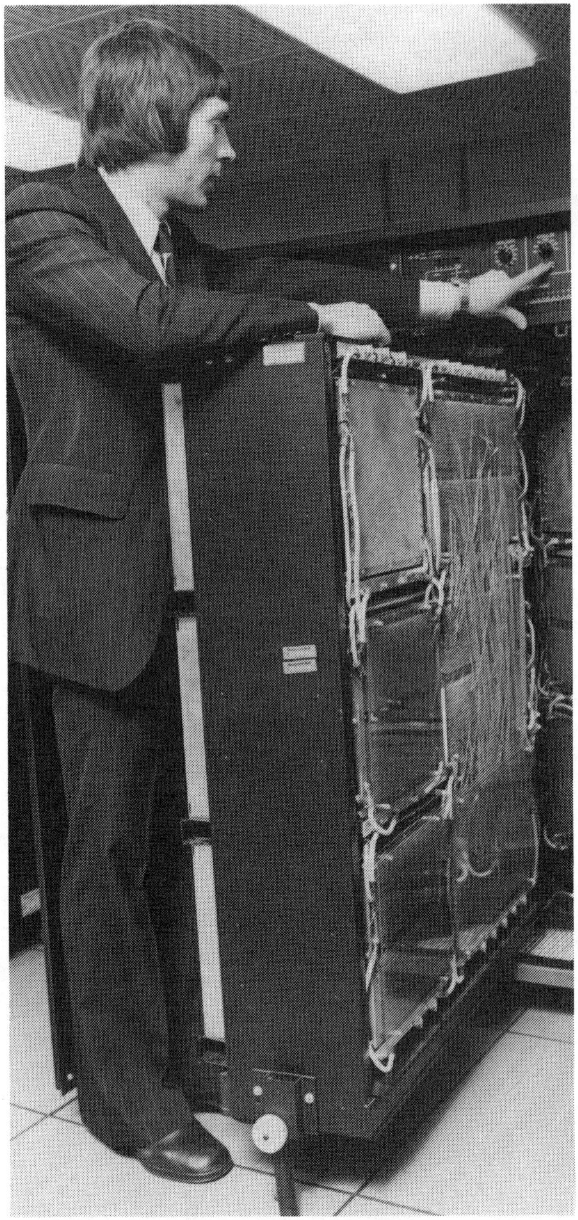

The main store of a Honeywell computer

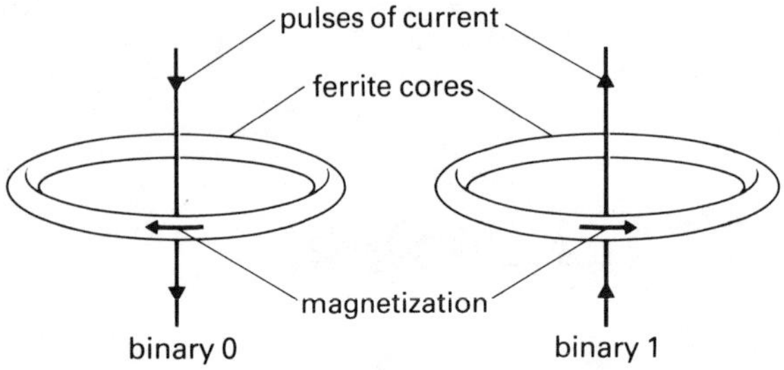

Fig. 4.3. Ferrite cores (enlarged)

Arrangement of cores in the memory

A computer memory contains several thousand cores. To avoid the problems of having a separate wire threading each core, they are arranged in **planes,** with wires along the rows and columns. There are two of these wires passing through each core. (See Figure 4.4.)

To change the magnetization of a core, pulses of half the threshold size are sent along the two wires which pass through the core. These half pulses combine to change the magnetization of the required

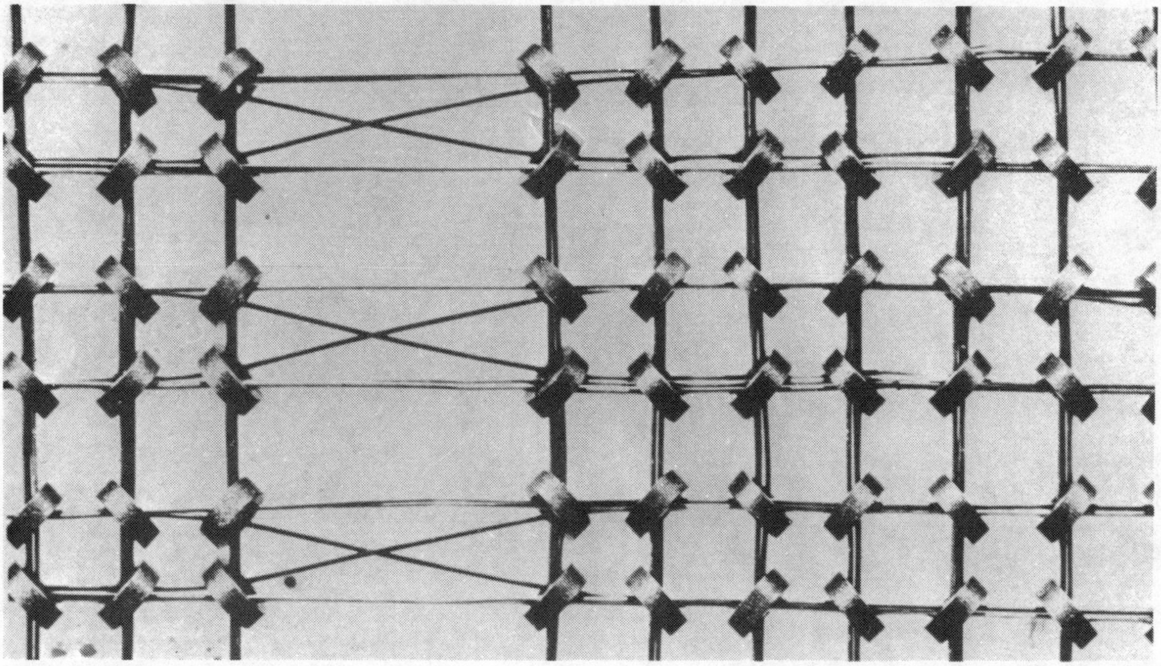

Part of a plane of ferrite cores in a computer memory

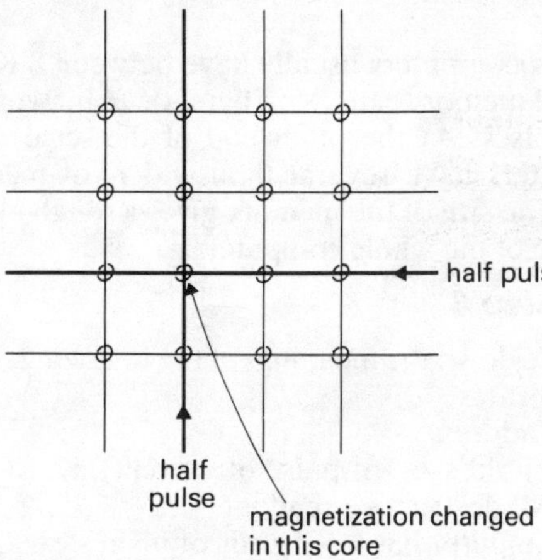

Fig. 4.4. A plane of ferrite cores

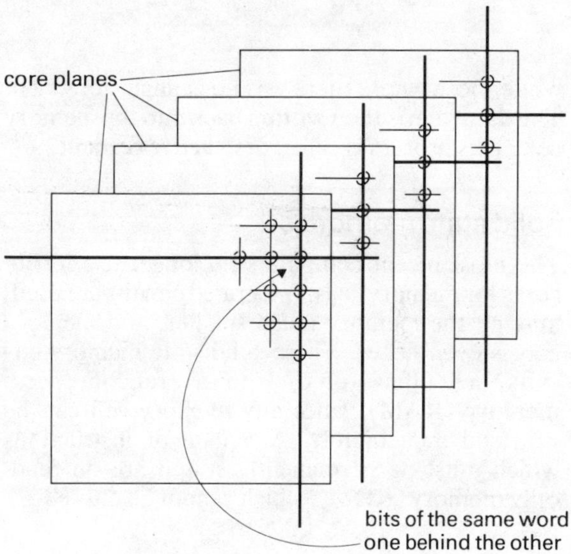

Fig. 4.5. The arrangement of core planes in a computer memory

core, but do not effect any other cores they pass through.

The planes are arranged one behind the other, one plane for each bit of a word. The bits of the same word are in line behind each other, in corresponding positions in the planes.

Reading and writing

An item of data is stored, or **written** in a cell in the memory by sending half pulses down the appropriate wires, as previously described. This process overwrites the previous data item stored in the cell.

A data item is copied, or **read,** from a cell in the memory by sending pulses in such a way as to set all the bits of the word to store 0. Other wires, not shown in the sketch, detect which cores changed magnetization. These cores originally stored a 1,

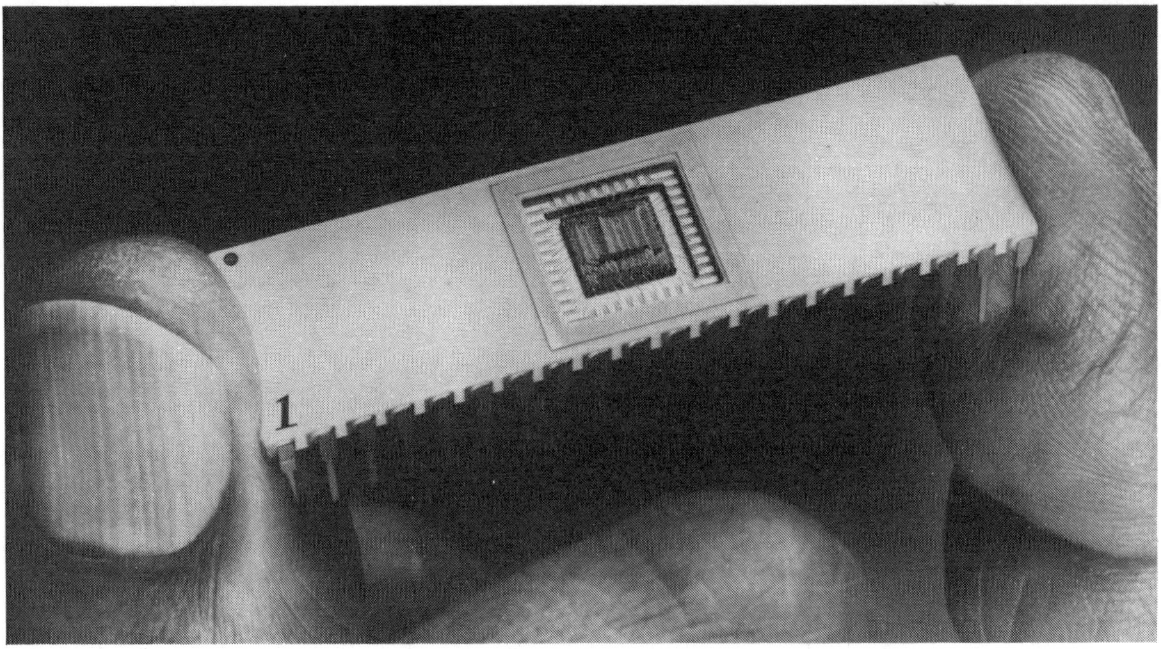
A Ferranti microprocessor. Chips like this have replaced ferrite cores in computer memories

while those where there was no change stored a 0. The data item is then written back into the memory cell. This process is called **destructive readout.**

Solid state memories

The most recent computers no longer use ferrite cores for memory cells. Integrated circuits are used, making the memory much smaller, and memory access even faster. These solid state memory circuits are often referred to as random-access memory (RAM), since any memory cell can be accessed immediately. Any data or instructions which must be permanently stored are on read-only memory (ROM), which cannot be altered.

The size of computer memories

In most computers with ferrite core memories, the core planes have 32 rows, each of 32 cores, making a total of $32 \times 32 = 1024$ cores per plane. The number 1024 is called **one K.** If the computer has 24 bits in a word, there will be 24 of these planes. The K unit is used for computers with ferrite core memories, or with integrated circuit memories. In some computers, memory size is quoted as a number of words, in others as a number of bytes.

Microcomputers usually have between 8 K and 32 K of memory cells, 8 bit bytes or 16 bit words in most cases. At the other end of the scale, large computers have several thousand K of memory cells. The size of the memory gives a rough idea of the size of the whole computer.

Exercise 4

1 Write down the meanings of the following words or phrases:
cell; address;
threshold size (of pulse of current); K; ROM; RAM; destructive readout.

2 A computer has 4 K words of main store. Each word comprises 24 bits. How many bits are there in the whole memory?

3 How many wires are needed to thread a plane containing 1 K cores?

4 Why are two half pulses of current used to change the magnetization of a core?

5 Why is a computer memory called an immediate access store?

6 An address is a set of words and numbers which locates a house. An address also locates a word in a computer memory. A telephone number locates one telephone in a town.
Make a list of some more numbers or codes which locate other information.

5

Input of data

This chapter describes ways in which data is supplied to a computer. Preparation of data for input often takes as long as, or longer than, the processing of the data.

Data for input into a computer must usually be stored on a **medium** which the computer can read. These input media include punched cards, paper tape, documents with characters in magnetic ink, and documents which can be read directly by optical means.

Various **devices** read the data from these media, changing it into pulses of electricity for processing.

Punched cards

One of the oldest storage media, punched cards have 80 columns, each of which can store one character. Holes are punched in the card, giving a binary coding. A hole represents a 1, no hole a 0.

The commonest codes for A, B and C are:

A 1 0 0 1 0 0 0 0 0 0 0 0
B 1 0 0 0 1 0 0 0 0 0 0 0
C 1 0 0 0 0 1 0 0 0 0 0 0

There are twelve rows for holes, and thus twelve bits in each code. The other codes are shown in the diagram below (Figure 5.1). The code for each character must be read down the column below the character.

Data is usually arranged in **fields** on a card. A field is an area usually of a fixed width, containing one item of information. For example, a card containing the catalogue number, description, VAT rate and price of an item might be set out as shown in Figure 5.2.

The cards containing one program or one set of data are called a **deck.**

Punching and verifying

Data is put onto cards by means of a **card punch,** which has a keyboard rather like that on a typewriter, but with capital letters only. Cards are fed in automatically, and the punch can be set to move directly to certain columns.

After punching, the cards are usually put through the card punch a second time to be checked, or **verified.** The machine is set to verify mode, and the

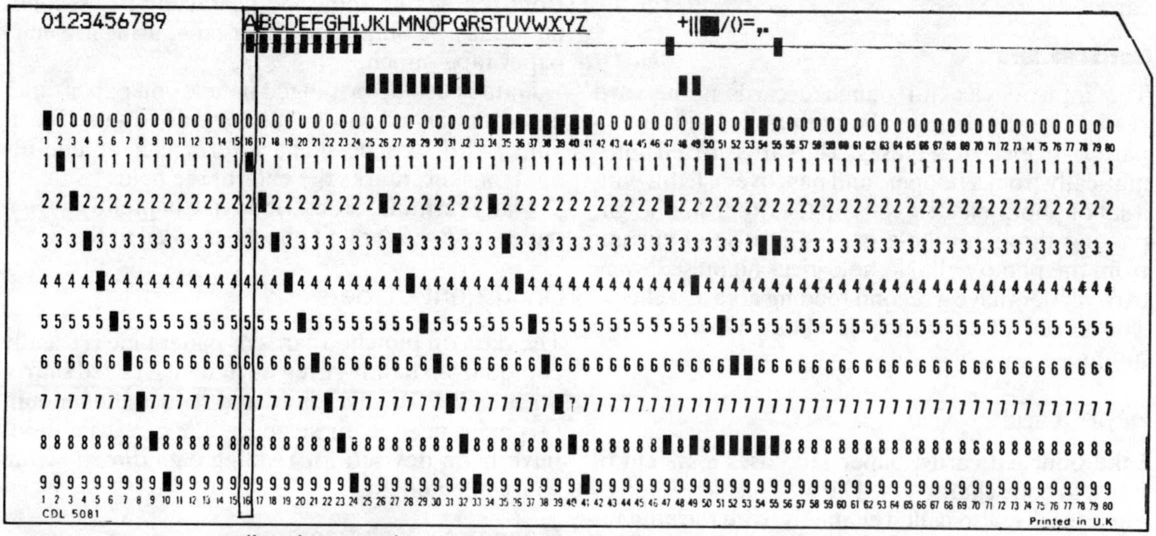

reading downwards
A = 100100000000

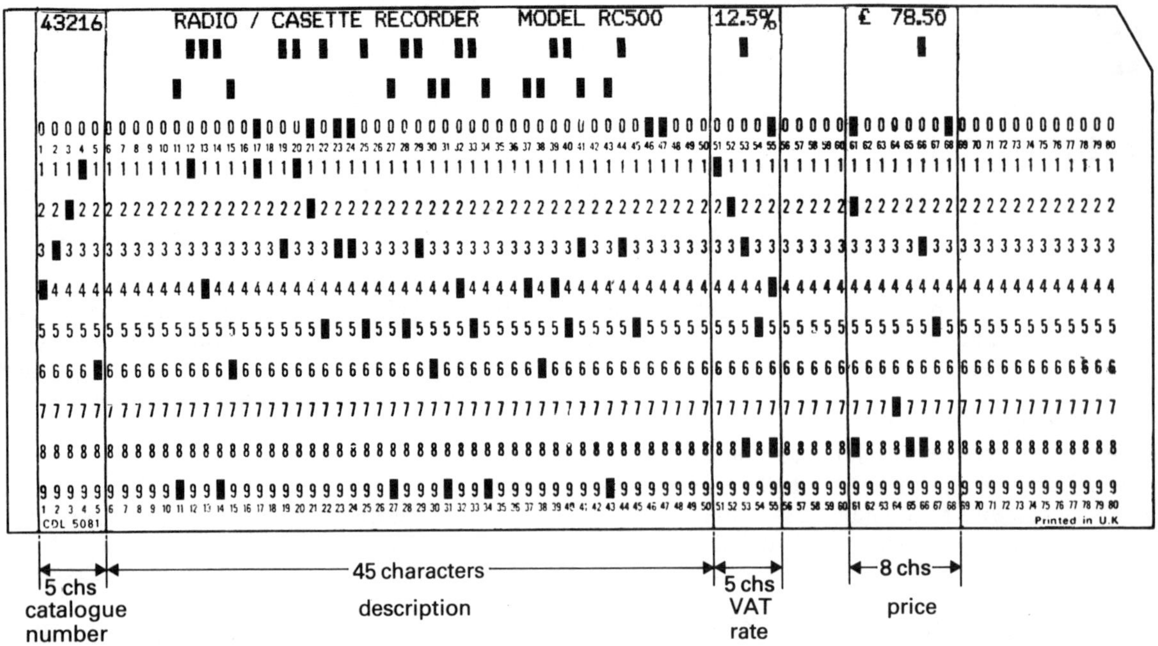

data is punched again. If the key pressed is the same as the character already on the card, the card moves to the next character position. If there is a different character, the keys are locked to indicate a possible error. If necessary, a new card must then be punched and verified.

A different kind of card punch can be used as an output device. It has no keyboard, and the information from the CPU is punched directly onto cards.

Card readers

The input device for punched cards is the **card reader,** which changes the pattern of holes into a pattern of electrical pulses. The cards are fed automatically from a hopper, and pass over a light, with a set of photo-electric cells on the other side. Light passing through a hole causes a pulse of current from the photo-cell. No hole gives no pulse. Some card readers have a second reading area as a check. The speed of operation is about 400 cards per minute.

Paper tape

Like punched cards, paper tape uses a system of holes to code characters. The tape has six, seven or eight **tracks,** also called channels, with the area for each character, called a **frame,** running across the tracks. One track is often a parity track. A hole is punched in this track so that the total number of holes in each frame is even, for **even parity** (and odd for **odd parity**).

Paper tape is prepared on a **paper tape punch,** which has a keyboard like a card punch. It is input into a computer by means of a **paper tape reader.** A paper tape reader either uses photo-electric cells like a card reader, or small metal contacts to 'feel' the holes. In either case, a pattern of electric pulses is produced. Reader speeds vary considerably – from ten to one thousand characters per second. Data may be output on paper tape, using a special paper tape punch.

Data is usually arranged in fields on paper tape, as with punched cards, but these are often of variable width. A special character, called an end-of-field marker, marks the ends of the fields.

Many terminals (described in Chapter 8) have a paper tape reader and punch attached to them.

Document readers

The data on punched cards or paper tape is usually copied from handwritten documents, called **source documents.** To save time, and reduce the amount of paper needed to store data, several methods have been devised for reading data directly from source documents.

Magnetic ink characters

Most commonly used on cheques, these are characters printed in a special ink containing iron filings,

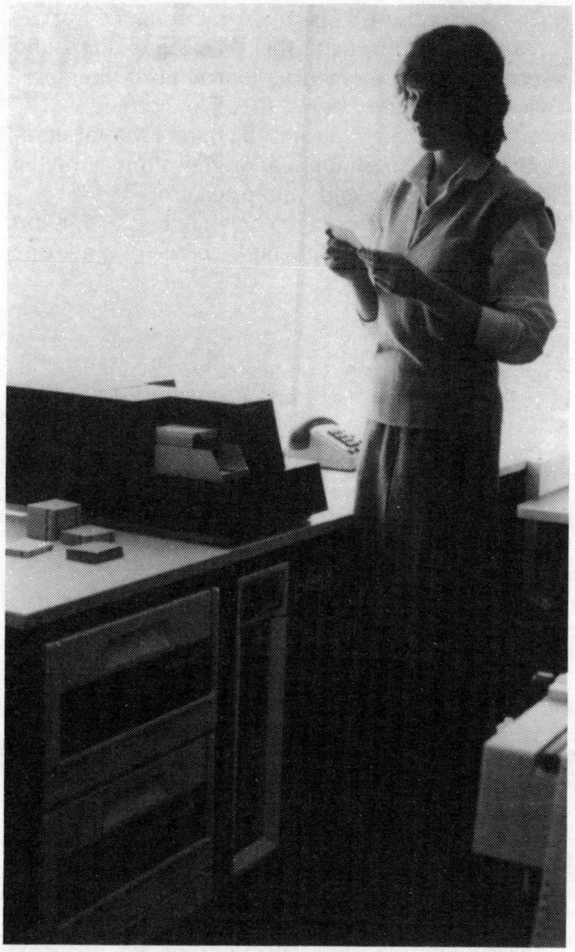

A Honeywell punched card reader in use

which can be magnetized. They read by a device called a **magnetic ink character reader.** This magnetizes the ink and then detects the combinations of magnetized and unmagnetized areas making up a character. The process is called **magnetic ink character recognition** (MICR).

Mark sense documents

These are pieces of paper, or cards the same size as punched cards, with small areas which may be shaded with a soft pencil. A mark sense reader shines a light on these areas. It detects the amount of light reflected, and produces a pulse of current if the area is shaded. Again this gives a binary coding of the data.

Common uses for mark sense documents include multiple choice tests, football pool coupons and recording gas or electricity meter readings.

Optical character recognition (OCR)

Optical character readers can recognize characters printed in ordinary ink, by the pattern of light they reflect.

Direct data entry (DDE)

With paper becoming more and more expensive, an increasingly popular input device is the **key-to-disc,** or **direct data entry** system.

A keyboard, somewhat like that on a typewriter, is connected to a visual display screen (like a small TV screen) and a magnetic disc. As data is typed, it is displayed on the screen and copied onto the magnetic disc. Data can easily be deleted or inserted, making verification quite simple.

Many computer installations are changing from punched card or paper tape input to direct data entry.

Buffers

All input and output devices contain storage spaces for the data being input or output at the time. These storage spaces are called **buffers.** For example, the buffer in a card reader can store 80 characters, the amount of data on one card. The characters are stored in the buffer until they are needed by the CPU.

Buffers are needed because all input and output

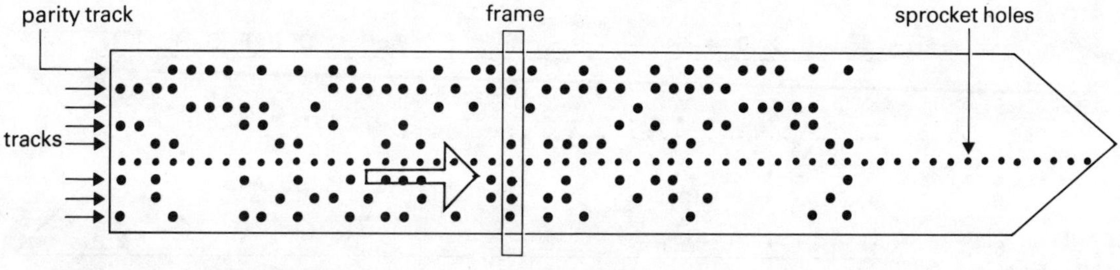

Fig. 5.3. A section of eight track paper tape

devices are much slower than a CPU. They enable the CPU to carry on processing while data is being input or output.

Exercise 5

1 Write down the meanings of the following words or phrases:
medium; device; field; deck; verify; track; frame; source documents; MICR; OCR; direct data entry; buffer;

2 What are the advantages and disadvantages of key-to-disc input systems?

3 Decide on suitable field widths, and draw specimen cards to contain the following data:
(a) Your name, address, post code and telephone number.
(b) Your name, date of birth, form, and the subjects you are taking (perhaps use a code for subjects).
(c) A person's name, works number, national insurance number, tax code, ordinary and overtime pay rates, and ordinary and overtime hours worked in a week.
(d) The name of a place, its Ordnance Survey map grid reference, the date, maximum and minimum temperature, barometric pressure, relative humidity, wind speed and direction.
(e) The record of a sale: the date, account number of the customer, catalogue number of the article, number sold, and price.

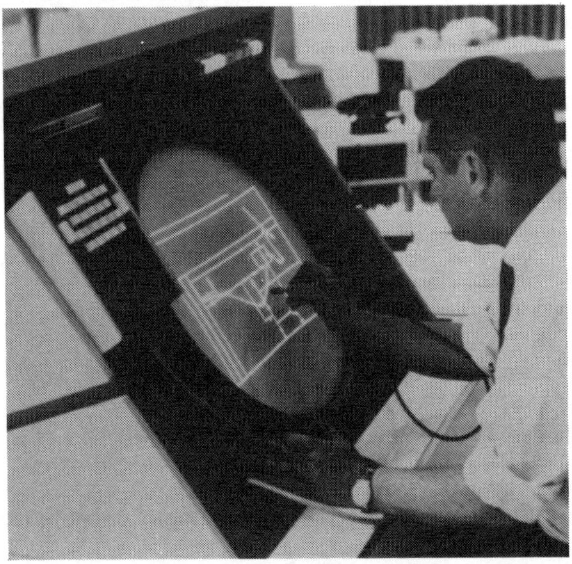

A light pen in use for data input on an ICL graphics terminal

4 The piece of paper tape shown in Figure 5.4, has three characters punched correctly and one punched incorrectly.

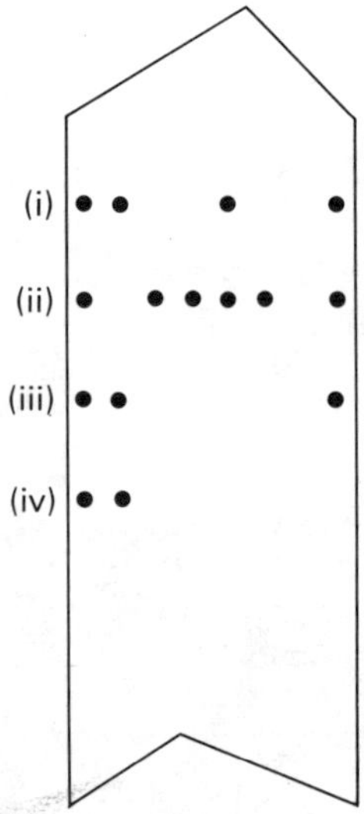

Fig. 5.4.

Using the idea of a parity check, say
(a) which of (i), (ii), (iii) or (iv) is the incorrect character.
(b) whether the tape has odd or even parity. (MREB 76)

5 Figure 5.5 shows the punchings used for some of the characters of an eight-channel paper tape code. The characters have been written above their corresponding punchings. Channel 8 is used for the parity bit. Draw a similar diagram to Figure 5.5 showing a piece of paper tape on which only the characters 7 and J and K have been punched. (EAEB 76 I)

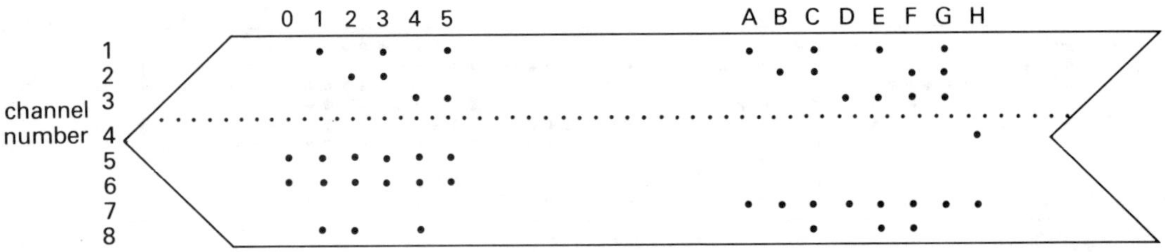

Fig. 5.5.

6

Output of data

This chapter describes how the results of data processing are output by a computer.

Output from a computer is usually printed on paper. It is often called **printout.** Several printing devices are commonly used, in most cases line printers or dot matrix printers. Output devices recently developed include computer output on microfilm (COM) systems, and laser beam printers. This chapter contains brief descriptions of these devices.

Line printers

The most common output device is a **line printer** – so called because it prints an entire line in one operation. There are two main types, the drum or barrel printer and the chain printer.

The drum printer

The drum printer has a rapidly rotating cylinder with a complete row of each character across its surface. Printing a line (usually 120 characters) takes one complete revolution of the drum. As the required character moves past the print position, a hammer strikes the paper against it (with an inked ribbon in between). Thus any **A**'s in a line are printed first, then any **B**'s, etc. At the end of the revolution of the drum, the paper moves on to the next line. For example, the word DATA will be printed in the following order:

```
 A A
DA A
DATA
```

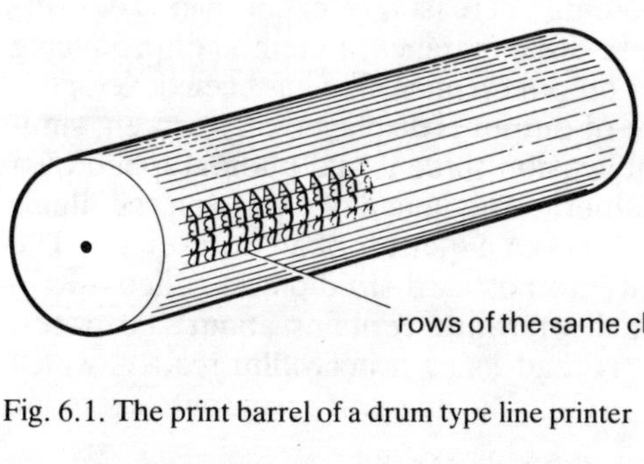

Fig. 6.1. The print barrel of a drum type line printer

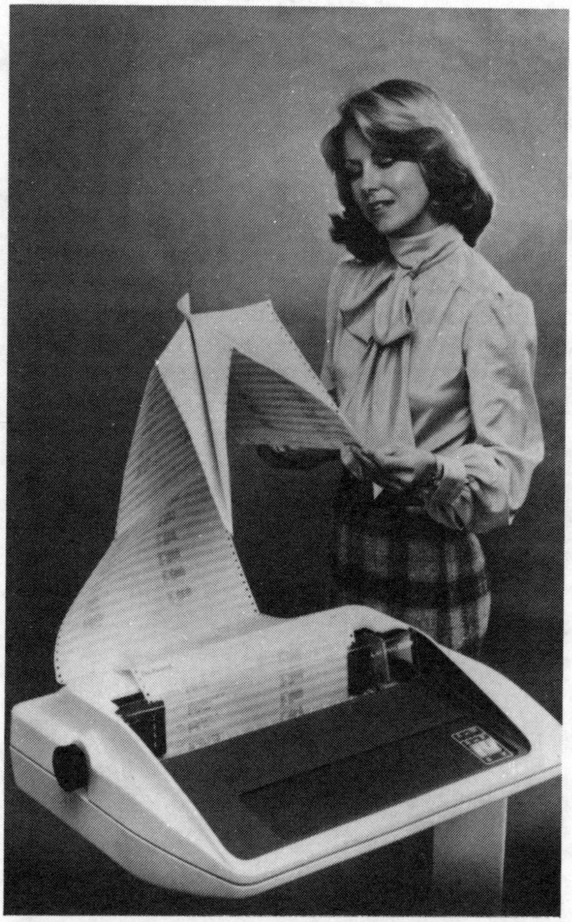

A Data General line printer in use

The chain printer

A chain printer has a rapidly moving chain carrying several sets of characters across the paper. As any character comes level with its required printing position, a hammer strikes the paper against it.

More common letters occur more frequently on the chain, shortening the average time taken for a letter to reach its printing position. As soon as a line is complete, the paper moves on.

Both types of line printer move the paper by means of sprockets fitting into holes along the sides of the paper. Speeds vary from 400 to 1200 lines per minute.

Specially printed stationery (such as blank cheque forms) is often used to avoid having to use the line printer for constant information. The layout of the output is designed to match the preprinted areas.

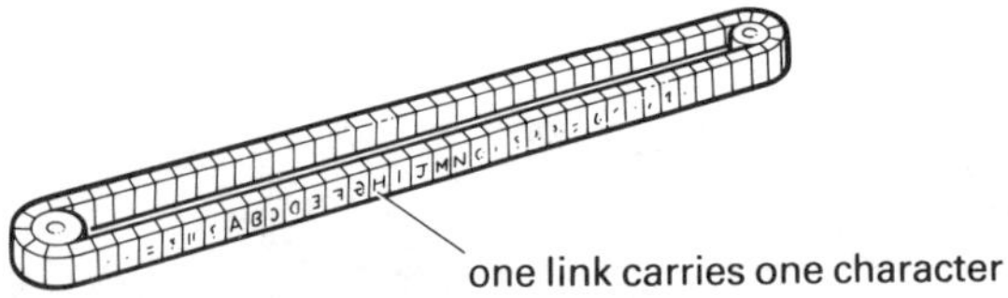

Fig. 6.2. The print chain of a chain type line printer

Dot matrix printers

Dot matrix printers are faster than typewriters, but not as fast as line printers. Each character is formed by a series of dots. The dots are produced by fine needles, which are arranged in a matrix, usually with five columns and seven rows. Different combinations of needles make up different characters. The diagram (Figure 6.3) shows how this is done.

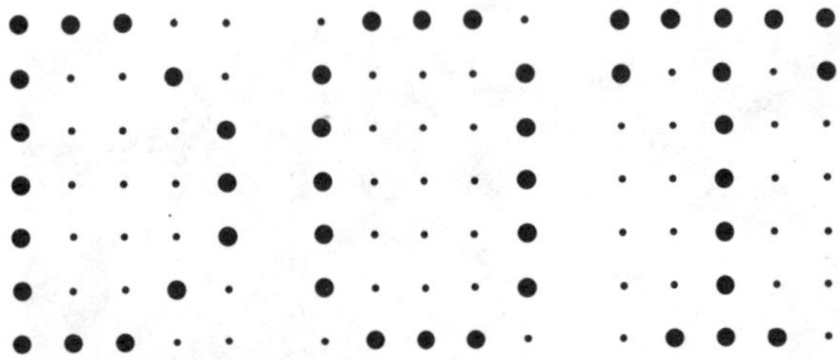

Fig. 6.3. Some characters formed by combinations of dots

Dot matrix printers operate at about 100 characters per second. At 120 characters per line, this is equivalent to 50 lines a minute.

Graph plotters

Graphs, architects' plans, engineering drawings and maps can be produced directly from program results by graph plotters (sometimes called **digital plotters**). There are two types of plotter: drum plotters and flat bed plotters.

In a drum type plotter, a roll of special paper moves forwards and backwards through the plotter, and a pen moves across the paper. In this way, lines of any direction, or letters can be drawn.

In a flat bed plotter, the paper is held still while the pen moves in all directions. In both types of plotter, the pen or the paper moves in small steps, rather than continuously, giving rise to the name digital plotter.

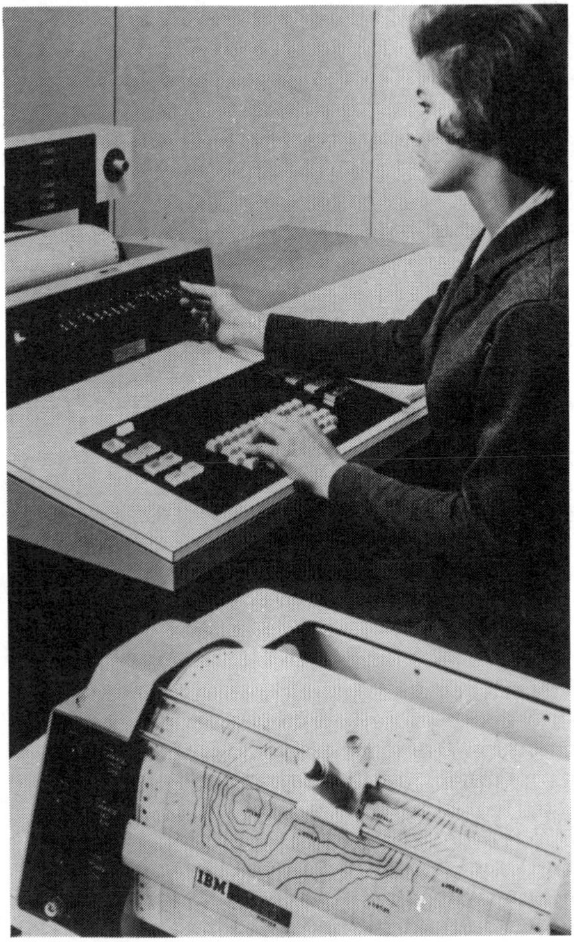

An IBM digital plotter at work

A digital plotter is, by computer standards, a very slow device. A complete graph or drawing can take several minutes to produce.

Computer output on microfilm (COM)

The main disadvantage of printed output is the large quantity of paper that is used. Paper is bulky, and becoming increasingly expensive. To overcome these disadvantages, a method of producing computer output on microfilm has been developed.

A page of output is displayed on a screen, similar to a television screen, and photographed by a special camera. The image of a page on the film is very small, about a quarter of an inch square. The film is cut into postcard-sized pieces called **microfiches,** each of which contains about 200 pages. The film is read using a **microfilm** reader, which projects an enlarged image of a page onto a screen.

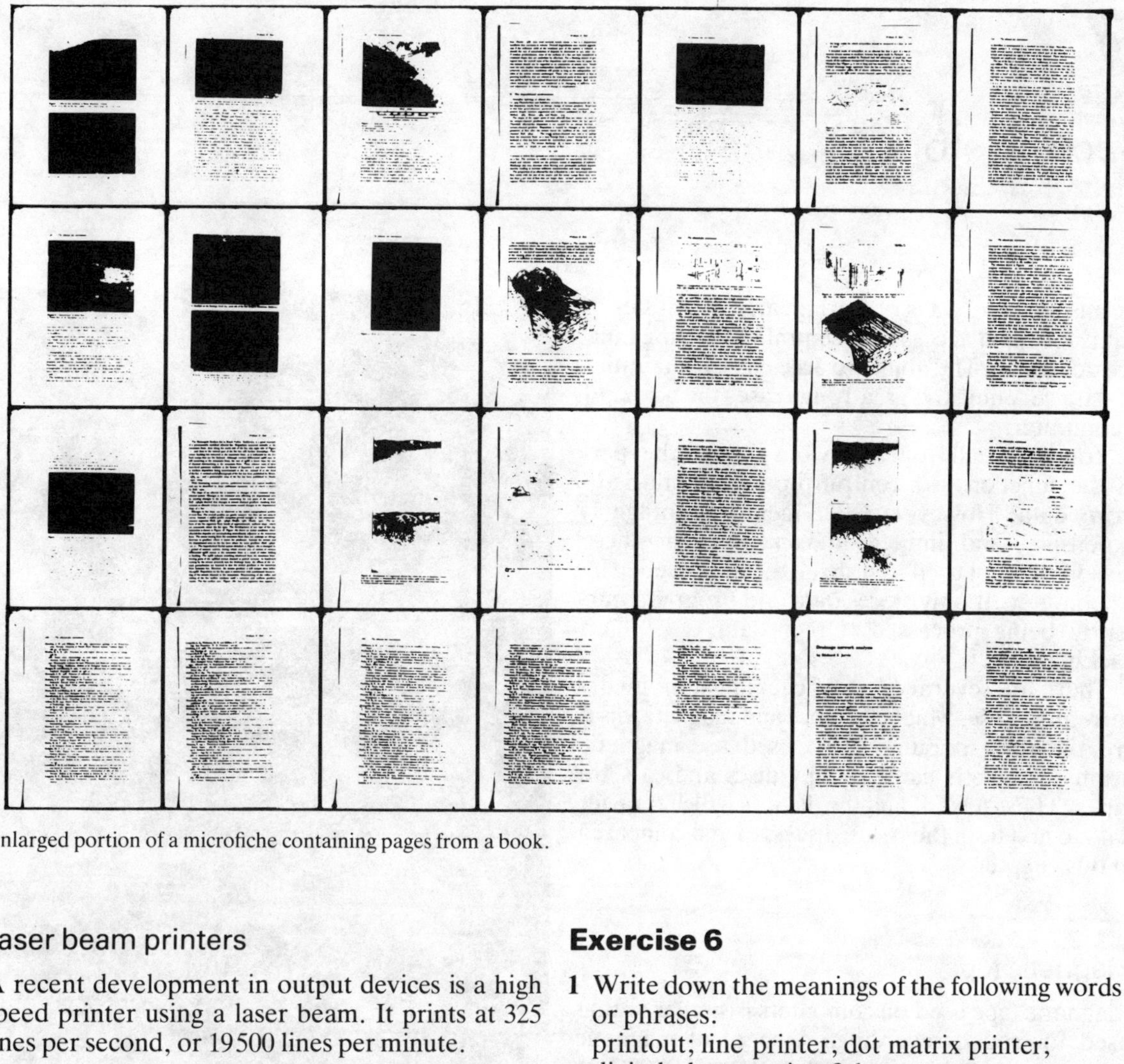

Enlarged portion of a microfiche containing pages from a book.

Laser beam printers

A recent development in output devices is a high speed printer using a laser beam. It prints at 325 lines per second, or 19500 lines per minute.

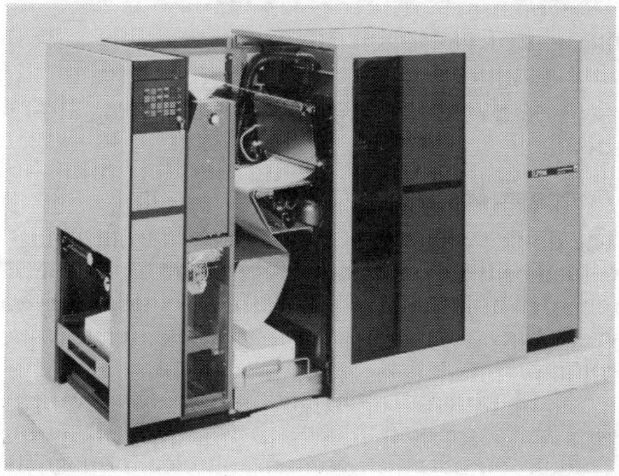

An ICL laser beam printer

Exercise 6

1 Write down the meanings of the following words or phrases:
printout; line printer; dot matrix printer; digital plotter; microfiche.

2 Show how the phrase OUTPUT DEVICE would be printed on a drum type line printer. Would the order of printing be the same for a chain type printer?

3 Part of a computer output has only one number on each of several lines:

1
2
3 etc.

Would this be printed more quickly on a drum type or a chain type line printer?

4 Make a list of some documents which are printed by a line printer on pre-printed stationery.

5 Why does a line printer work much more quickly than a typewriter?

6 What, in your opinion, are the advantages of computer output on microfilm?

7

Backing store

In this chapter, ways of storing large quantities of data, for rapid access by a central processing unit, are described. The ability to access large quantities of data very quickly, greatly increases the power of a computer.

You will recall from a previous chapter that part of the function of a central processing unit is to store data. However, CPU memory storage is expensive, and limited in capacity. For these reasons it is not used to store all the data needed by a computer. It only stores data and programs currently being processed. Other data is kept on **backing store.**

There are several types of backing store media currently in use. Magnetic tapes and magnetic discs are the most popular. Also used are magnetic drums, magnetic cards, floppy discs and cassette tapes. These media, and the devices which transfer data to and from them, are discussed and compared in this chapter.

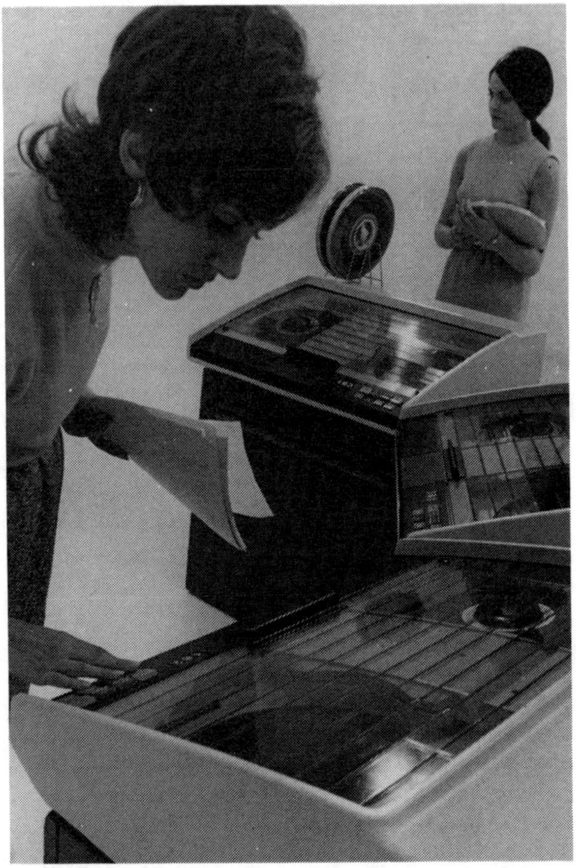

IBM magnetic tape units

Magnetic tape

Magnetic tape used on computers is similar to that used for sound recording. A spool of magnetic tape is normally half an inch wide and 2400 feet long. It is made of plastic, coated with iron oxide, or a similar substance, which can be magnetized.

Data is stored in a binary code, usually a character code (see Chapter 3). Each bit is represented by a small area on the tape which can be magnetized in one of two directions to store a 0 or a 1. The areas storing the bits of one data item are in line across the width of the tape.

The **packing density** of the data is up to 1800 characters per inch. This means that a complete magnetic tape can store nearly fifty million characters. Because the spacing of the data is so close, magnetic tape must be kept at a fairly constant temperature. Too much expansion or contraction makes it impossible to read.

Data is stored in **blocks** on the tape, separated by gaps. The gaps are to allow the tape to be started or stopped, as data can only be read from or written onto the tape when it is moving at full speed.

Magnetic tape units

The device which transfers data to or from a magnetic tape is called a **magnetic tape unit,** or **magnetic tape drive.** Details of the design of these devices vary, but they all have the following features in common:

There are spools for the tape, and wheels which pass the tape over a read, a write and an erase head, each of which contains an electro-magnet. The speed of the tape is very precisely controlled.

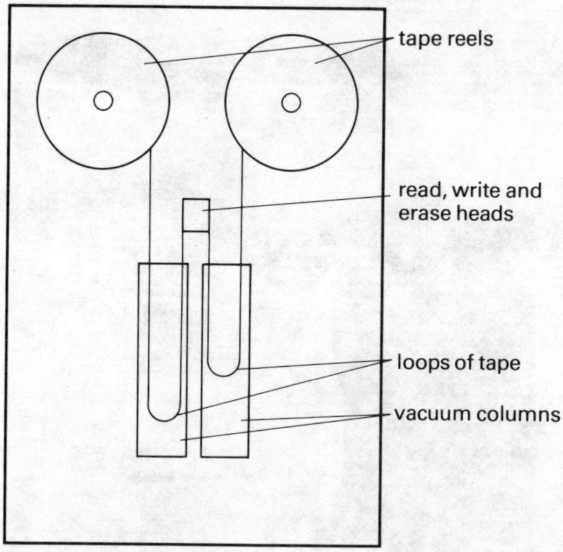

Fig. 7.1. A magnetic tape unit

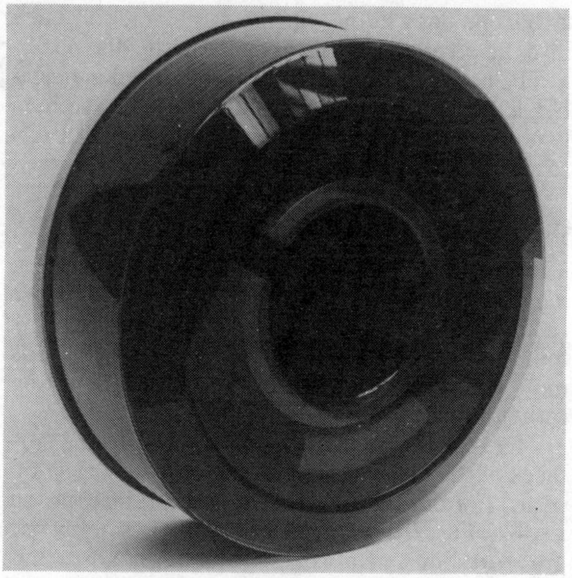

An exchangeable magnetic disc pack

Most magnetic tape drives have loops of tape in vacuum columns to allow for the extremely rapid acceleration or deceleration as the tape starts or stops.

Data is transferred at 100000 characters per second or more. However, it might take a minute or longer to locate the required data if the tape has to be wound forwards or backwards.

To guard against accidentally erasing data, spools have a **write permit ring.** If the ring is removed, it prevents any new data being recorded on that spool of tape.

Magnetic discs

Owing to their high speed to access to data, and decreasing price, magnetic discs are becoming the most common backing store medium.

Magnetic discs are made of metal, very precisely machined, coated with a substance that can be magnetized. The discs are either used singly, or in packs, usually of ten, mounted on one shaft. Some disc packs are fixed in place in their disc drives, while others can be removed. The latter type are called **exchangeable disc packs.**

As with magnetic tapes, small areas are magnetized in one direction or the opposite direction to store a 0 or a 1. These areas are arranged around the disc in circular **tracks.** The tracks are often divided into blocks, or **sectors,** with gaps in between.

In a disc pack, bits of the same data item (usually a character) are positioned one above each other in corresponding positions on each disc surface.

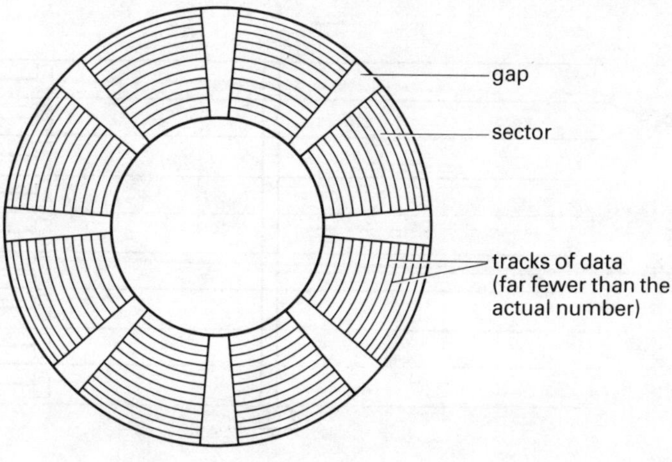

Fig. 7.2. Data layout on a magnetic disc

Adjacent data items, on the same track in each disc, lie on an imaginary **cylinder** in the disc pack.

The amount of data stored is measured in **megabytes.** A megabyte is one million bytes, one byte generally storing one character. Disc packs can store up to 300 megabytes.

Disc drives

The device which transfers data to or from a magnetic disc is called a **disc drive.** It rotates a disc or disc pack at 2000 revolutions per minute or more. For disc packs, a set of **read/write heads** moves across the disc surfaces, on a mounting rather like the fingers of a hand. See Figure 7.3.

The read/write heads are very close to the surfaces of the discs, sometimes floating on a cushion of air. For this reason, discs must never be exposed to dust. Disc drives are closed, and discs not in use are stored in special covers. The air in most computer rooms is filtered.

Disc drives can be used to read or record data. It takes one tenth of a second, on average, to locate an item of data. Reading or writing then takes place at 150000 characters per second or more.

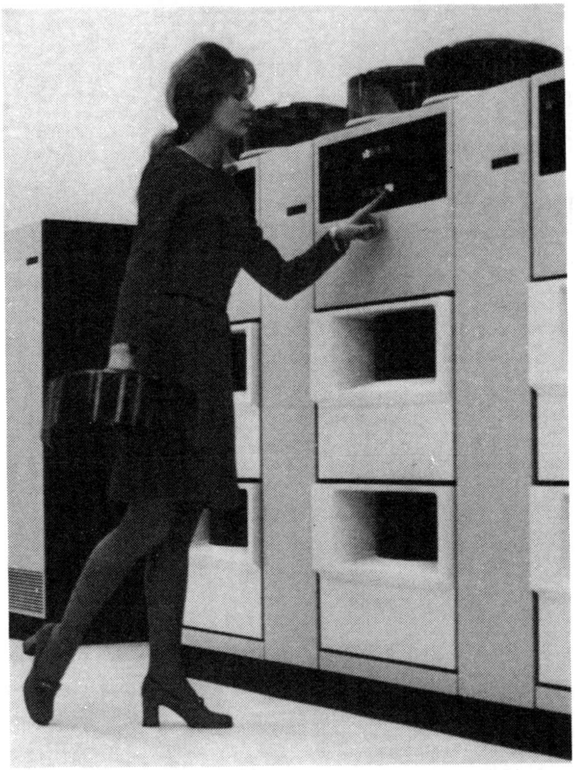

IBM magnetic disc drives

Magnetic drums

Magnetic drums are metal cylinders, coated with a substance which can be magnetized. Data is recorded by means of small magnetized spots, as with magnetic tapes and discs. The spots are arranged in circular tracks around the drum. The tracks may be divided into sectors.

The drive for a magnetic drum has one read/write head for each track. Data is transferred at up to 1500000 characters per second. The capacity of magnetic drums varies from half a megabyte to ten megabytes.

Magnetic cards

Magnetic cards are made from flat plastic, coated with a magnetizable substance. A number of cards are housed in a **magazine.** The method of coding data is similar to that used for magnetic tape. A magnetic card reader extracts the required card from the magazine, moves it rapidly past a set of read/write heads, and returns it to its place in the magazine.

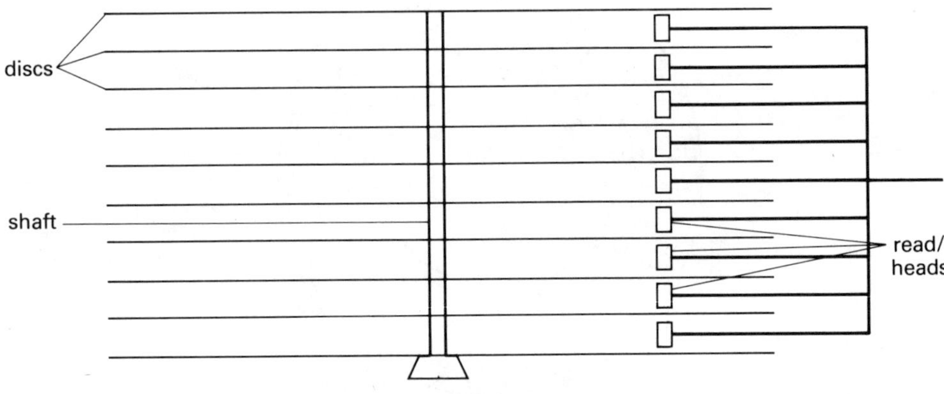

Fig. 7.3: Side view of a magnetic disc pack in a disc drive

The total storage capacity of all the cards in one reading device is very high, up to 5000 megabytes. However, access time is relatively slow, approximately half a second in most cases.

Floppy discs

A relatively new backing store medium, floppy discs are small discs made of a flexible material, coated with a magnetizable substance. The layout of data, and the method of reading and writing, are similar to those used by ordinary magnetic discs. Typical storage capacities of floppy discs vary from a quarter to a half of a megabyte.

Cassettes

Ordinary audio cassette tapes, or specially made tapes that resemble them very closely, can be used to store data in digital form. Data is read or written by cassette tape recorders which closely resemble ordinary audio cassette recorders. Cassette tapes are most frequently used as backing store by microcomputers. The speed of transfer of data is much less than that of conventional magnetic tape. See Table 7.1.

A comparison of backing store capabilities

The backing store media mentioned vary considerably in storage capacity, speed of transfer of data and price. All these factors must be taken into account in selecting the backing store medium for a particular computer application.

There is another important consideration – whether the medium provides **serial access** or **random access** to the stored data.

A serial access medium is one where the time taken to reach a data item depends on its position on the medium. Magnetic tape is a serial access medium. The time taken to reach an item on the tape depends on its distance along the tape from the place currently over the read/write heads.

Advantages and disadvantages of backing store media

A random or direct access medium is one where the time taken to locate a data item is largely independent of its position on the medium. Magnetic discs are a direct access medium. The time taken by the read/write heads to locate a data item does not depend very much on the position of the data item on the disc.

The nature of the computer application usually

Table 7.1

Storage medium	Capacity (megabytes)	Average access time (milliseconds)	Character Transfer Rate (megabytes per second)
magnetic tape	48	up to several minutes	0.02 to 0.3
magnetic disc	2 to 300	100 to 25	0.1 to 0.8
magnetic drum	0.5 to 10	25 to 5	0.2 to 1.5
magnetic cards	400 to 5000	200 to 600	0.2 to 1.0
floppy discs	0.25 to 0.5	40 to 400	0.02 to 0.06
magnetic tape cassettes	0.02 to 0.1	up to several minutes	10 to 800 characters per second
CPU memory	0.008 to 10	1.8 to 0.1 microseconds	0.5 to 10

Note 1 millisecond = 1 thousandth of a second
1 microsecond = 1 millionth of a second
1 megabyte = 1 million bytes

The above figures are only approximate. Improved performance figures for these media are frequently announced.

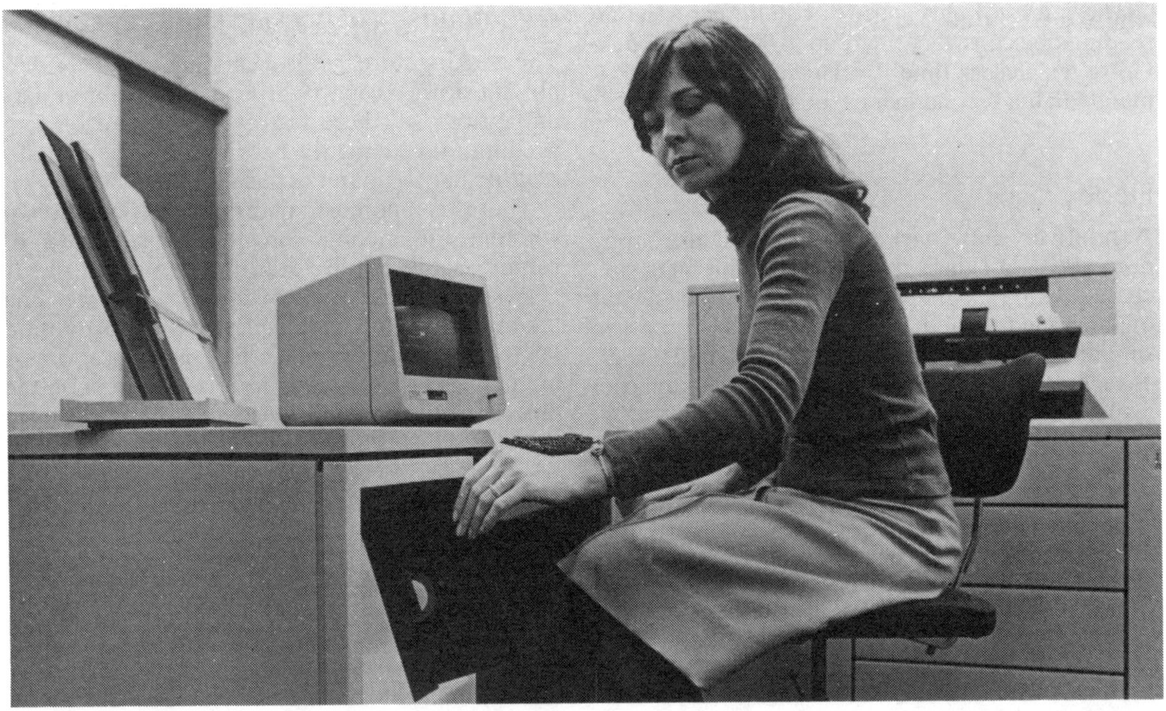

A floppy disc in use in an IBM office computer system

dictates whether serial access, or random access or both are required. If cost is the main factor, then magnetic tapes will store the same volume of data much more cheaply than magnetic discs. The choice between floppy discs and cassette tapes usually arises when microcomputers are used. Once again cost and serial or random access must be taken into consideration.

Magnetic drums played a significant part in the development of computers, but have now been largely superseded by magnetic discs. Magnetic drums are not usually exchangeable, and have a far smaller storage capacity than magnetic discs, though their access time to a data item is faster.

Magnetic cards have the advantages of being a random access medium with very high storage capacity, but are far slower than magnetic discs. They are not very widely used.

Exercise 7

1 Write down the meanings of the following words or phrases:
exchangeable disc pack; random access;
serial access; packing density; block; track;
write permit ring; megabyte; magazine; sector;
cylinder.

2 Classify all the storage media described in this chapter under the headings **serial access** and **random access.**

3 The data for a telephone directory is to be stored on magnetic discs.
(a) An entry in the directory comprises a surname, initials, address and telephone number. Estimate the number of bytes needed per entry (one byte stores one character).
(b) Using your estimate from part (a), calculate the number of bytes needed for 2.5 million entries.
(c) How many 30 megabyte discs will this require?
(d) Using a key-to-disc input system, how long would this data take to type at 4 characters per second?

4 Why must magnetic tapes and discs be kept at a fairly constant temperature?

5 A punched card can store 80 characters. How many punched cards would be needed to store the same data as a 40 megabyte disc?

6 Would serial or direct access be more suitable for:
(a) Storing a list of names in alphabetical order, ready for printing also in alphabetical order.
(b) Storing bank account files, which may be accessed in any order.
(c) Storing a number of short programs, any of which may be accessed at any time.
(d) Storing the data for the pay slips of a number of employees?

8

Terminals

Although computers process data very quickly, much time can be lost sending the data to and from the computer, and preparing the data for input. In many cases, much more efficient use is made of a computer by having **terminals** for input and output.

A terminal is a device which enables a person to have direct access to a computer. Terminals can be close to a computer, or linked to it from long distances by telephone lines. The latter type of terminals are called **remote access** terminals.

Because they are connected to the CPU of a computer, terminals are called **on-line** devices. Devices such as card punches, not connected to the CPU of a computer, are called **off-line** devices.

This chapter describes the types of terminals commonly in use, and how they are linked to computers. The way in which computer time is shared among a number of terminals is described in Chapter 15. The types of data processing which can be done on computers with terminals are described in Chapter 17.

Types of terminal

Three types of terminal are available: teletype-writers, visual display units and graphical display units.

Teletypewriter

A teletypewriter (called teletype for short) is similar to an electric typewriter, although most models use capital letters only. Input data and programs are typed on the keys and transmitted to the computer. Output is typed automatically by the computer, at about ten characters per second.

Visual display unit

A visual display unit (or VDU) has a keyboard like

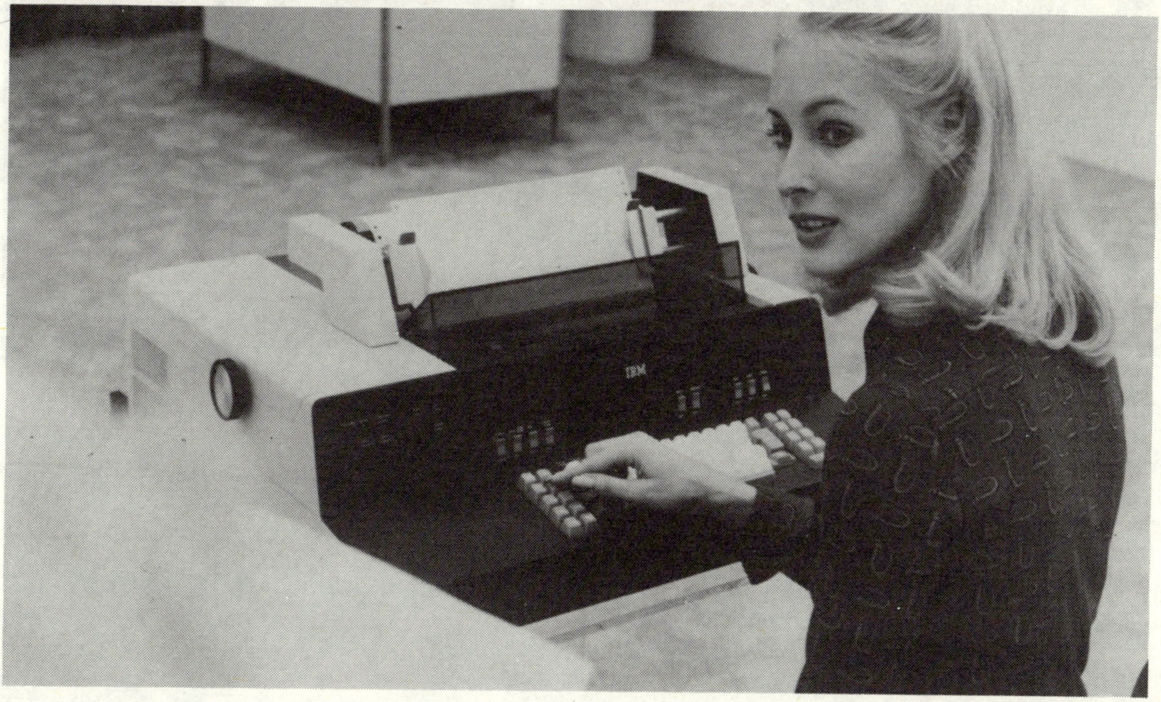

An IBM terminal in use

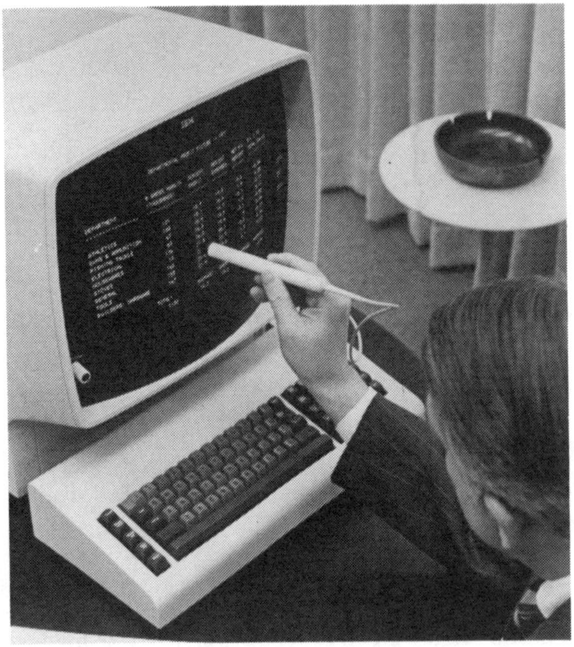

An IBM visual display unit

a teletype. Instead of being printed on paper, characters are displayed on a screen similar to that in a television set. Output on a VDU is often faster than on a teletype, and most have simple facilities for making corrections. The only disadvantage of a VDU is that no printed record (called **hard copy**) is produced.

Graphical display unit

A graphical display unit resembles a VDU, and can be used like one. However, in addition to characters, the screen can display lines and shaded areas. Graphical display units can display pictures, maps, graphs, and engineering and architectural drawings, particularly of three dimensional shapes which can be made to rotate. Most graphical display units have a **light pen** which can be used to draw lines onto the screen.

Linking terminals to computers

A problem in linking remote access terminals to computers is that the binary pulses they both use

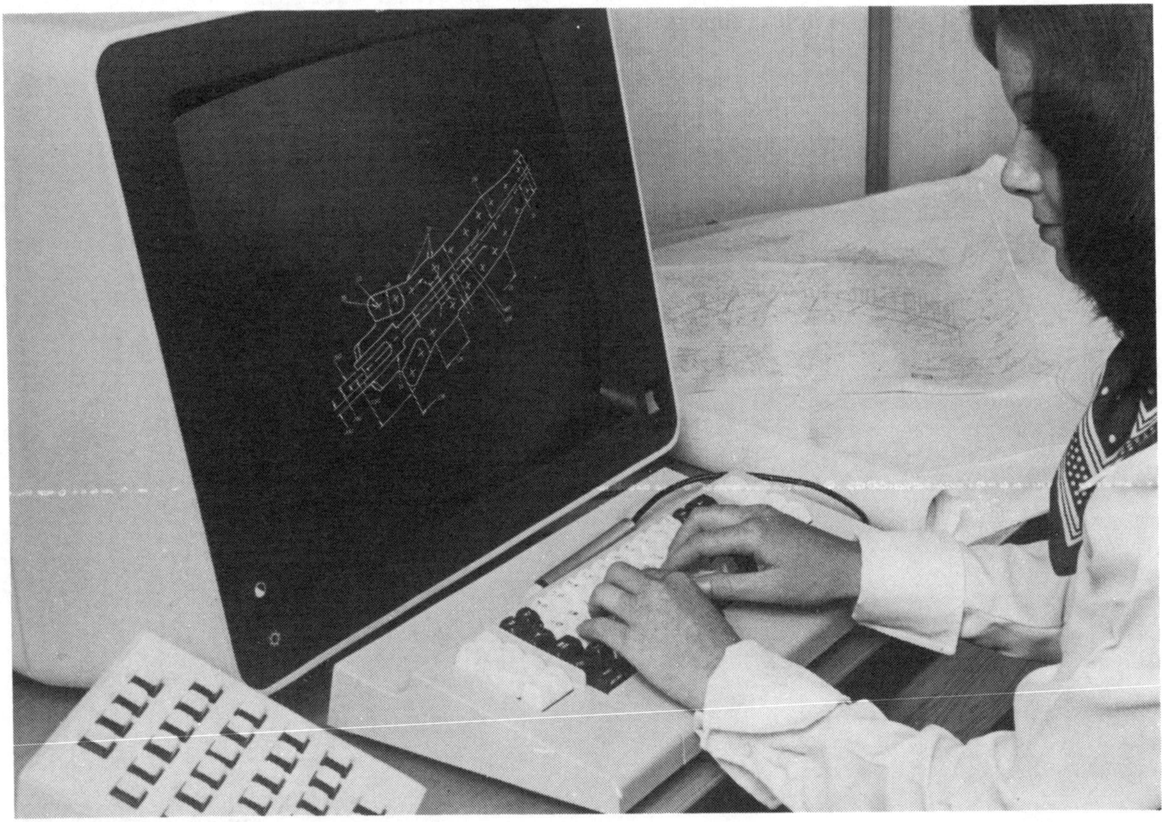

An IBM graphical display unit being used for computer-aided design

do not travel well down telephone lines. The slightest amount of interference in the telephone line would cause wrong characters to be transmitted.

To overcome this problem, terminals are connected to telephone lines via devices which change a stream of binary pulses into a wave of varying frequency, and vice versa. A similar device links the other end of the telephone line to the computer.

There are two types of these devices. A **modem** (for **mo**dulator/**dem**odulator) generates an electrical wave which is fed directly into the telephone line. An **accoustic coupler** generates a sound wave, which is then picked up by the telephone receiver. See Figure 8.1. The speed of transmission of data along a telephone line is measured in **bauds.** One baud is one bit per second. In most cases, transmission speeds are between 100 and 1000 bauds.

Exercise 8

1 Write down the meanings of the following words or phrases:
terminal; on-line; teletype; VDU; hard copy; light pen; interface; modem; baud.

2 What is the speed of input of data on a teletype?

3 Would a teletype, VDU or graphical display unit be more suitable for
(a) correcting a new program,
(b) drawing in a railway network on a map,
(c) running an accounts program,
(d) a library book information service,
(e) designing a motor car body,
(f) checking if an airline seat reservation can be made,
(g) recording sales?

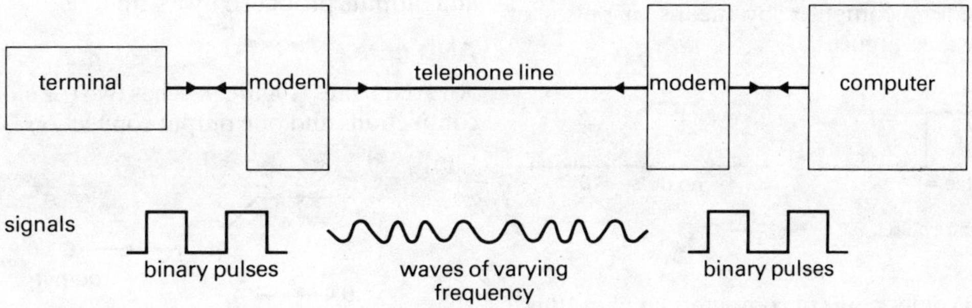

Fig. 8.1: Linking a terminal to a computer

9

Computer logic

Section A

This is the first of four chapters which deal with the way in which data is processed inside a computer. In this chapter, elementary ideas of computer logic are introduced. It will be seen that a few simple logical processes can be build up in various combinations to carry out all the processing tasks that a computer performs.

You will recall that data and control instructions move inside a computer by means of pulses of electricity. See Figure 9.1.

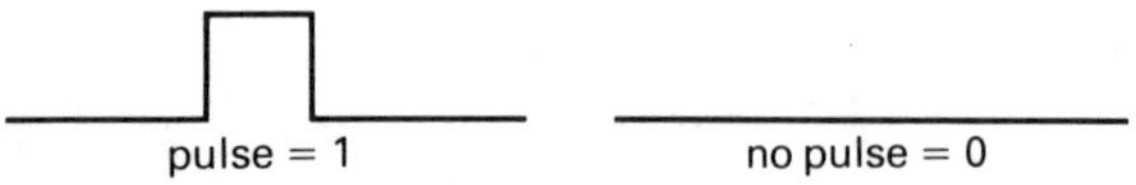

Fig. 9.1: Binary pulses

Certain components of computers combine these pulses as if they were following a set of rules. These components are called **logic elements.** Computer logic is the combination of inputs and outputs produced by logic elements.

Logic hardware

Processing of data is done on a large number of electrical circuits in the CPU of a computer. The hardware devices which do the processing are transistors or integrated circuits. An integrated circuit, often called a **chip,** is a very small circuit including a number of transistors. At the end of this chapter is a short section which gives a brief introduction to the structure and functioning of transistors.

In common with most computer components, logic elements are bistable devices. They have only two stable output states, representing 0 and 1 respectively.

Gates

The commonest use of logic elements is to act as switches, although they have no moving parts. They open to pass on a pulse of electricity, or close to stop it. For this reason they are known as **gates.**

The three commonest types of gates are introduced in this section. They are AND, OR and NOT gates. Two more types, NOR and NAND gates, are introduced in a later section of this chapter.

The way these gates work is described by **operation tables,** sometimes called **truth tables.** An operation table shows the combinations of inputs and outputs produced by a gate.

AND gate

An AND gate (Figure 9.2) has two (or more) input connections and one output connection.

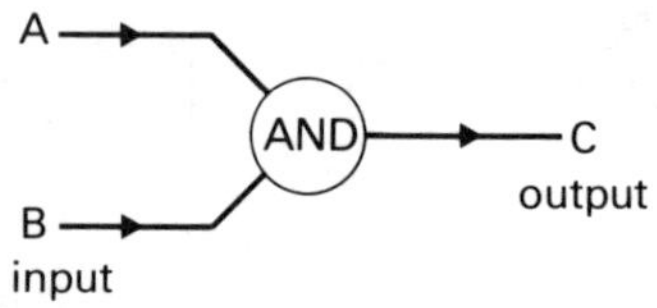

Fig. 9.2: A two input AND gate

Operation table

Input		Output
A	B	C
0	0	0
0	1	0
1	**0**	**0**
1	1	1

For example, the line of the table in bold type means that if there is a pulse at input A, and none at input B, there will no pulse at output C. A pulse is produced at output C if there is a pulse at input A *and* at input B. This gate may be described by the expression:

C = A AND B

OR gate

An OR gate (Figure 9.3) also has two (or more) input connections and one output connection.

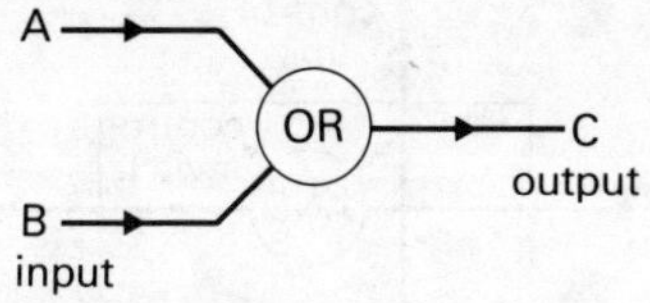

Fig. 9.3: A two input OR gate

Operation table

Input		Output
A	B	C
0	0	0
0	1	1
1	0	1
1	1	1

A pulse is produced at output C if there is a pulse at input A *or* at input B, or at both inputs. This gate may be described by the expression:

C = A OR B

NOT gate

A NOT gate has one input and one output. (Figure 9.4.)

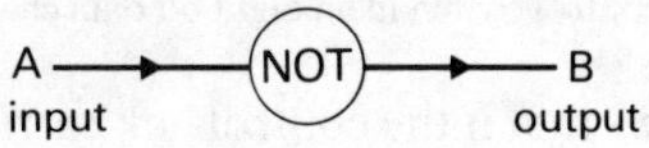

Fig. 9.4: A NOT gate

Operation table

Input	Output
A	B
1	0
0	1

The input signal is reversed. The expression for a NOT gate is:

B = NOT A

Other ways of writing logic expressions are introduced in the next section of this chapter.

Combinations of gates

All the logical and arithmetic operations done by computers are carried out by combinations of the logic elements mentioned previously. These combinations are called **logic circuits.** Some of these combinations are extremely complex.

The operation table for a combination of logic elements is worked out by following all the possible sets of input signals through the logic circuit.

Example 1

In Figure 9.5 the input combination A = 1, B = 0, C = 1 is followed through the circuit. A similar process gives the other outputs.

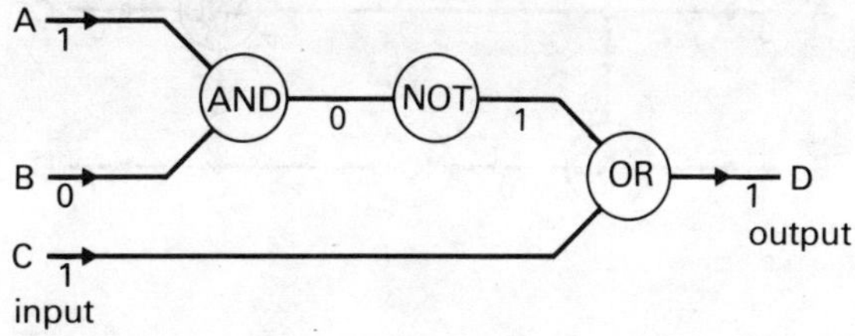

Fig. 9.5

Operation table

Input			Output	
A	B	C	D	
0	0	0	1	
0	0	1	1	
0	1	0	1	
0	1	1	1	
1	0	0	1	
1	0	1	1	shown in Figure 9.5
1	1	0	0	
1	1	1	1	

Example 2

In Figure 9.6 the input combination A = 0, B = 0, C = 1 is followed through the circuit. A similar process gives the other outputs.

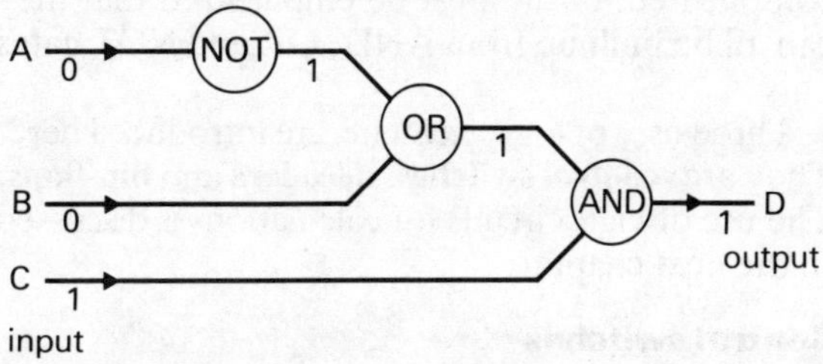

Fig. 9.6

Operation table

Input			Output	
A	B	C	D	
0	0	0	0	
0	0	1	1	shown in Figure 9.6
0	1	0	0	
0	1	1	1	
1	0	0	0	
1	0	1	0	
1	1	0	0	
1	1	1	1	

Example 3

In Figure 9.7 the input combination A = 0, B = 1 is followed through the circuit.

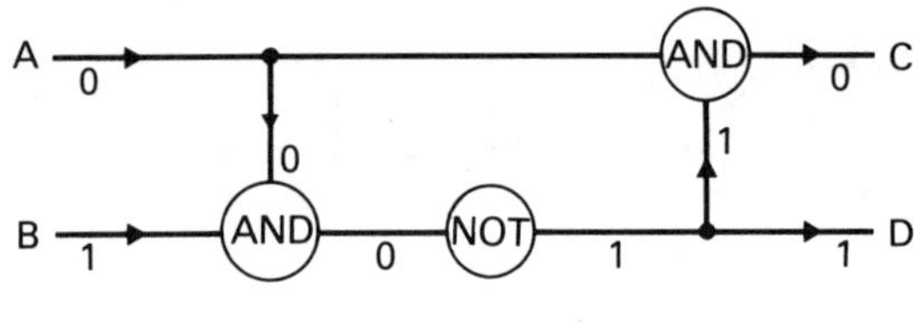

Fig. 9.7

Operation table

Input A	Input B	Output C	Output D	
0	0	0	1	
0	1	0	1	shown in Figure 9.7
1	0	1	1	
1	1	0	0	

These examples show how logic elements can be combined. You will notice that the combinations of inputs in the operation tables are obtained by counting in binary.

Some uses of logic elements

Logic elements are used in computers for storing certain data, doing calculations, making decisions and controlling the flow of data. Most of the logic circuits which perform these tasks are extremely complicated, but it must be emphasized that they can all be built up from AND, OR and NOT gates only.

Three uses of logic elements are introduced here. They are: **control switches, decoders** and **flip-flops.** The use of logic circuits for calculations is discussed in the next chapter.

Control switches

In many places in a computer, the flow of data is controlled by a switch. Data channels in a computer usually carry one word at a time. There is a wire for each bit of the word.

A **control switch** consists of a set of AND gates, one for each bit of the word. One input of each AND gate is connected to the control link, and the other is connected to a wire in the data channel. See Figure 9.8.

A control switch works as follows:

If one input to an AND gate is 1, the other input is copied to the output. But if one input is 0, the ouput is always 0. Check this from the operation table for an AND gate.

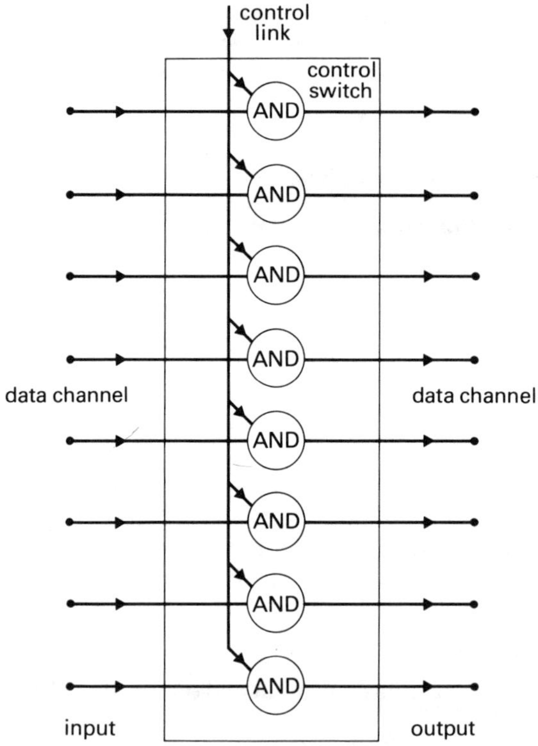

Fig. 9.8: A control switch in an eight bit data channel

It follows that if the control link carries the value 1, all the inputs in the data channel are copied to the outputs. The control switch is on. If, on the other hand, the control link carries a 0, all the outputs are 0. The control switch is off.

Decoders

A **decoder** is a hardware device which recognises a certain pattern of bits in a word, or part of a word. It outputs a 1 when this pattern is input, and a 0 for all other patterns.

For example, a decoder to recognise the bit pattern 1 0 1 is shown in Figure 9.9.

The output is 1 for the input pattern 1 0 1 and 0 for all other inputs. Check this yourself.

Decoders in most computers have one output for each possible combination of inputs. For example three input bits require eight outputs for the eight possible input patterns. Decoders are used in a computer to locate cells in the memory (**address decoders**) and to respond to different instructions (**operation decoders**).

Flip-flops

Logic elements can be combined to store data. The combination is called a **flip-flop** because a single

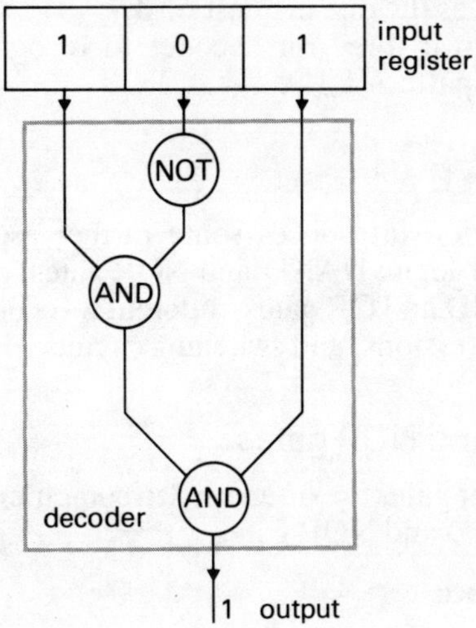

Fig. 9.9: A three bit decoder

input pulse can cause it to flip from one output state to another.

The actual combination of logic elements is not shown here, but the effect is as follows (Figure 9.10):

A flip-flop has two input connections and two output connections. A single pulse at the S input causes a train of pulses at the 1 output. The train continues until there is a single pulse at the R input. The train then is sent from the 0 output, until there is a single pulse at the S input.

One flip-flop stores a single bit. A set of flip-flops, called a **register,** stores a complete word. All computers use flip-flops to store data while it is being processed, and new computers use flip-flops instead of ferrite cores in the memory. Pocket calculators use flip-flops to store numbers.

Summary

The most important ideas which have been introduced in this section are as follows:

☐ Logic elements are components of a computer which combine binary pulses according to a few rules of logic. The hardware forming logic elements are transistors or integrated circuits.

☐ Logic circuits contain combinations of logic elements to carry out some specific task.

☐ The combination of inputs and outputs for a logic element or logic circuit is described by an operation table.

☐ A combination of logic elements can be described by a logic expression.

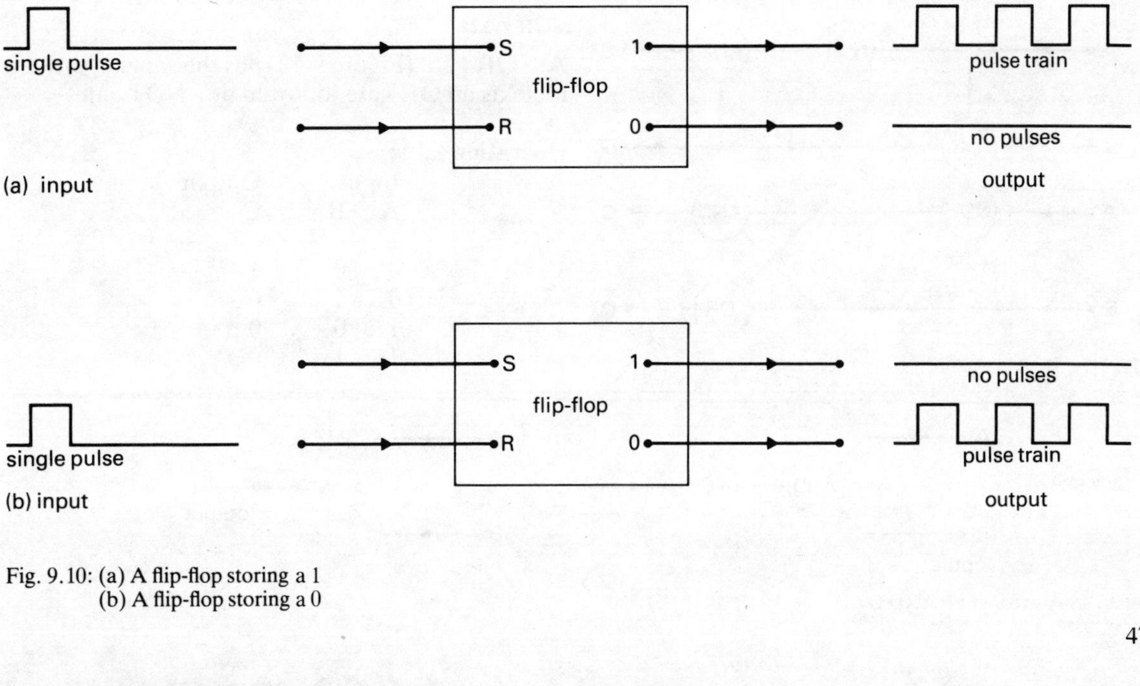

Fig. 9.10: (a) A flip-flop storing a 1
(b) A flip-flop storing a 0

Exercise 9a

1 Write down the meanings of the following words or phrases:
logic element; chip; gate; truth table;
control switch; decoder; flip-flop; logic circuit;
register.

For questions **2–7** work out operation tables for the logic circuits shown in Figure 9.11.

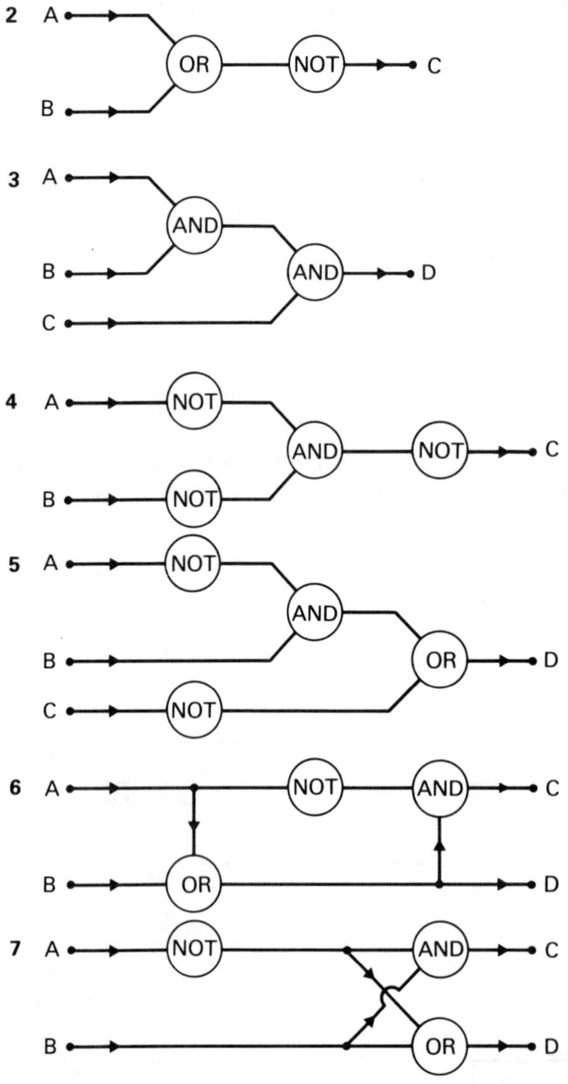

Fig. 9.11

8 Which single gate could replace all the gates in question **4**?

9 Draw another logic circuit having the same effect as the one in question **3.**

10 Design a three bit decoder to recognize the input pattern 1 1 0.

Section B

This section introduces some further aspects of computer logic: NAND and NOR gates, multiple input AND and OR gates, different ways of writing logic expressions, and switching circuits.

NAND and NOR gates

Two other gates are often used in computers. They are NAND and NOR gates.

NAND gate

A NAND gate (Figure 9.12) has the same operation table as an AND gate followed by a NOT gate.

Operation table

Inputs A	Inputs B	Output C
0	0	1
0	1	1
1	0	1
1	1	0

Compare this operation table with the one for an AND gate.

NOR gate

A NOR gate (Figure 9.13) has the same operation table as an OR gate followed by a NOT gate.

Operation table

Inputs A	Inputs B	Output C
0	0	1
0	1	0
1	0	0
1	1	0

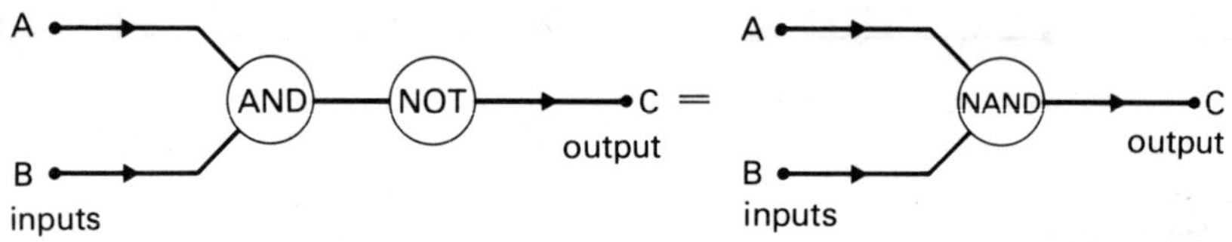

Fig. 9.12: A two input NAND gate

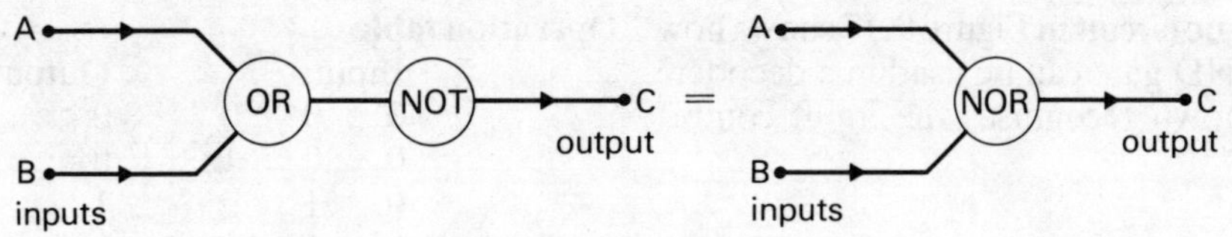

Fig. 9.13: A two input NOR gate

Compare this operation table with the one for an OR gate.

Figure 9.14 shows a logic circuit containing a NAND and a NOR gate.

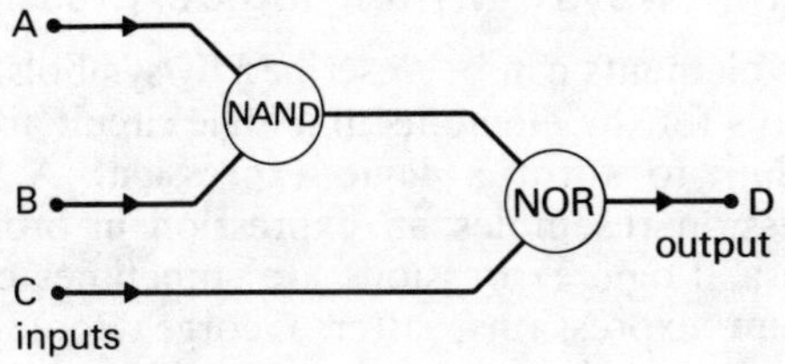

Fig. 9.14

Operation table

Inputs A	B	C	Output D
0	0	0	0
0	0	1	0
0	1	0	0
0	1	1	0
1	0	0	0
1	0	1	0
1	1	0	1
1	1	1	0

Multiple input AND and OR gates

AND and OR gates with more than two inputs are frequently used in computers. Their operation tables are extensions of the ones for two-input gates.

Three input AND gate (Figure 9.16)

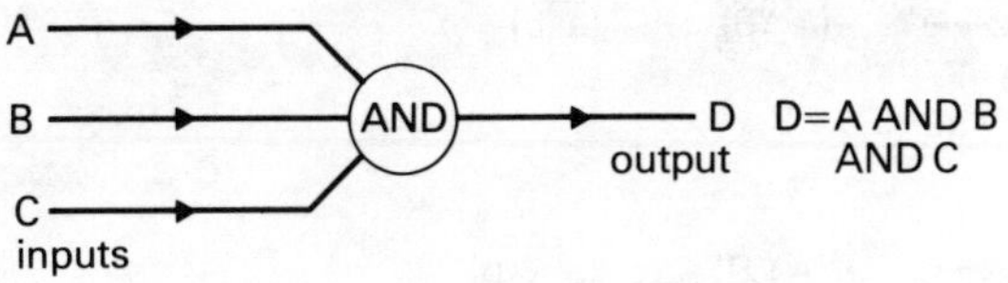

Fig. 9.15: A three input AND gate

The operation table has eight combinations of inputs.

Operation table

Inputs A	B	C	Output D
0	0	0	0
0	0	1	0
0	1	0	0
0	1	1	0
1	0	0	0
1	0	1	0
1	1	0	0
1	1	1	1

Output D carries a 1 if there is a 1 at input A *and* input B *and* input C.

Three input OR gate (Figure 9.17)

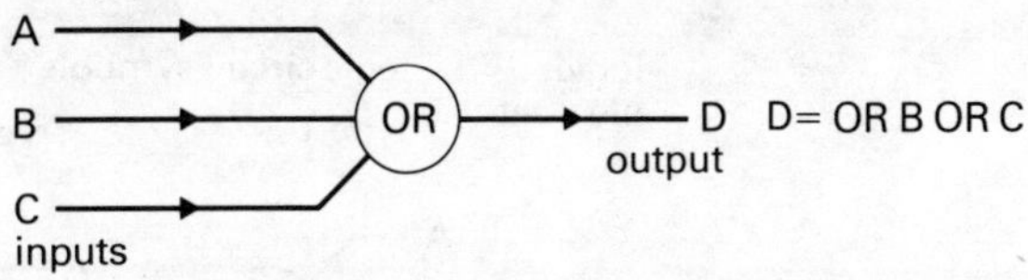

Fig. 9.16: A three input OR gate

Operation table

Inputs A	B	C	Output D
0	0	0	0
0	0	1	1
0	1	0	1
0	1	1	1
1	0	0	1
1	0	1	1
1	1	0	1
1	1	1	1

Output D carries a 1 if there is a 1 at input A *or* input B *or* input C.

For any number of inputs, the definitions of AND and OR gates are as follows:

An AND gate has a 1 output if *all* its inputs are 1, and a 0 output otherwise.

An OR gate has a 1 output if *any* of its inputs are 1, and a 0 output otherwise.

Example The logic circuit in Figure 9.17 shows how a three input AND gate can be used in a decoder. The decoder shown recognises the input combination 0 1 0.

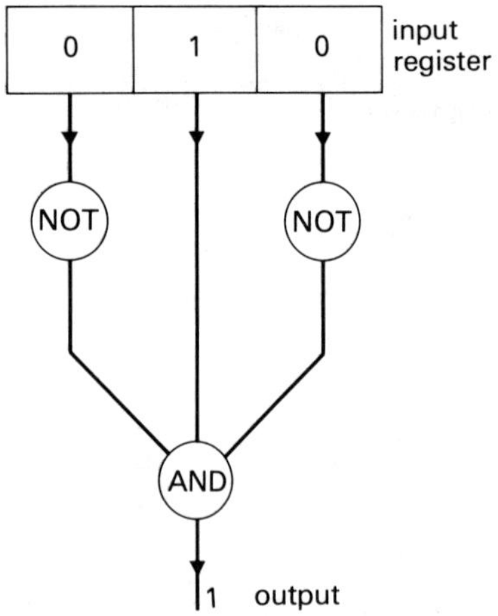

Fig. 9.17: A three bit decoder

Operation table

Inputs			Output
0	0	0	0
0	0	1	0
0	1	0	1
0	1	1	0
1	0	0	0
1	0	1	0
1	1	0	0
1	1	1	0

Different ways of writing logic expressions

Logic elements can be described by symbols. The symbols for the elements in a logic circuit are put together to form a **logic expression.** A logic expression resembles an expression in ordinary algebra. Logic expressions are sometimes called **Boolean** expressions, after George Boole, the founder of mathematical logic (see Chapter 21).

Unfortunately there are several different sets of symbols for logic elements. The most common sets of logic symbols are shown in Figure 9.18.

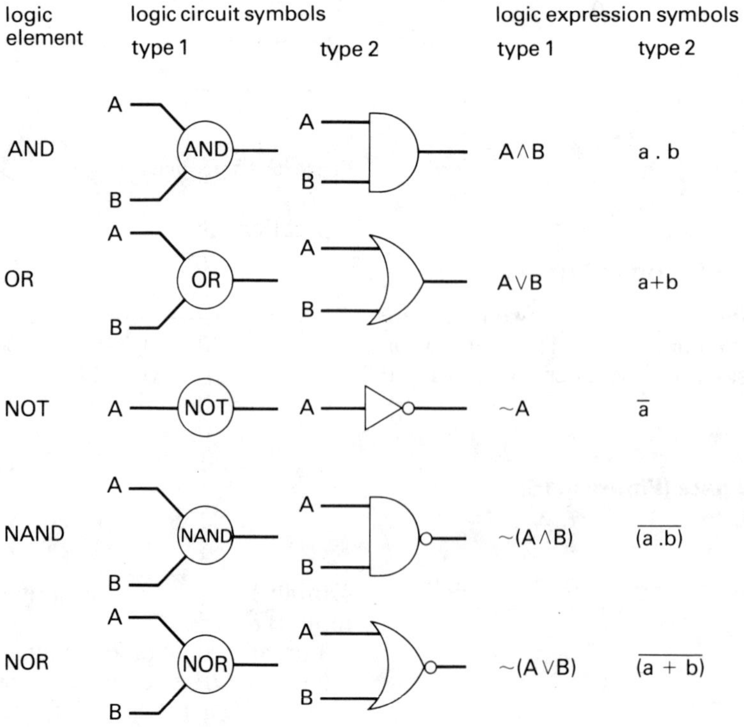

Fig. 9.18: Logic symbols

The following are examples of logic circuits, and the expressions which describe them, using all the different sets of symbols. Notice how brackets are used to show the order in which logic elements occur in the circuits.

Example 1
Circuit

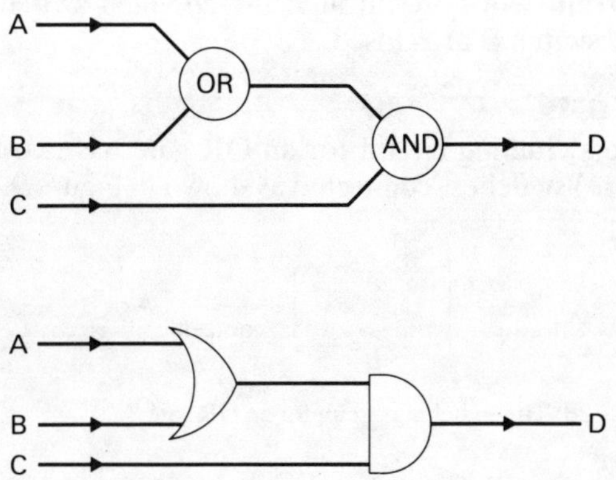

Fig. 9.19

Expression

D = (A OR B) AND C
$D = (A \vee B) \wedge C$
$d = (a + b).c$

Example 2
Circuit

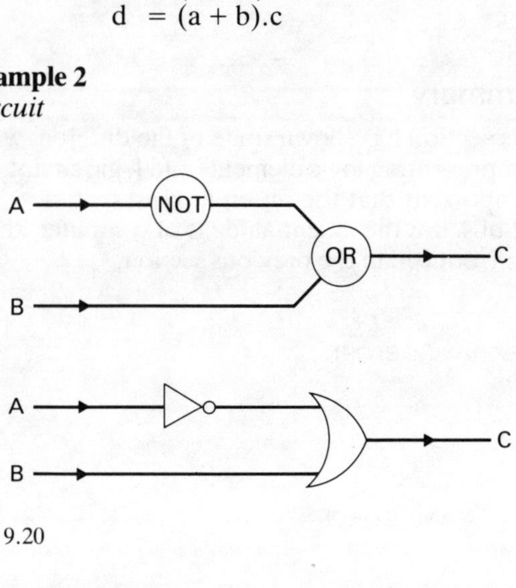

Fig. 9.20

Expression

C = (NOT A) OR B
$C = (\sim A) \vee B$

$c = (\bar{a}) + b$

Compare these expressions with the ones for a NOR gate.

Example 3
Circuit

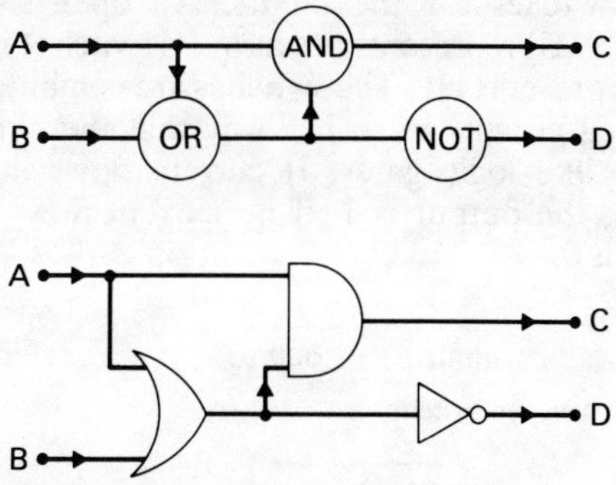

Fig. 9.21

Expressions

C = A AND (A OR B)
D = NOT (A OR B)

$C = A \wedge (A \vee B)$
$D = \sim(A \vee B)$

$c = a.\ (a + b)$

$d = \overline{(a + b)}$

Example 4
Circuit

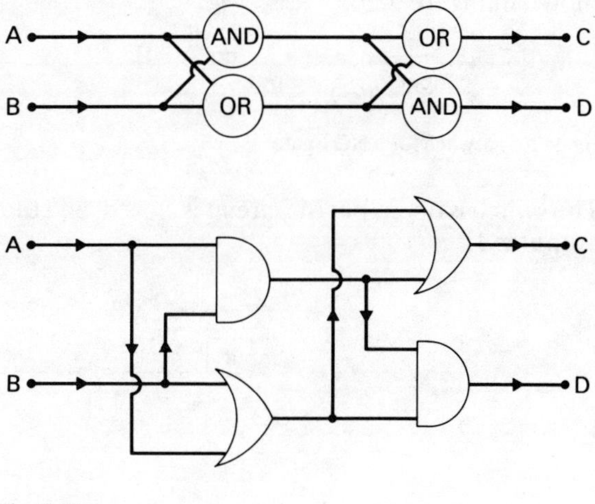

Fig. 9.22

Expressions

C = (A AND B) OR (A OR B)
D = (A AND B) AND (A OR B)

$C = (A \wedge B) \wedge (A \vee B)$
$D = (A \wedge B) \wedge (A \vee B)$

$c = (a.b) + (a + b)$
$d = (a.b) . (a + b)$

Switching circuits

Another way of representing computer logic is by using switches for the inputs. An open switch (Figure 9.23) represents a 0, a closed switch (Figure 9.24) represents a 1. The switches are combined in **switching circuits** in such a way that the circuits behave like logic gates. If current flows in the circuits, the output is 1, if no current flows, the output is 0.

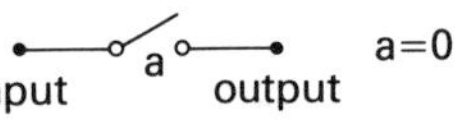

Fig. 9.23: An open switch

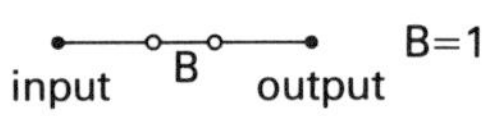

Fig. 9.24: A closed switch

NOT gate

A single switch represents a NOT gate as shown in Figure 9.25.

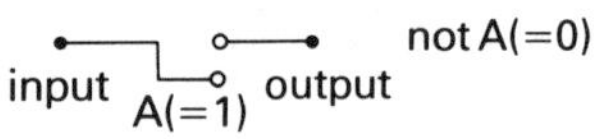

Fig. 9.25: A switch for a NOT gate

If the switch is in the closed position (as shown), the circuit is open, and the output is 0.

A NOT gate in the open position is drawn as shown in Figure 9.26.

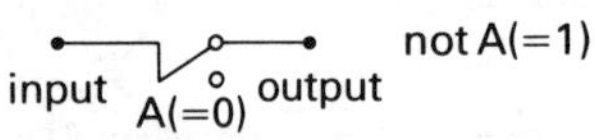

Fig. 9.26: A switch for a NOT gate

The switch is open, but the circuit is closed, and the output is 1.

AND gate

The switching circuit for an AND gate has two (or more) switches, connected as shown in Figure 9.27.

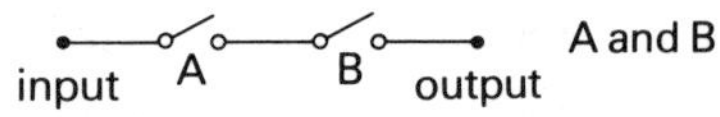

Fig. 9.27: The switching circuit for an AND gate

Current will flow through the circuit if switch A *and* switch B are closed.

OR gate

The switching circuit for an OR gate has two (or more) switches, connected as shown in Figure 9.28.

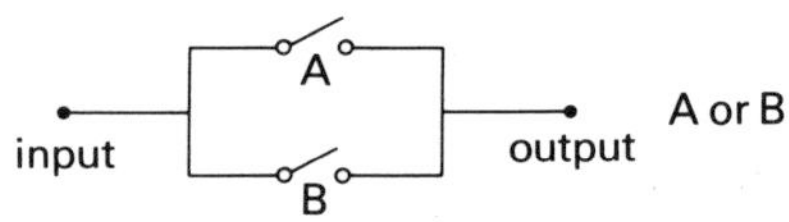

Fig. 9.28: The switching circuit for an OR gate

Current will flow through the circuit if switch A *or* switch B is closed.

Combinations of logic gates

Switching circuits can represent combinations of logic gates. Figure 9.29 shows some examples.

Summary

This section has shown some of the different ways of representing logic elements and logic circuits. It is important that the different representations do not obscure the essential ideas of computer logic, as introduced in the previous section.

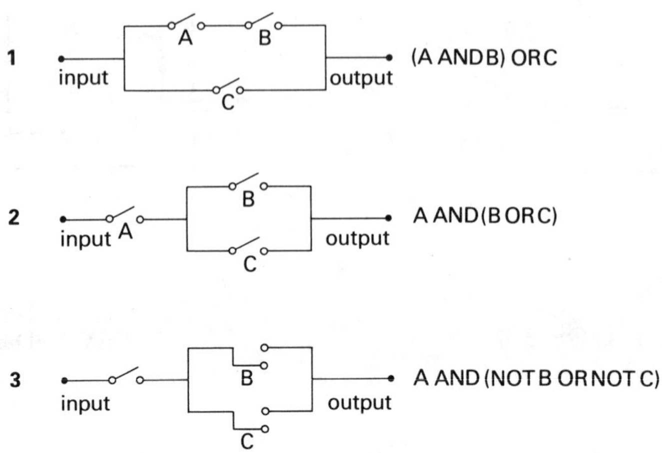

Fig. 9.29

* Transistors

All present day computers depend on circuits containing transistors for their operation. Transistors can function as amplifiers, or as logic elements.

There are several types of transistor, but all are made of **semiconductor** materials. Semiconductor materials are crystals, often of silicon, with a carefully controlled amount of impurities in them.

The impurities cause a surplus of electrons (**n-type semiconductor**) or a shortage of electrons (**p-type semiconductor**) in the crystal. This allows a certain amount of current to pass through the semiconductor – not as much as in a conductor like copper, but more than in an insulator like plastic. This current can be precisely controlled by other currents in the transistor.

The commonest type of transistor contains three very small pieces of semiconductor material, connected as shown in Figure 9.30.
This is an *n-p-n* transistor. The flow of electrons across the boundaries between the *n* and the *p* types of semiconductor (the *p-n* **junction**) determines the way the transistor operates.

Integrated circuits consist of larger crystals of semiconductor material connected together to have the same effect as a number of separate transistors. Large scale integrated (LSI) circuits are equivalent to thousands of transistors.

Exercise 9b

1 Using whichever set of symbols you prefer, write logic expressions for the logic circuits in questions **2** to **7** of Exercise 9a.

2 Draw logic circuits for these logic expressions. Use whichever type of symbols you prefer:

(a) $D = (A \vee \sim B) \wedge C$,

$d = (a + \overline{b}).c$

(b) $D = \sim((A \vee B) \vee C)$,

$d = (\overline{(a + b) + c)}$

(c) $D = A \vee (\sim(B \wedge C))$,

$d = a + \overline{b.c})$

(d) $D = (\sim A \wedge B) \vee (A \wedge \sim B)$,

$d = (\overline{a}.b) + (a.\overline{b})$

3 Work out operation tables for the logic circuits in question **2.**

4 Draw switching circuits for these logic expressions: (a) (A OR B) AND C; (b) A AND B AND C; (c) A OR B OR C; (d) (A AND B) OR (C AND D); (e) (A AND B) AND (C OR D).

5 Write logic expression for the switching circuits shown in Figure 9.31.

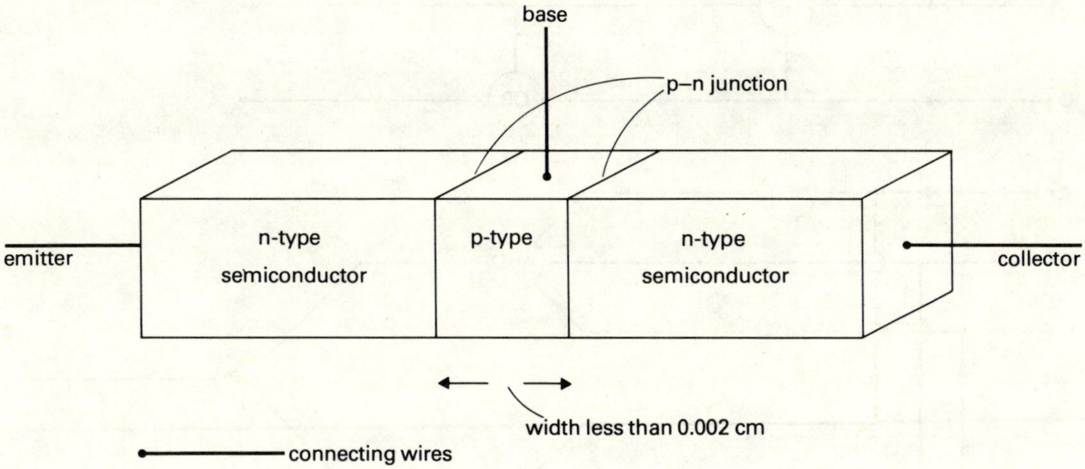

Fig. 9.30: A transistor

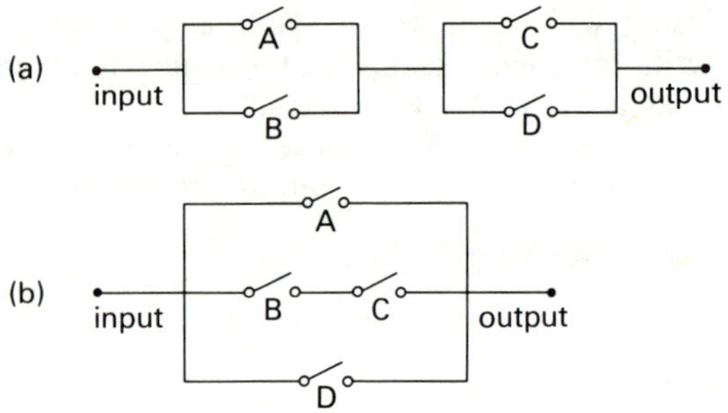

Fig. 9.31

6 Draw operation tables for the logic circuits shown in Figure 9.32.
In part (c), show the combinations of signals at D, E and F. Suggest a use for this logic circuit.

7 Fill in the chart to show what the signal is at each of C, D and F for the given values of A and B in Figure 9.33.

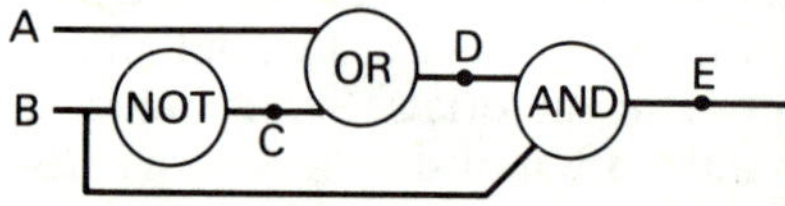

A	B	C	D	E
0	0			
0	1			
1	0			
1	1			

Fig. 9.33

What single gate would produce the same output at E as these three gates? (MREB 76)

8 Write out the truth table for an AND gate which has inputs X and Y and output R.

Three registers in a computer are called A, B and C. Each holds 8 bits. The three bits at the

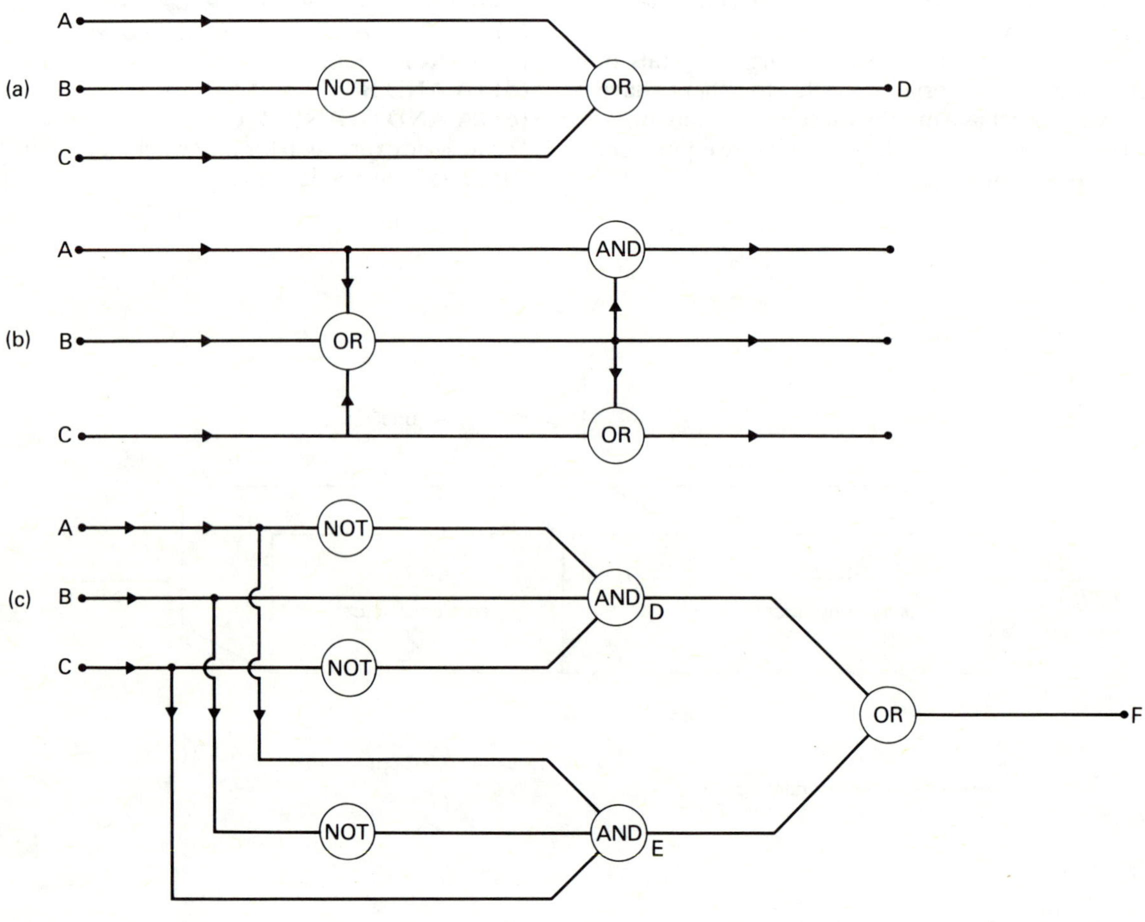

Fig. 9.32

left-hand end of register A are to be copied into the three left-hand bits of register C leaving the rest of register C set to zeros.

Register A contains the bit pattern
1 0 1 0 1 0 1 0.

(a) Describe, with the aid of a diagram, how this might be done using all three registers and AND gates.

(b) Show clearly the bit pattern needed in register B. (EAEB 76 II)

9 Construct a truth table (4 rows) to show the truth value of $(A \wedge (\sim B)) \vee ((\sim A) \wedge B)$. (UCLES 76 I)

10 (a) Draw a switching circuit for an OR gate.
(b) Write down the Boolean expression for the circuit shown in Figure 9.34.

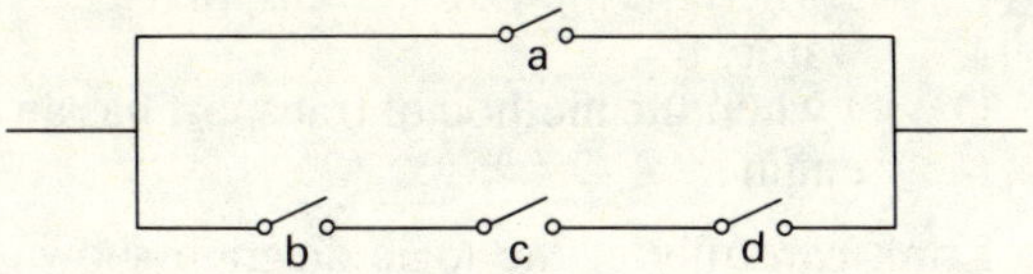

Fig. 9.34

(c) Examine the logic circuit shown in Figure 9.35 which has inputs A, B and C and outputs X and Y.

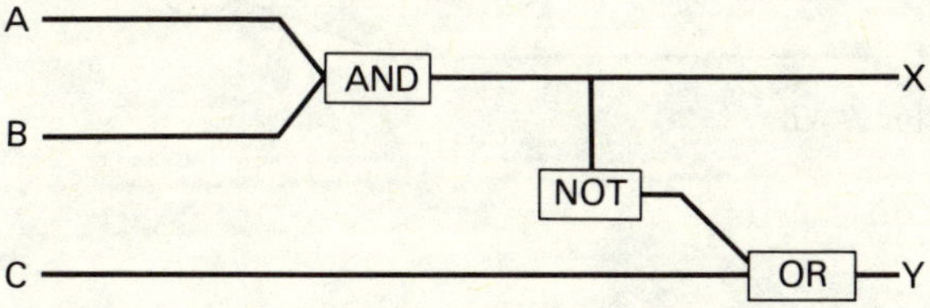

Fig. 9.35

(i) State the Boolean expressions for X and Y.
(ii) Draw the truth table for this logic circuit to show the outputs X and Y for all possible inputs at A, B and C. (YREB 76 I)

11 Consider the logic circuits in Figure 9.36, where the inputs are A and B and the output is C.

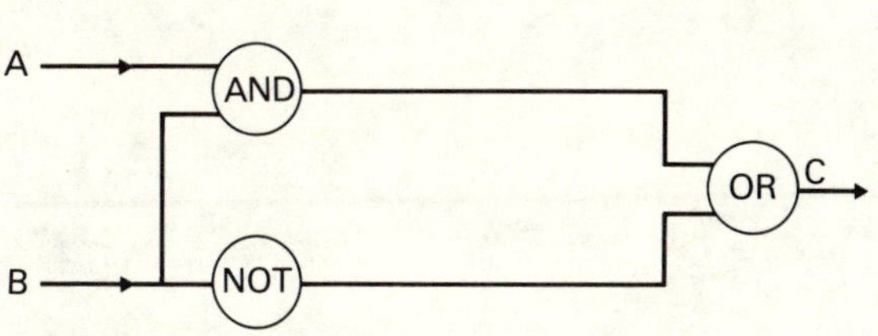

Fig. 9.36

(a) Write down the Boolean expressions for the following: (i) The output from the AND gate, (ii) The output from the NOT gate, (iii) The output C from the OR gate.
(b) What is the output at C if in the logic circuit above (i) A is 1 and B is 0, (ii) A is 0 and B is 1, (iii) A is 1 and B is 1, (iv) A is 0 and B is 0.
(c) Draw a logic circuit diagram to represent the output Z which is obtained from inputs W, X and Y when

Z = (W AND X) OR (X AND Y)

(YREB 77 I)

12 (a) Copy and complete the table below for the logic diagram in Figure 9.37.

Input 1	Input 2	Output 1	Output 2
0	0		
0	1		
1	0		
1	1		

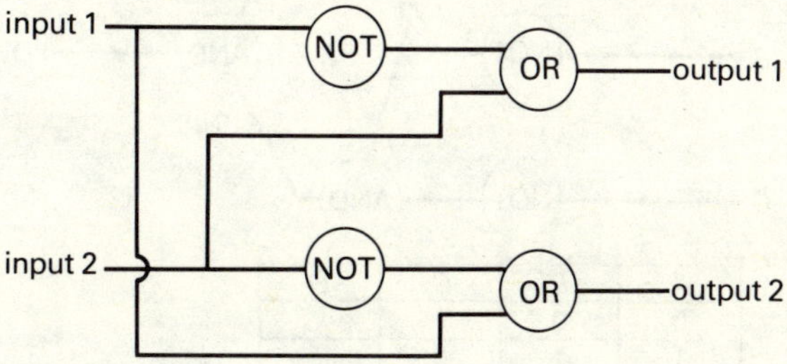

Fig. 9.37

(b) Hence or otherwise construct a logic diagram using two NOT gates, two OR gates and one AND gate, which has two inputs and one output and operates so that the output is 1 if the two inputs are the same and is 0 if they are different.
(c) If the two OR gates of your circuit in (b) were both replaced by AND gates and the AND gate replaced by an OR gate how would the circuit now operate? (WMEB 75 I)

13 In the following question, select the correct answer from the ones given in (a) to (e).

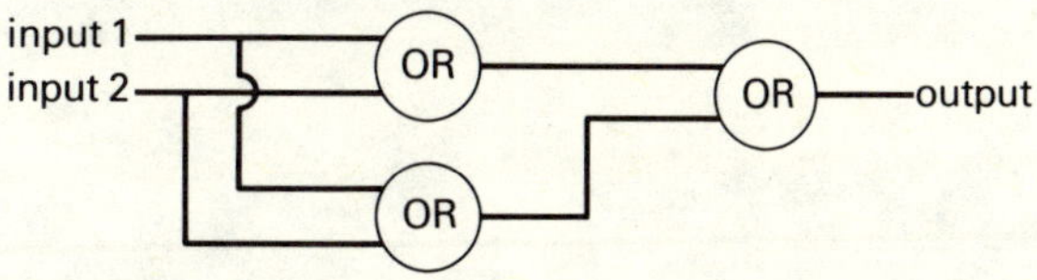

Fig. 9.38

The circuit shown in Figure 9.38 operates in the same way as:
(a) an OR gate, (b) an AND gate,
(c) a NOT gate, (d) a half adder,
(e) a full adder. (WMEB 76 I)

14 A safety system on a machine uses three switches A, B and C. The motor receives a stop signal X if switch A is closed (B and C being open), or if switch C is closed (A and B being open), or if A, B and C are all closed.

Draw a truth table showing all possible states of the switches and whether the motor is running or stopped.

Also draw a logic network using AND, OR, NOT gates with A, B and C as inputs and the stop signal X as output. (JMB 78 specimen)

15 Using the circuit in Figure 9.39, fill in the outputs at D in the table, given the inputs A, B C in the table. (WJEC(O) 75)

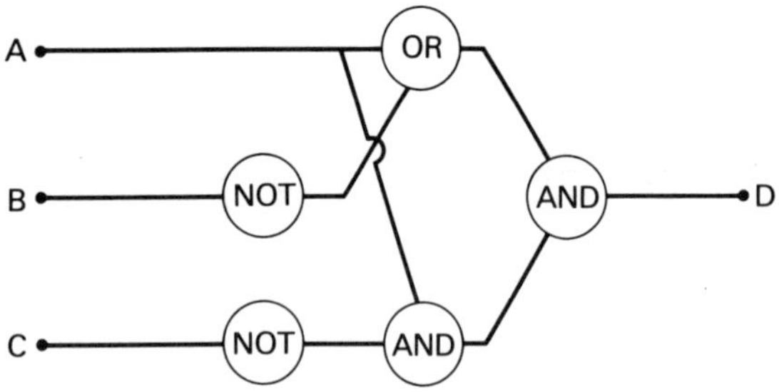

A	*B*	*C*	*D*
0	0	1	
1	1	0	

Fig. 9.39

(a) The inputs P, Q, and R to the AND gate.
(b) The input S to the NOT gate.
(c) The inputs B and C to the OR gate.
What method of transport is represented? (YREB 78 II)

16 The following list gives methods of transport by land, sea and air:

aeroplane; bicycle; car; cruiser; hovercraft; submarine.

Descriptions of the way these vehicles travel are coded as follows:

A = 1 when the method of transport has wheels.
B = 1 when the method of transport has wings.
C = 1 when the method of transport floats on water.
D = 1 when the method of transport has an engine.

Look carefully at the logic diagram shown in Figure 9.40 and complete the statements for output E = 1.

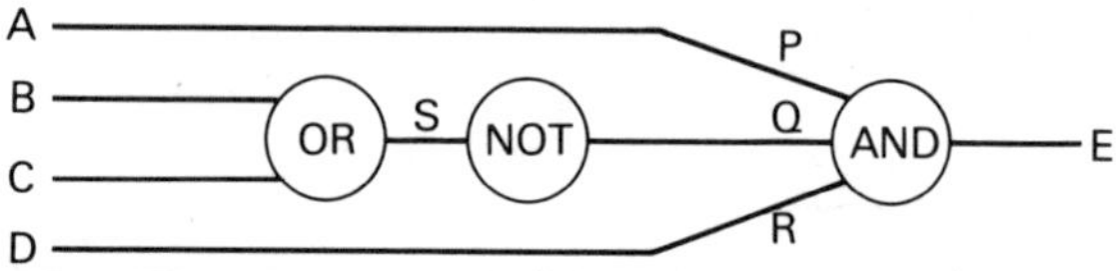

Fig. 9.40

10

Computer arithmetic

Section A

Computers can do arithmetic in two different ways. Some operations are performed directly by hardware devices. Other operations are done by repeating and combining the arithmetic and logic operations performed by the hardware. The second type of operation is controlled by a sequence of instructions permanently stored in the computer.

Generally speaking, simpler operations like addition are done by hardware, and more complicated ones like raising to powers and calculating logarithms are done by sequences of permanently stored instructions. Each type of computer has its own mixture of the two types of operations. In most cases it is true to say that the larger and faster the computer, the more arithmetic operations are done by hardware.

Virtually without exception, all computers do addition by hardware. This chapter describes how logic elements introduced in the previous chapter can be combined to form circuits which add binary numbers. Then some indication is given of how subtraction, multiplication and division can be done by combining addition with other simple logic operations. The second part of the chapter describes how errors can occur in arithmetic operations done on computers.

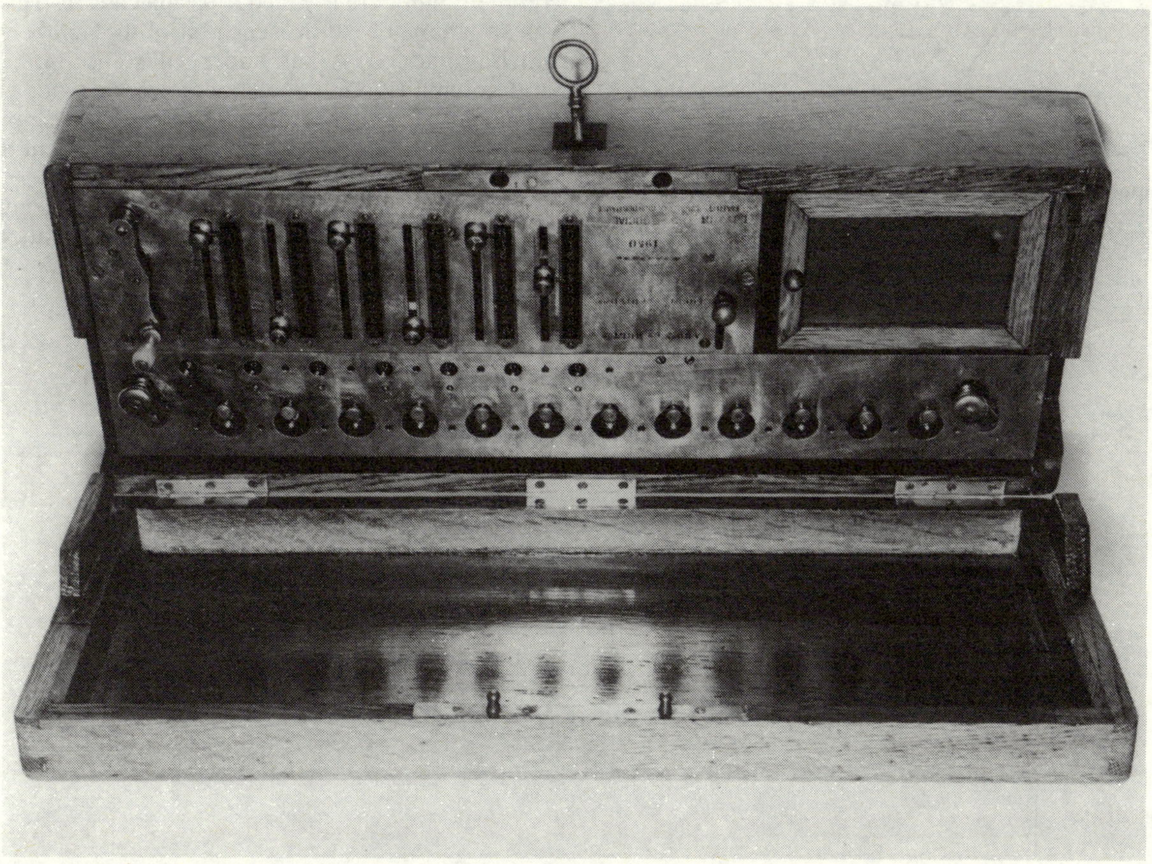

A Thomas Arithmometer, built in 1820. This is a very early predecessor of a modern computer

Addition

The logic circuits which do addition are described below in some detail.

Half adder

You will recall the rules for adding two binary digits:

$0 + 0 = 0$
$0 + 1 = 1$
$1 + 0 = 1$
$1 + 1 = 1\ 0$ i.e. 0 carry 1

These rules provide the operation table for a logic circuit to add two binary digits:

Input		Output	
A	B	sum	carry
0	0	0	0
0	1	1	0
1	0	1	0
1	1	0	1

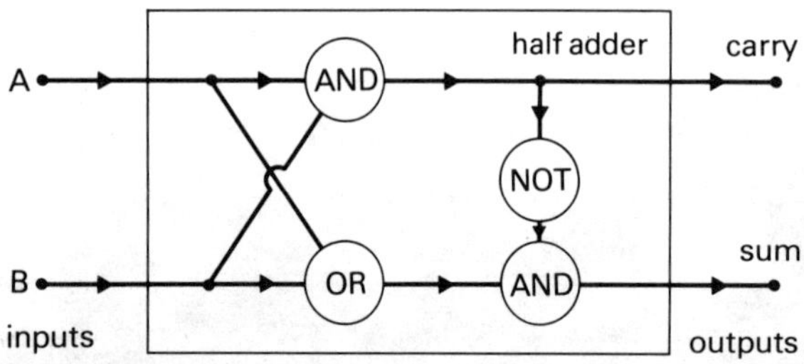

Fig. 10.1: A logic circuit for a half adder

Comparing inputs and outputs, you will notice that an AND gate will do the carry, and a modified OR gate will do the sum. One logic circuit which matches these requirements is shown in Figure 10.1.

Logic expressions for the sum and carry outputs are as follows:

Sum $= (A \vee B) \quad (\sim(A \wedge B))$
Carry $= A \wedge B$

This logic circuit is called a **half adder** because it cannot include a digit carried from a previous column.

Full adder

A **full adder** is a logic circuit which adds two binary digits, and then adds on a third digit carried from a previous column. A full adder is made of two half adders, connected as shown in Figure 10.2.

Notice that a full adder has three inputs and two outputs.

Parallel adder

The device which many computers use to add two complete numbers is called a **parallel adder.** This has an adding circuit for each bit of the numbers which are added. A half adder will suffice in the units column (though a full adder is often used, as explained below). There is a full adder in each of the other columns. The carry from one column is input into the adder in the next column.

When two numbers are added, there is a delay until all the carry bits have passed from one adder

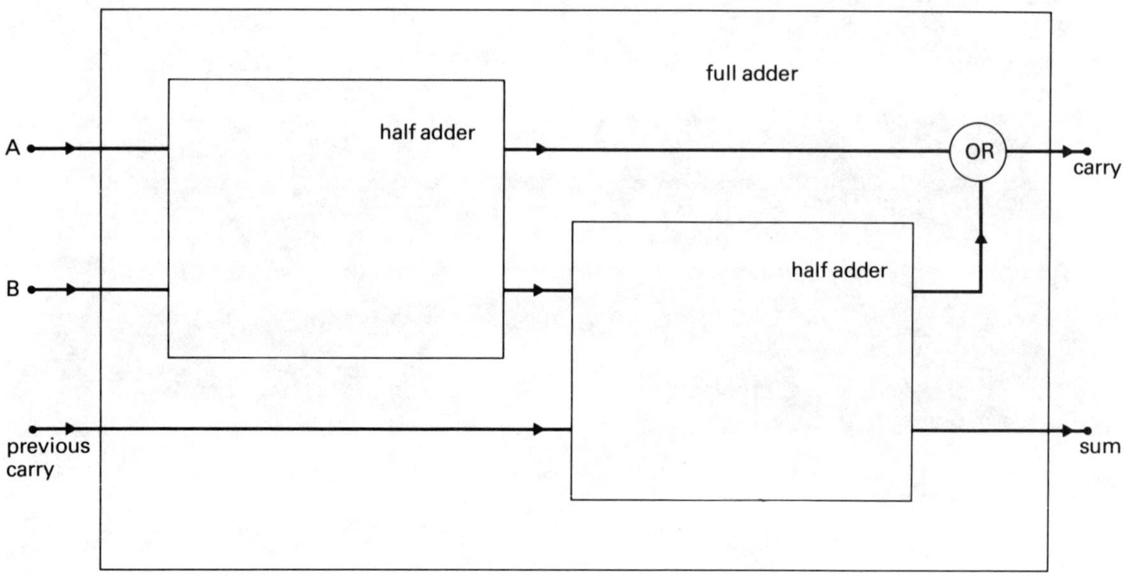

Fig. 10.2: A full adder

to the next. Some computers have additional circuits to reduce this delay.

The carry from the last column is stored in a separate **overflow bit.** If the overflow bit contains a 1, it sometimes (but not always) indicates that an error has occurred. Errors are discussed later in this chapter.

A full adder is often used in the units column, to allow a 1 to be added very easily, using the previous carry input. This is very convenient when finding the twos complement of a number, or subtracting using complements.

Figure 10.3 shows an eight bit parallel adder. It has a full adder in the units column, and a connection for a 1 input. An adder of this type is used in the IMC-1 model computer.

Serial adder

Another device which adds all the bits of two complete numbers is called a **serial adder.** Unlike a parallel adder, it adds one pair of bits at a time. Other logic circuits are used to **shift** the input numbers and the sum one place after each addition. The carry from one addition is stored in a **delay register** until the next pair of bits is input. The delay register can also be used to add 1 to a number. After all the bits have been added, it will contain the overflow bit. Figure 10.4 shows an eight bit serial adder.

Computers which have parallel adders usually do all their processing one byte or word at a time. They are called **parallel computers.** On the other hand, computers which have serial adders usually do all their processing one bit at a time. They are called **serial computers.**

Other arithmetic operations

A parallel or serial adder is the basic calculating circuit of most computers. As well as addition, it is used for subtraction, multiplication and division. The next few paragraphs give a very brief description of how these other operations are done.

Subtraction

As described in Chapter 3, subtraction is done by finding the complement of the second number and adding it to the first.

Finding the twos complement of a number is done by changing the zeros to ones and ones to zeros, and then adding 1. A set of NOT gates, as shown in Figure 10.5, will change the zeros to ones and ones to zeros.

The 1 input of a parallel adder then adds 1,

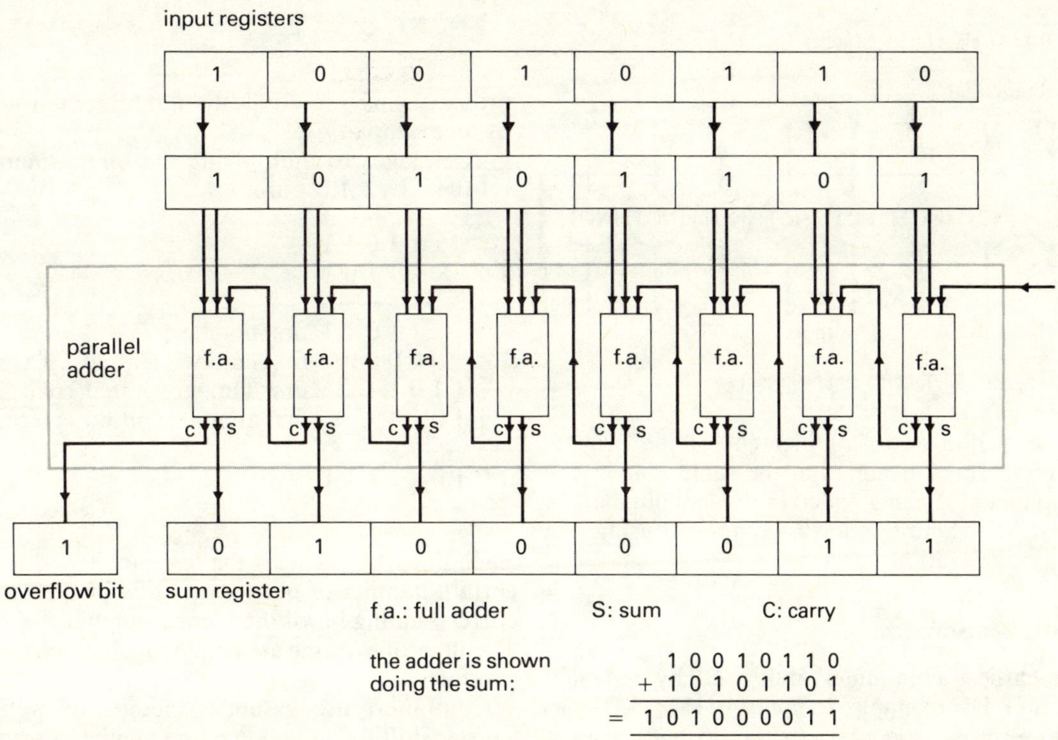

Fig. 10.3: An eight bit parallel adder

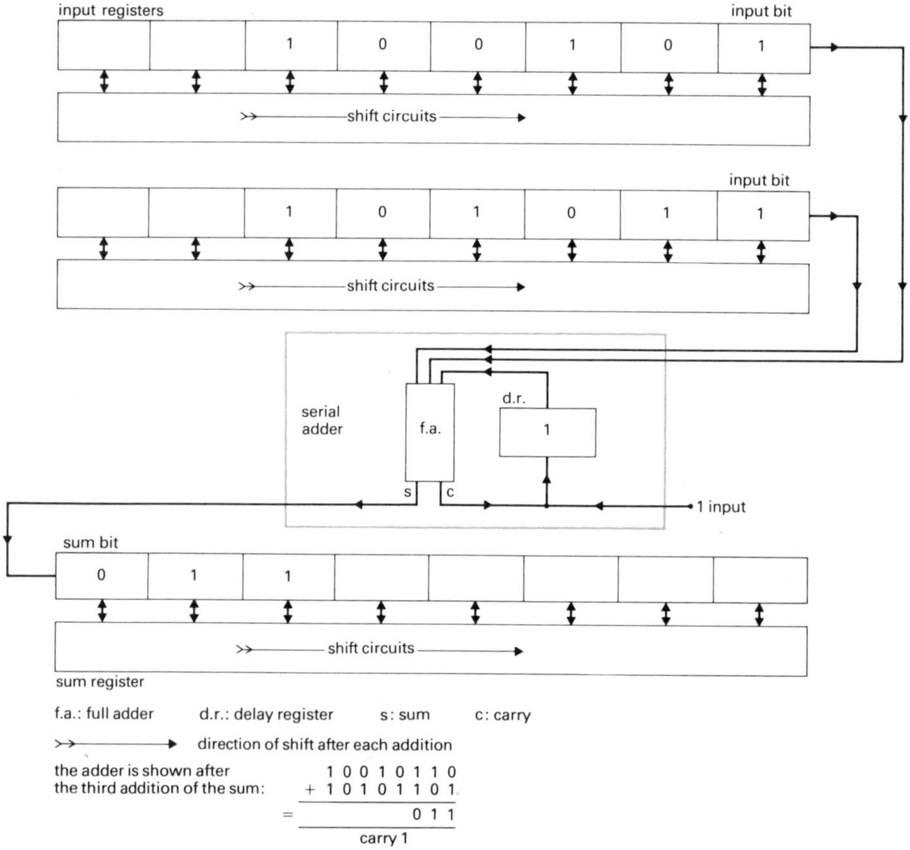

Fig. 10.4: An eight bit serial adder

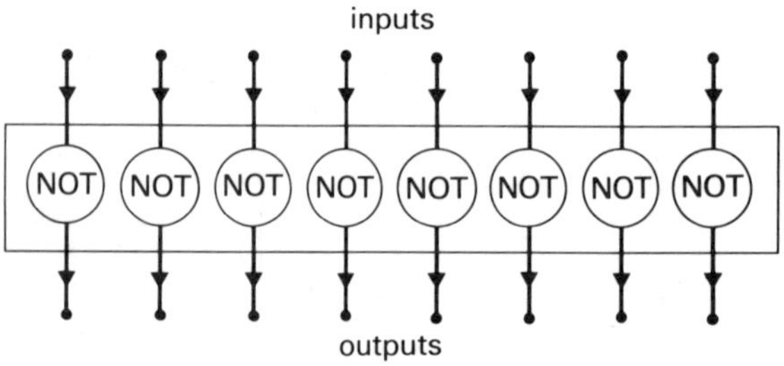

Fig. 10.5: A parallel set of eight NOT gates

providing the twos complement of the original number. The 1 is added at the same time as the complement is being added to the first number. In this way, the subtraction is completed using one addition operation.

Multiplication

The earliest computers multiplied by repeated addition. For example, to multiply 31 by 8, 31 was added 8 times. Modern computers do multiplication by **shifting** and addition. The method is based on ordinary binary multiplication. It is best introduced by an example.

The stages of multiplying the binary numbers 1 1 0 1 1 by 1 1 0 1 are:

```
          1 1 0 1 1
      ×     1 1 0 1
      -------------
          1 1 0 1 1   first number,                 × 1
        0 0 0 0 0     first number, shifted 1 place,  × 0
      1 1 0 1 1       first number, shifted 2 places, × 1
    1 1 0 1 1         first number, shifted 3 places, × 1
  -----------------
  1 0 1 0 1 1 1 1 1
  -----------------
```

Each line of working is the first number, shifted a certain number of places, or a row of zeros if the corresponding bit of the second number is a zero. The lines of working are added together to give the product.

Computers use a similar method of multiplication, shifting and adding one number according to the bits of the other.

You will notice that the product is much longer than either input number. In general, a product can be up to twice the length of the input numbers. Products must often be stored in **double length words,** otherwise errors arise. This situation is discussed in more detail in the second section of the chapter.

Division

Division is done on a computer by repeated shifting, comparison and subtraction. The subtraction is done by complementation and addition. Errors can arise when the two numbers do not divide exactly.

All by addition

You will now realize that a computer with a serial or parallel adder, a set of NOT gates and logic circuits to do shifting, can add, subtract, multiply and divide. This is the way that many computers do their arithmetic. However, several more complicated aspects of computer arithmetic have not been discussed, for example, multiplication and division of negative numbers, or calculations with numbers in binary coded decimal form.

Exercise 10a

1 Write down the meanings of the following words or phrases:
half adder; full adder; parallel adder;
overflow bit; serial adder; delay register;
double length word.

2 Copy and complete this operation table for a full adder:

Input A	B	previous carry	Output sum	carry
0	0	0	0	0
0	0	1	1	0
0	1	0	...	...
...	...	...	...	...

(8 lines altogether)

3 The sketch of a half adder in Figure 10.6 shows which wires carry pulses of current when the inputs are 0 and 1.
Copy the sketch and colour the wires for the inputs 1 and 1.

4 (a) Combine the sketches of a half adder and a full adder to show all the AND, OR and NOT gates of a full adder.
(b) Choose a pattern of zeros and ones for the inputs. Colour the wires on your sketch to show how the pulses from this pattern of inputs pass through the adder.

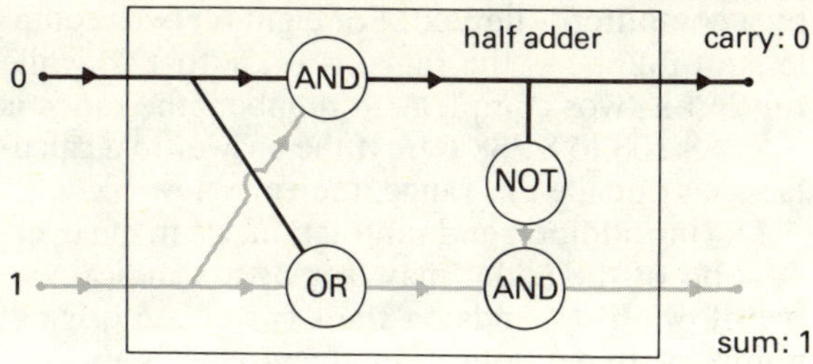

Fig. 10.6

5 An **exclusive OR gate** (Figure 10.7) has the following pattern of inputs and outputs.

Input A	B	Output C
0	0	0
0	1	1
1	0	1
1	1	0

C = A EOR B

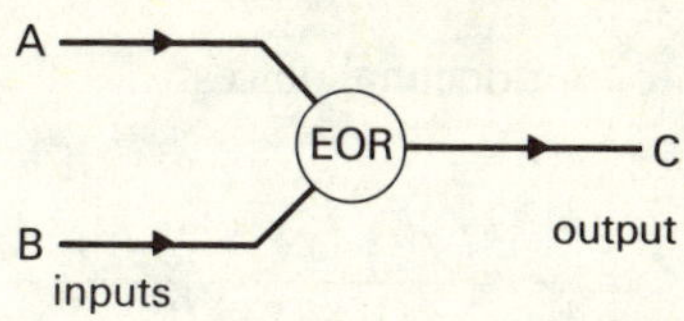

Fig. 10.7: An exclusive OR gate

Design a half adder containing an exclusive OR gate.

***6** Copy the sketch of a parallel adder. Colour the wires carrying pulses of current for the input numbers 0 1 1 0 0 1 0 1 and 1 0 0 1 1 1 0 1.

***7** What is the maximum length of the answer when two six bit binary numbers are multiplied together? Give an example to illustrate your answer.

Section B

Errors

Although the logic elements of a computer hardly ever go wrong, there are a few ways in which errors can arise in computer arithmetic. The commonest ways are **overflow, truncation** and **rounding.**

Overflow

Because a fixed number of bits is used to store a number, the range of numbers that can be stored by a computer is limited. For eight bit twos complement numbers, the range is -128 to 127, while for 24 bit twos complement numbers the range is $-8\,388\,608$ to 8 388 607. If the answer to a calculation is outside this range, then **overflow** occurs.

During addition and subtraction, a 1 in the overflow bit of the adder may or may not indicate an overflow. It depends on the signs of the original numbers. In multiplication, the product is always a double length number. Overflow occurs if an attempt is made to store the product in a storage area which is too small for it.

If overflow occurs, the computer usually outputs an **error message.** It stops processing the program in which the error has occurred.

Truncation errors

Fractions such as two thirds cannot be represented exactly as decimals. Similarly, not all fractions can be stored exactly on a computer.

Truncation errors occur when a fraction is cut off after a certain number of decimal (or binary) places. For example, in base ten:

$$\tfrac{2}{3} = 0.6666$$

truncated to four decimal places.

In base two:

	$\frac{1}{2}$	$\frac{1}{4}$	$\frac{1}{8}$	$\frac{1}{16}$	$\frac{1}{32}$	$\frac{1}{64}$
$\frac{2}{3}$ = 0 .	1	0	1	0	1	0

truncated to six binary places.

Truncation errors also occur in division if the two numbers do not divide exactly.

Rounding errors

To reduce the truncation error, fractions in base ten are **rounded** by raising the last figure by one if the following figure would have been five or more. For example:

$$\tfrac{2}{3} = 0.6667$$

rounded to four decimal places.

In binary, the last figure is raised by one if the next figure would have been a one. For example:

$$\tfrac{2}{3} = 0.1\,0\,1\,0\,1\,1$$

rounded to six binary places.

In some computers, fractions are rounded automatically.

Floating point numbers

Errors can occur when numbers are changed into their floating point form, or when calculations are done using floating point numbers.

For example, changing 9 to an eight bit floating point number:

$$9 = \tfrac{9}{16} \times 16 = \tfrac{9}{16} \times 2^4$$
$$\tfrac{9}{16} = 0.1\,0\,0\,1$$

which must be truncated to three binary places for storage.

Thus 9 is stored as:

	mantissa				exponent			
	$\pm$	$\frac{1}{2}$	$\frac{1}{4}$	$\frac{1}{8}$	$\pm$	4	2	1
9 =	0	1	0	0	0	1	0	0

The floating point form actually stores the number 8.

Floating point calculations

Calculating with floating point numbers can give rise to errors. For example, multiplying 7 by 5 using 8 bit floating point numbers:

	mantissa				exponent			
	$\pm$	$\frac{1}{2}$	$\frac{1}{4}$	$\frac{1}{8}$	$\pm$	4	2	1
$7 = \frac{7}{8} \times 8 = \frac{7}{8} \times 2^3 =$	0	1	1	1	0	0	1	1
$5 = \frac{5}{8} \times 8 = \frac{5}{8} \times 2^3 =$	0	1	0	1	0	0	1	1

The fraction parts are multiplied and the powers of two added:

```
  mantissa      exponent
    0.1 1 1       0 1 1
  ×  .1 0 1     + 0 1 1
   --------     -------
      1 1 1       1 1 0
    0 0 0       -------
  1 1 1
 ----------
 0.1 0 0 0 1 1
 ----------
```

The product is truncated to three binary places. The answer is:

mantissa				exponent				
$\pm$	$\frac{1}{2}$	$\frac{1}{4}$	$\frac{1}{8}$	$\pm$	4	2	1	
0	1	0	0	0	1	1	0	$= \frac{1}{2} \times 2^6 = 32$

The correct answer is $7 \times 5 = 35$. Once again an error has been introduced.

On computers with larger storage areas for floating point numbers, similar errors will occur, though they will be much smaller in proportion to the numbers used.

Rounding and truncation errors, and errors in floating point arithmetic are not usually detected by the computer. Error messages are not output when they occur.

Conclusion

You will now realize that a calculation performed on a computer will not always produce a completely accurate result. This section should help dispel the myth that 'the computer is always right'.

Exercise 10b

1 Write down the meanings of the following words or phrases:
overflow; truncation; rounding; error message.

2 For an eight bit twos complement number, the range of numbers that can be stored is −128 to 127. For a nine bit twos complement number, the range is −256 to 255.

Calculate the range of numbers that can be stored on:

(a) ten bit twos complement number,
(b) twelve bit twos complement number,
(c) sixteen bit twos complement number,
*(d) *n* bit twos complement number.

3 (a) Truncate these decimal numbers to three decimal places:

0.634 91, 23.8152, 0.000 479, 3.61

(b) Truncate these binary numbers to four binary places:

0.0 1 0 1 1 0, 1 0.0 1 1 0 0 1,
0.0 0 1 0 0 1 0, 1 0.0 0 1

(c) Round these decimal numbers to two decimal places:

0.619, 0.8028, 67.4153, 41.696

(d) Round these binary numbers to three binary places:

0.1 0 1 0 1, 1.0 1 0 1 0 1
1 0.0 1 1 1 1, 1.0 0 1

4 Calculate (in binary) .1 0 1 × .1 1 0. Truncate the answer to four binary places. How big is the error that has been caused?

***5** Calculate: $\frac{2}{3} - \frac{7}{12}$

(a) by subtracting the fractions, in base ten.
(b) by converting each fraction into a four bit, truncated binary fraction, subtracting, and converting the answer back to a base ten fraction.
(c) as part (b), but rounding the binary fractions.
(d) comment on the errors caused in parts (b) and (c).

***6** The following numbers are in floating point form:

mantissa				exponent			
±	$\frac{1}{2}$	$\frac{1}{4}$	$\frac{1}{8}$	±	4	2	1
0	1	1	1	0	1	0	0
0	1	1	0	0	0	1	0

(a) Multiply the numbers (multiply the fraction parts, add the powers of two). Truncate the answer into an eight bit floating point word.
(b) Convert the numbers and the answer to base ten, and comment on the error caused.

***7** Do the following calculations (a)–(e) using six bit, twos complement numbers. For each answer, state whether or not
(i) overflow has occurred (overflow bit = 1),
(ii) the six bit answer is correct.

Comment on these results.
(a) −1 + −1 (b) 13 − 24 (c) 18 + 15
(d) −25 + 17 (e) −11 + −29

8 (a) Write the number 641.37 in floating point form.
(b) (i) Express 0.2 (base 10) in base 2 correctly rounded to five binary places.
(ii) Working in base 10 arithmetic go through the flowchart in Figure 10.8. What will be the value of S when STOP is reached?
(iii) With 0.2 expressed in binary, to five binary places, go through the flowchart again. What will the value of S be this time? Give your answer in base 2.
(iv) Convert answer (iii) to base 10.
(v) Explain why answers (ii) and (iv) differ.
(EAEB 78 I)

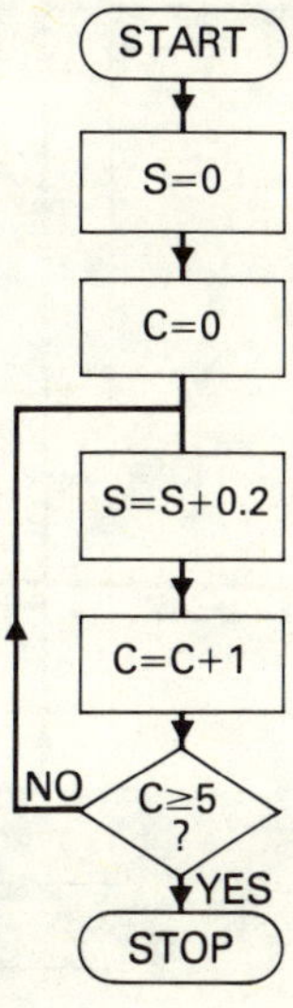

Fig. 10.8

11

Machine language

Section A

This chapter, and the one which follows it, give some idea of what happens inside the central processing unit of a computer. This chapter describes the working of the arithmetic and logic unit of a CPU, and the way in which instructions are stored during processing. Ideas introduced previously – about coding and storing data, the CPU, computer logic and computer arithmetic – are developed further. Much of the explanation makes use of the IMC-1 model computer.

The arithmetic and logic unit

The ALU is the part of a central processing unit where calculations are done and decisions are made. It contains several **registers** which store data items while they are being processed. The most important register is called the **accumulator.** One of the functions of the accumulator is to store answers to the steps of calculations. The ALU also contains a serial or a parallel adder, and other logic circuits.

The IMC-1 arithmetic and logic unit

Figure 11.1 shows the ALU of the IMC-1 model computer. You will notice that most of the components in it have been introduced in previous chapters.

The components of the arithmetic and logic unit of the IMC-1 are as follows:

The **accumulator** is an eight bit register which stores answers to steps of calculations, and numbers during input or output. (See page 47.)

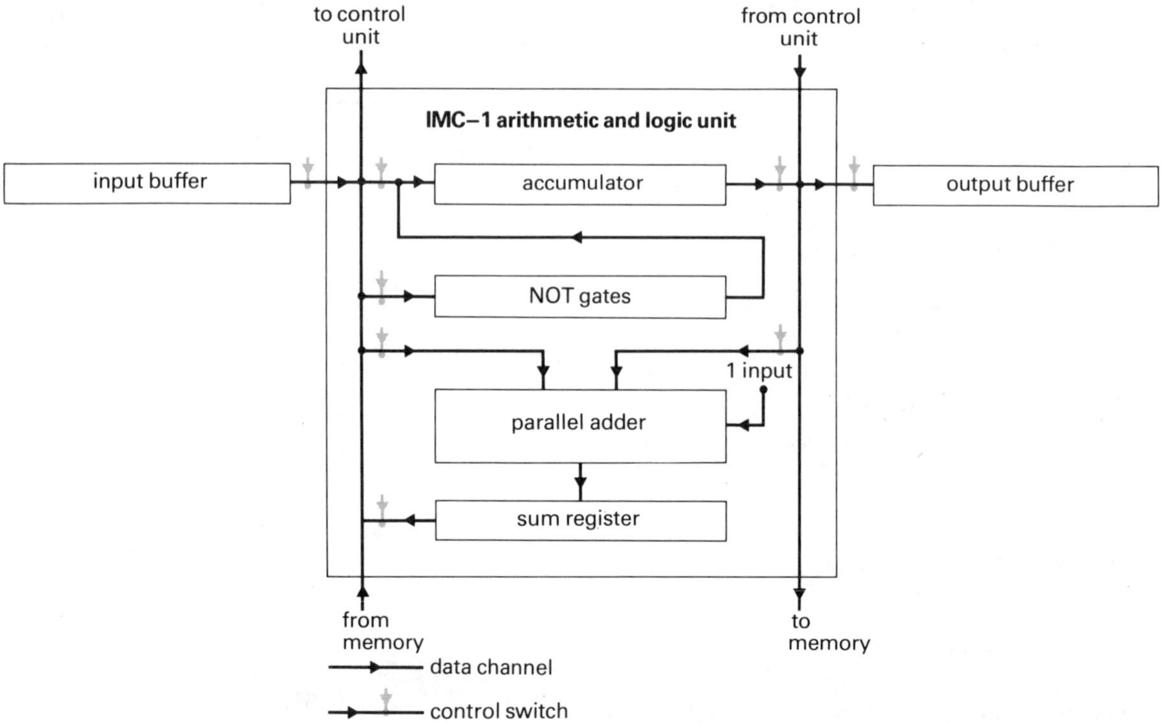

Fig. 11.1: The IMC-1 arithmetic and logic unit

A set of eight **parallel NOT gates.** These gates reverse all the bits of any word passing through them. One of their uses is in finding complements of numbers. (See page 59.)

An eight bit **parallel adder.** It adds two eight bit input numbers, and stores the result in the **sum register.** The parallel adder has a separate input for a 1 in the units column. This is used during subtraction by adding complements. (See page 58.)

Eight bit **input** and **output buffers.** These are connected to peripheral devices. They store input and output data respectively. (See page 31.)

Eight bit parallel **data channels.** These have eight wires, to carry all the bits of one word. They connect all the components of the ALU. They also connect the ALU to the memory, and to the control unit.

Several **control switches** in the data channels. (See page 46.) They are also connected to the control unit, by wires not shown in the diagram. the control unit opens various combinations of switches in response to different instructions.

Machine language

Instructions in a form which a computer can process directly are in a binary code called **machine language,** or **machine code.** A set of machine language instructions forms a machine language program.

Each type of computer has its own machine language, suited to the hardware of its CPU. Machine languages differ considerably between different types of computer, but they all have some features in common. Most important common features are:

- ☐ Machine code instructions are in binary.
- ☐ Most machine instructions refer to the accumulator.
- ☐ Machine instructions include an **operation code,** and (in most cases) a **memory address.** The operation code specifies the type of operation to be carried out. Operations include input, output, add or store in the memory. The memory address is a binary number which locates the memory cell to be used.

The following are examples of machine instructions, using ten bit words:

Example 1 Machine instruction 0 1 1 0 0 1 1 0 1 1

operation code 0 1 1 0: copy from memory to accumulator

memory address 0 1 1 0 1 1 = 27

This instruction means: copy the word in memory cell 27 into the accumulator.

Example 2 Machine instruction 0 1 0 1 0 1 1 0 1 0

operation code 0 1 0 1: add from memory into accumulator

memory address 0 1 1 0 1 0 = 26

This instruction means: add the number in memory cell 26 to the number in the accumulator, and store the answer in the accumulator.

Note: All the different operation codes form the **instruction set** of the computer.

The IMC-1 machine language

Although it is far simpler than any machine language used in practice, the IMC-1 machine language has many of the essential features of machine languages. An IMC-1 machine instruction consists of eight bits. Three bits are for the operation code, and five bits are for the memory address. Each operation has a code word. The instruction set is as follows:

Operation code	Code word	Interpretation
0 0 1	INP	copy number from input buffer to accumulator
0 1 0	OUP	copy number from accumulator to output buffer
0 1 1	LOA	copy number from memory to accumulator
1 0 0	STO	copy number from accumulator to memory
1 0 1	ADD	add number in memory to number in accumulator, and copy result into accumulator
1 1 0	NEG	negate (NOT) number from memory to accumulator
1 1 1	ADI	add number in memory to number in accumulator, add 1 at the 1 input, and copy result into accumulator
0 0 0	END	end of program

Each instruction causes a different combination of control switches to be opened by the control unit. Open switches allow data to pass from one register to another, or through processing circuits. This is explained in more detail in the next chapter.

An example of a complete IMC-1 machine instruction is:

operation code **memory address**
1 0 1 1 0 0 0 1

1 0 1 means ADD 1 0 0 0 1 = 17 in base ten

This instruction means: add the number in memory cell 17 to the number in the accumulator, and copy the result into the accumulator.

Not all IMC-1 machine instructions need a memory address. For example:

operation code **memory address**
0 0 1 0 0 0 0 0

0 0 1 means INP 0

This instruction means: copy the number in the input buffer into the accumulator.

Some examples of IMC-1 machine language programs

Some simple programs in IMC-1 machine language are shown below. The binary machine instructions are shown loaded in position in the IMC-1 memory. Also shown are the memory cells used by the programs for storing data.

The programs are then **dry run,** that is to say, the instructions are carried out by hand, and the results written down. The dry run demonstrates how they would work if they were actually run.

Example 1 Input and store two numbers. Add them together, and store and output their total.

The method used is as follows:

The two numbers are input and stored in the memory. The first number is loaded into the accumulator, and the second number added to it. The total is stored in the memory, and also output. See Figure 11.2. Notice how memory addresses in machine instructions correspond to actual addresses of data locations. For example, the memory address in the second machine instruction is 18. This locates the memory cell in which the first data number is stored, at address 18.

Notice also that the program does not start in the first cell in the memory.

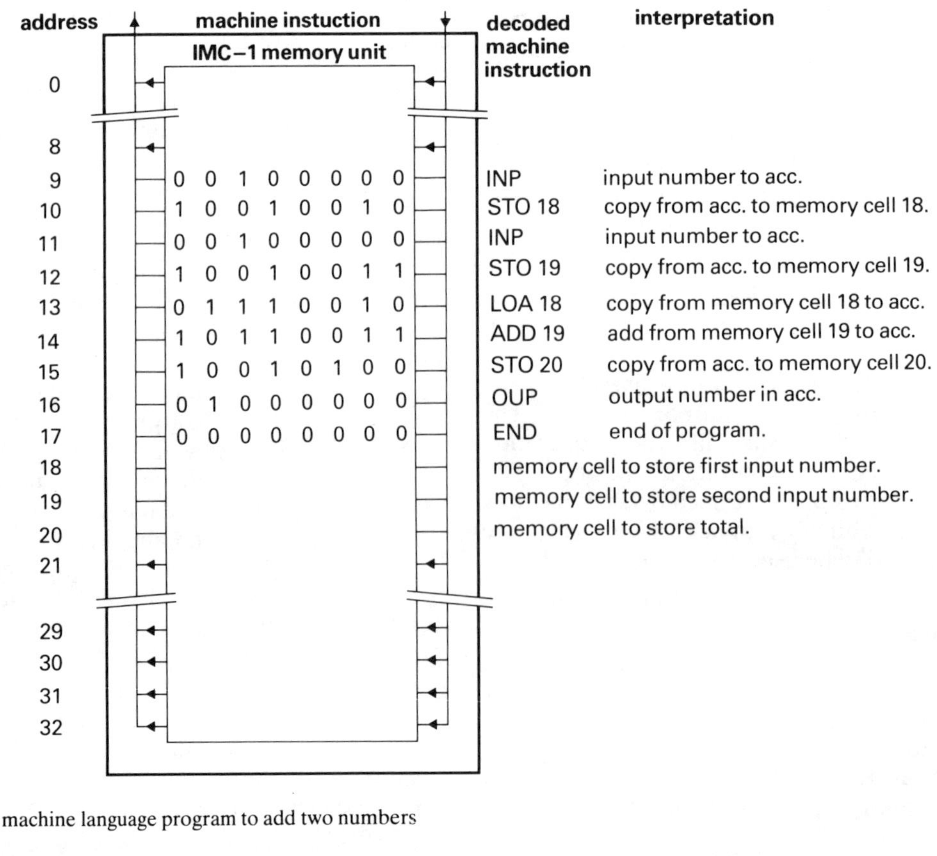

Fig. 11.2: A machine language program to add two numbers

Dry run

The numbers 0 1 0 1 1 0 0 1 (= 89) and 0 0 0 0 1 0 0 0 (= 8) are used as input data. The dry run is done in base ten. See Table 11.1 on the next page.

Example 2 Input and store two numbers. Subtract them, and store and output their difference.

The method is as follows:

The two numbers are input and stored in the memory. The second number is negated from the memory to the accumulator (in other words 1's become 0's and the 0's become 1's). This negated number is then added to the first number, with an extra 1 added at the 1 input.

Adding the extra 1 to the negated number produces the twos complement of the second number. Adding this complement to the first number is equivalent to subtracting the numbers.

The difference, now in the accumulator, is stored in the memory, and also output. This method is based on the twos complement subtraction method introduced in Chapter 3.

Note: Once again, it is important to notice how the memory addresses in machine instructions correspond to actual addresses of data locations. In this example, the data is not stored immediately after the program.

Dry run

The numbers 0 1 0 0 0 0 1 0 (= 66) and 0 0 0 0 1 1 0 0 (= 12) are used as input data. The dry run is done in binary, since the method uses the properties of twos complement numbers.

The number output is 0 0 1 1 0 1 1 0 (= 54). See Table 11.2 on the next page.

Summary

This section has introduced the essential features of the arithmetic and logic unit of a computer, as well as a simple machine language. It is important to appreciate how the machine language relates to the structure of the ALU, and how complicated machine language programs are, even for a simple process like adding two numbers.

An important point to notice is that instructions and data are stored together in the memory, and

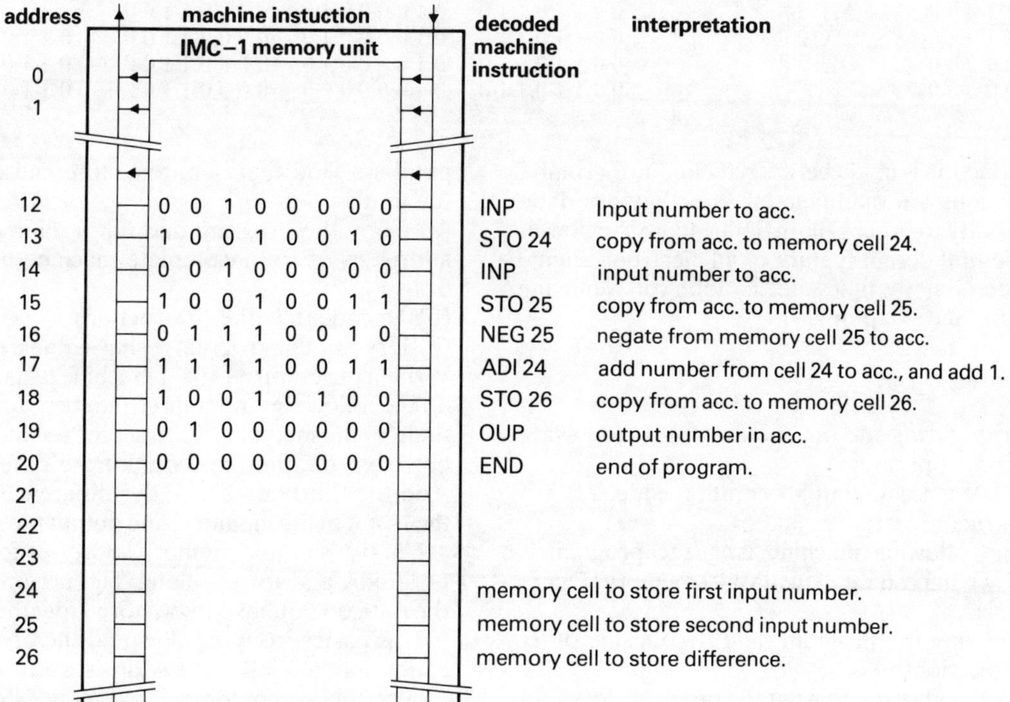

Fig. 11.3: A machine language program to subtract two numbers

Table 11.1

Binary machine instruction	Decoded machine instruction	Contents of accumulator and memory cells			
		Acc	Cell 18	Cell 19	Cell 20
0 0 1 0 0 0 0 0	INP	89			
1 0 0 1 0 0 1 0	STO 18	89	89		
0 0 1 0 0 0 0 0	INP	8	89		
1 0 0 1 0 0 1 1	STO 19	8	89	8	
0 1 1 1 0 0 1 0	LOA 18	89	89	8	
1 0 1 1 0 0 1 1	ADD 19	97	89	8	
1 0 0 1 0 1 0 0	STO 20	97	89	8	97
0 1 0 0 0 0 0 0	OUP	97	89	8	97
0 0 0 0 0 0 0 0	END	97	89	8	97

Table 11.2

Binary machine instruction	Decoded machine instruction	Contents of accumulator and memory data cells			
		Acc	Cell 24	Cell 25	Cell 26
0 0 1 0 0 0 0 0	INP	0 1 0 0 0 0 1 0			
1 0 0 1 1 0 0 0	STO 24	0 1 0 0 0 0 1 0	0 1 0 0 0 0 1 0		
0 0 1 0 0 0 0 0	INP	0 0 0 0 1 1 0 0	0 1 0 0 0 0 1 0		
1 0 0 1 1 0 0 1	STO 25	0 0 0 0 1 1 0 0	0 1 0 0 0 0 1 0	0 0 0 0 1 1 0 0	
1 1 0 1 1 0 0 1	NEG 25	1 1 1 1 0 0 1 1	0 1 0 0 0 0 1 0	0 0 0 0 1 1 0 0	
1 1 1 1 1 0 0 0	ADI 24	0 0 1 1 0 1 1 0	0 1 0 0 0 0 1 0	0 0 0 0 1 1 0 0	
1 0 0 1 1 0 1 0	STO 26	0 0 1 1 0 1 1 0	0 1 0 0 0 0 1 0	0 0 0 0 1 1 0 0	0 0 1 1 0 1 1 0
0 1 0 0 0 0 0 0	OUP	0 0 1 1 0 1 1 0	0 1 0 0 0 0 1 0	0 0 0 0 1 1 0 0	0 0 1 1 0 1 1 0
0 0 0 0 0 0 0 0	END	0 0 1 1 0 1 1 0	0 1 0 0 0 0 1 0	0 0 0 0 1 1 0 0	0 0 1 1 0 1 1 0

no distinction is made between them. Furthermore, instructions are manipulated as if they are data. This ability to process both data and instructions is an essential design feature of all electronic digital computers. It was first stated by John von Neumann in 1946. (See Chapter 21.)

Exercise 11a

1 Write down the meanings of the following words or phrases:
register; accumulator; operation code; instruction set; dry run.

2 The following machine language program is shown in position in the IMC-1 memory (Figure 11.4).
(a) Copy the program, and decode the other instructions.
(b) Briefly explain what the program does.
(c) Dry run the program, using suitable data.

3 Part of a machine language program is shown in Figure 11.5, in position in the IMC-1 memory. Its purpose is to input and store three numbers, add them up, and store and output the total.
(a) Copy the program and fill in the memory addresses of the incomplete machine instructions.
(b) Decode the other instructions.
(c) Dry run the program, using suitable data.

*4 Write a program in IMC-1 machine language to do the following: Input three numbers and store them in the memory. Subtract the second number from the first, and output the difference. Add the third number to this difference, store the result in the memory, and output the result.

Choose suitable memory addresses for your program, and for the data. The program and the data do not have to be stored together.

It is easiest to write down all the operation codes first, and fill in the addresses afterwards.

5 In a certain computer instructions are stored in cells (locations) each of which has 12 bits. In a cell containing an instruction the first 4 bits reading from the left are the operation code. The remaining 8 bits give the address of the

address binary	decimal	machine instruction	decoded machine instruction
0 1 0 1 0	10	0 0 1 0 0 0 0 0	INP
0 1 0 1 1	11	1 0 0 1 0 0 0 0	STO 16
0 1 1 0 0	12	1 0 1 1 0 0 0 0	
0 1 1 0 1	13	1 0 0 1 0 0 0 1	
0 1 1 1 0	14	0 1 0 0 0 0 0 0	
0 1 1 1 1	15	0 0 0 0 0 0 0 0	
1 0 0 0 0	16		storage for data
1 0 0 0 1	17		storage for data

Fig. 11.4

address binary	decimal	machine instruction	decoded machine instruction
1 0 0 0 0	16	0 0 1 0 0 0 0 0	INP
1 0 0 0 1	17	1 0 0 1 1 1 0 0	STO 28
1 0 0 1 0	18	0 0 1 0 0 0 0 0	
1 0 0 1 1	19	1 0 0	
1 0 1 0 0	20	0 0 1	
1 0 1 0 1	21	1 0 0	
1 0 1 1 0	22	0 1 1 1 1 1 0 0	
1 0 1 1 1	23	1 0 1	
1 1 0 0 0	24	1 0 1	
1 1 0 0 1	25	1 0 0	
1 1 0 1 0	26	0 1 0	
1 1 0 1 1	27	0 0 0 0 0 0 0 0	
1 1 1 0 0	28		
1 1 1 0 1	29		
1 1 1 1 0	30		
1 1 1 1 1	31		

Fig. 11.5

data cell whose contents are used in the operation. For example:

Binary pattern	Op code	Address of data cell
011000101101	0110	0010 1101
	DIVIDE	45

The following operation codes are used:

0 0 0 1 LOAD a copy of the contents of the addressed cell into the accumulator

0 0 1 0 STORE a copy of the contents of the accumulator in the addressed cell

0 0 1 1 ADD a copy of the contents of the addressed cell to the contents of the accumulator and leave the answer in the accumulator

0 1 0 0 SUBTRACT a copy of the contents of the addressed cell from the contents of the accumulator and leave the answer in the accumulator

0 1 0 1 MULTIPLY the contents of the accumulator by a copy of the contents of the addressed cell and leave the answer in the accumulator

On a copy of the diagram below (Figure 11.6)
(a) decode the sequence of binary instructions,
(b) work out the sequence of instructions and insert the values which will appear in each data cell after the instruction has been executed.

binary instruction	decoded instruction: op. code	decoded instruction: address	accumulator	cell 17	cell 18	cell 19	cell 20
			0	+4	−12	+9	0
0 0 0 1 0 0 0 1 0 0 0 1	LOAD	17	+4	+4	−12	+9	0
0 1 0 1 0 0 0 1 0 0 1 1							
0 0 1 0 0 0 0 1 0 1 0 0							
0 0 1 1 0 0 0 1 0 1 0 0							
0 0 1 0 0 0 0 1 0 0 0 1							
0 0 0 1 0 0 0 1 0 0 1 0							
0 1 0 1 0 0 0 1 0 0 1 0							
0 1 0 0 0 0 0 1 0 1 0 0							
0 1 0 0 0 0 0 1 0 0 0 1							
0 0 1 0 0 0 0 1 0 0 1 1							

(The last five columns are headed "accumulator and data cell contents".)

Fig. 11.6

The first line has been done for you. (EAEB 76 I)

6 The diagram below shows a program instruction for a simple computer that is designed with a fixed wordlength of 14 bits.

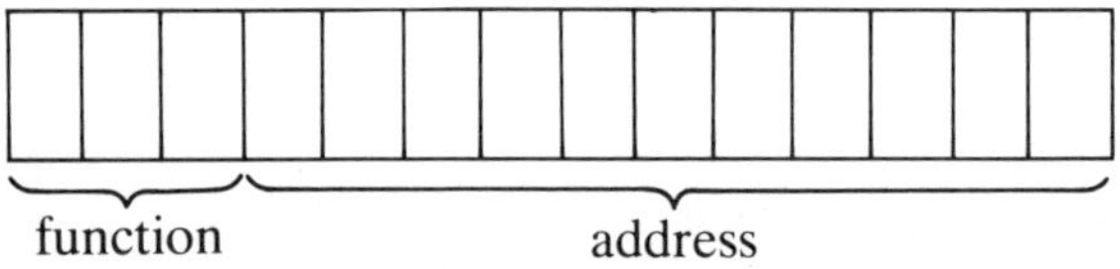

(a) Of how many DIFFERENT functions is the machine capable?
(b) How many directly addressable locations are available? (AEB 78 specimen)

7 In a certain computer instructions and data are stored in 8 bit locations. For an instruction the three left hand bits are the operation code. The remaining five bits give an address.

	Op code	Address
Example of an instruction:	0 1 0	0 1 1 0 1
	STO	13

The first three operation codes are:

0 0 0	HAL	Halts execution of the program.
0 0 1	LOA	Loads a copy of the contents of the addressed location into the accumulator.
0 1 0	STO	Stores a copy of the contents of the accumulator in the addressed location.

(a) Complete the table of operation codes in Figure 11.7. The codes follow sequentially.

(b) Complete the table in Figure 11.8 by writing in the binary coding of the instructions.

(c) Work through the program using the table in Figure 11.8. Enter the values which will appear in the accumulator and data locations as the instructions are executed.

(d) Why would an instruction such as ADD 45 not be possible? (EAEB 78 I)

Section B: Further aspects of machine languages

Some further aspects of machine languages are now introduced, namely **indirect addressing** and **address modification** (or **indexing**). They have been excluded from the IMC-1 machine language for simplicity, but are very important in machine languages in practice.

* Indirect addressing

The method of accessing data by the memory address part of a machine instruction, as described earlier, is called **direct addressing.** Most computers can also access data by **indirect addressing.**

When indirect addressing is used, the memory address part of a machine instruction locates a cell in the computer memory. This cell contains the address of the data item required by the machine instruction. Figure 11.10 shows an example of this using 12 bit words.

000	HAL	halts execution of the program.
001	LOA	loads a copy of the contents of the addressed location into the accumulator
010	STO	stores a copy of the contents of the accumulator in the addressed location.
	ADD	adds a copy of the contents of the addressed location to the contents of the accumulator. Leaves the results in accumulator.
	SUB	substracts a copy of the contents of the addressed location from the contents of the accumulator. Leaves the results in the accumulator.
	JIN	jump to execute the addressed location if the contents of the accumulator are negative.
	JEQ	jump to execute the addressed location if the contents of the accumulator are zero.
	JUM	jump to execute the addressed location.

Fig. 11.7

address	contents	binary coding
1	LOA 12	
2	SUB 13	
3	JEQ 11	
4	STO 12	
5	LOA 14	
6	ADD 13	
7	STO 14	
8	ADD 15	
9	STO 15	
10	JUM 1	
11	HAL 0	
12	+3	0 0 0 0 0 0 1 1
13	+1	0 0 0 0 0 0 0 1
14	+1	0 0 0 0 0 0 0 1
15	+1	0 0 0 0 0 0 0 1

Fig. 11.8

accum-ulator	location 12	location 13	location 14	location 15
	3	1	1	1

Fig. 11.9

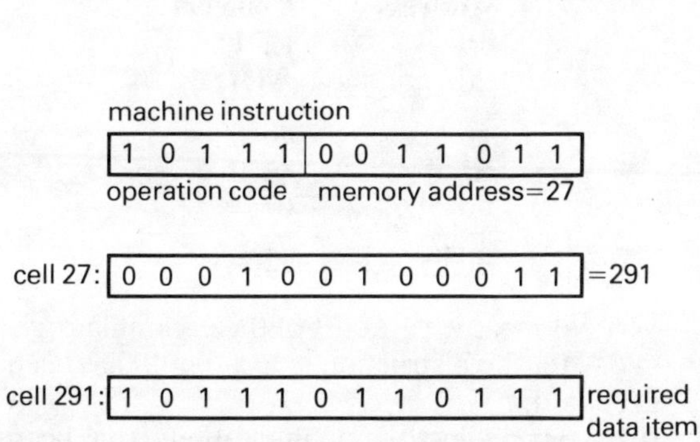

Fig. 11.10: Indirect addressing

Indirect addressing has several advantages. One is that the machine instruction memory address only occupies part of a word. The address that it accesses, however, occupies a complete word.

Provided that the address decoder is large enough to decode a complete word, the number of memory cells that can be accessed by a machine instruction is greatly increased by indirect addressing.

Another advantage of indirect addressing is that data is often organized into complex structures like lists or matrices. Indirect addressing simplifies the programs which process data in these structures.

* Address modification

On most computers, the memory address part of a machine instruction can be modified by adding to it the number stored in a special register called the **index register.** For example, using twelve bit words: (Figure 11.11)

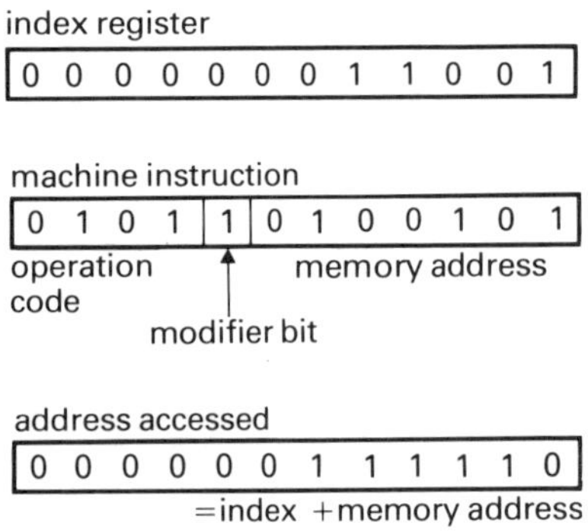

Fig. 11.11: Address modification

This process is called **address modification.** It is controlled by one bit of the machine instruction, called the **modifier bit.** It stores a 1 if the memory address is to be modified, and a 0 if there is no modification.

As with indirect addressing, the uses of address modification include increasing the number of memory cells addressed by a machine instruction, and simplifying access to structured data. To distinguish it from a modified or indirect address, the direct address of a data item is sometimes called its **absolute address.**

Machine languages in practice

The machine languages of the majority of computers are extremely complicated. Most computers have several accumulators, several index registers (or registers which can either be accumulators or index registers) and large instruction sets.

For example, in ICL 1900 series computers, which use 24 bit words, 7 bits are for the operation code, 3 bits are for the accumulator address, 2 bits are for the index register and 12 bits are for the memory address. A computer of this sort has an instruction set of $2^7 = 128$ machine language instructions.

The instruction sets of most computers include operations which transfer control to other parts of the program. Some operations will only transfer control under certain conditions, for example if the accumulator contains zero. Instructions of this type are discussed in Chapter 13.

Exercise 11b

1 Write down the meanings of the following words or phrases:
indirect addressing; address modification; index register; modifier bit.

*__2__ A computer has twelve bit machine instructions, arranged as follows (Figure 11.12):

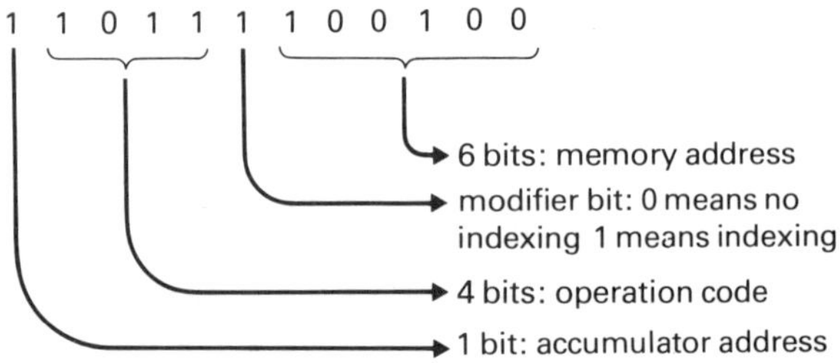

Fig. 11.12

(a) How many different operation codes are there?
(b) How many accumulators does the computer have?
(c) How many memory cells can be addressed directly (with no indexing)?
(d) If the index register has twelve bits, what is the largest address it can contain?
(e) How many memory cells can be addressed with indexing?

3 The machine language of a computer includes the following instructions:

LDI x : Load the number with indirect address x onto the accumulator.
ADI x : Add the number with indirect address x to the number in the accumulator.

The memory of the computer includes the following:

Address	Contents
19	LDI 57
20	ADI 56
56	4048
57	4050
4048	673
4050	126

Write down the contents of the accumulator:
(a) After the instruction in location 19 has been executed.
(b) After the instruction in location 20 has been executed.

4 A certain computer's machine language contains the following instructions:

FETCH n: Copy the contents of the location whose absolute address is n into the accumulator.

SUB n: Subtract the number contained in the location whose absolute address is n from the accumulator.

STORE n: Copy the contents of the accumulator into the location whose absolute address is n.

BNEG n: Branch (jump) to location n if the number in the accumulator is negative.

STOP: End of program.

The following instructions are stored in locations 17 to 21 inclusive:

location 17	FETCH 66
location 18	BNEG 21
location 19	SUB 69
location 20	STORE 69
location 21	STOP

Before these instructions are executed, the accumulator contains +75.

What will be the contents of the accumulator and locations 66 and 69 after execution if, before execution

(a) location 66 contains +21, location 69 contains −78,

(b) location 66 contains −21, location 69 contains +78? (OLE 78 I)

12

Processing a program

This chapter completes the description of the working of the central processing unit of a computer. The essential features of the control unit of the CPU are introduced, and the steps in the processing of a machine language program are described. Once again, much of the explanation makes use of the IMC-1 model computer. A diagram of the complete IMC-1 is included in this chapter.

The control unit

The **Control Unit** is the part of a central processing unit which co-ordinates the step-by-step running of the whole computer. By means of the control switches in data channels at various points throughout the computer, the control unit regulates the flow of data and instructions to and from the memory, during input and output, to and from backing store and within the CPU itself. The control unit is also responsible for the timing of all the operations done by the computer.

The IMC-1 control unit

Figure 12.1 shows the control unit of the IMC-1 model computer.

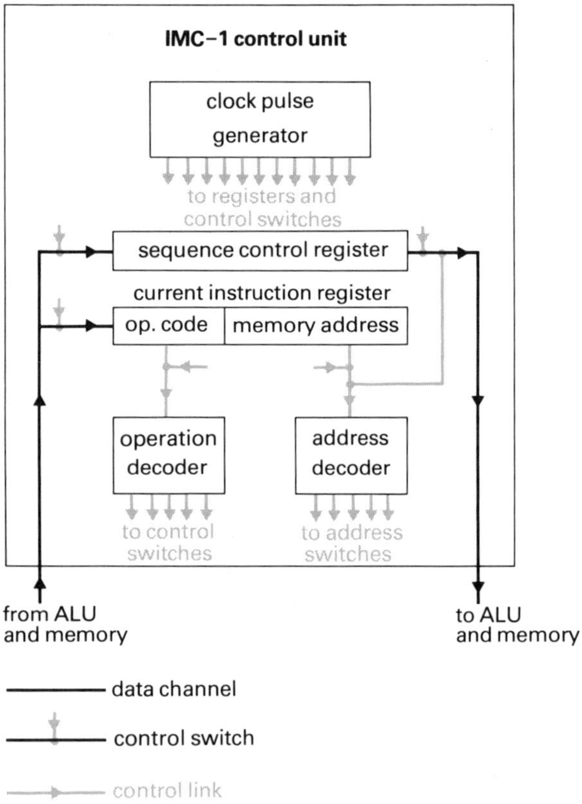

Fig. 12.1: The IMC-1 control unit

The components of the control unit of the IMC-1 are as follows:

Clock pulse generator:
The clock pulse generator sends out pulses of electricity at regular intervals to registers and control switches in the computer. These pulses regulate the timing of the whole computer.

Sequence control register:
An eight bit sequence control register (SCR), also known as a **program counter.** This controls the order in which machine instructions are processed. At any time, the SCR contains the address of the next machine instruction to be processed.

Current instruction register:
An eight bit current instruction register (CIR). This stores a copy of the machine instruction being processed at the time. The first three bits of the CIR contain the operation code, and the other five bits store the memory address.

Operation decoder:
A three bit operation decoder. It is connected to the three bits of the CIR which contain the operation code. The operation decoder recognizes the different operation codes, and sends pulses to various control switches in the computer, depending on the operation. (See page 46.)

Address decoder:
A five bit address decoder. It is connected to the five bits of the CIR which contain the memory address. When it has decoded an address, the address decoder sends a pulse to the control switches attached to the memory cell with that address. This enables data to be stored in or copied from the memory cell addressed. (See page 46.)

For simplicity, most of the control links in the IMC-1 have not been included in the diagrams. Every control switch has a control link from the clock pulse generator and one from the operation decoder or the address decoder.

The IMC-1 complete

The three parts of the central processing unit of the IMC-1, namely the memory, the ALU and the control unit, have now been introduced. Figure 12.2 shows how they fit together to form the complete IMC-1.

You will notice how the data channels link up to form **data highways** connecting all the units of the CPU. For simplicity, the control links between the three parts have been omitted.

Instruction cycles

This section describes some of the steps involved in processing a machine language instruction. The steps are repeated as each machine instruction is processed. Together they make up the **instruction cycle** of the computer.

The three most important steps of an instruction cycle are the **fetch, execute** and **reset** steps. These steps are explained using the IMC-1 model computer, and a machine language program introduced in the previous chapter.

At the start of a program, the sequence control register is loaded with the address of the first instruction of the program.

Fetch

The first part of the instruction cycle fetches the machine instruction to be processed from the memory to the current instruction register. The sequence control register contains the address of this instruction. This address is decoded in the address decoder to locate the instruction, which is then copied into the current instruction register.

Execute

The machine instruction in the current instruction register is carried out. The operation decoder determines the type of operation, and sends pulses to the appropriate control switches. If the instruction contains a memory address, the address decoder accesses the memory cell with this address. This locates the data item which is referred to by the instruction.

Reset

The reset step prepares the CPU for the next machine instruction in the program. In most cases, this requires the address in the sequence control register to be increased by 1. In the IMC-1, the 1 input and the parallel adder are used for this.

Not all machine instructions require a reset step. For example, the 0 0 0 (end of program) instruction of the IMC-1 has no need for a reset step. In actual machine languages, instructions which transfer control to other parts of a program do not require reset steps. In most computers, the reset step is carried out by an adder in the control unit, at the same time as the execute step.

Continuing the cycle

After the reset step, the sequence control register contains the address of the next instruction of the program. This instruction is fetched, and the cycle continues.

The IMC-1 instruction cycle

The diagram below (Figure 12.3) shows the IMC-1 with the first example program from the previous chapter loaded in its memory. The steps of the instruction cycle which process the first instruction of this program are now described. The description uses binary numbers only, to emphasize that this is the way computers actually work.

Fetch

At the start of the program, the sequence control register stores the address of the first instruction, namely 0 1 0 0 1. The clock pulse generator sends a pulse to open control switch A. This sends the address from the SCR to the address decoder. The address decoder opens switch B, at address 0 1 0 0 1, while the clock pulse generator opens switch C. This copies the first instruction, 0 0 1 0 0 0 0 0, from the memory to the current instruction register.

Execute

The machine instruction in the current instruction register is carried out. Control switch D is opened by a clock pulse to decode the operation code. In this case it is 0 0 1: INP (copy from input buffer to accumulator). The operation decoder sends pulses

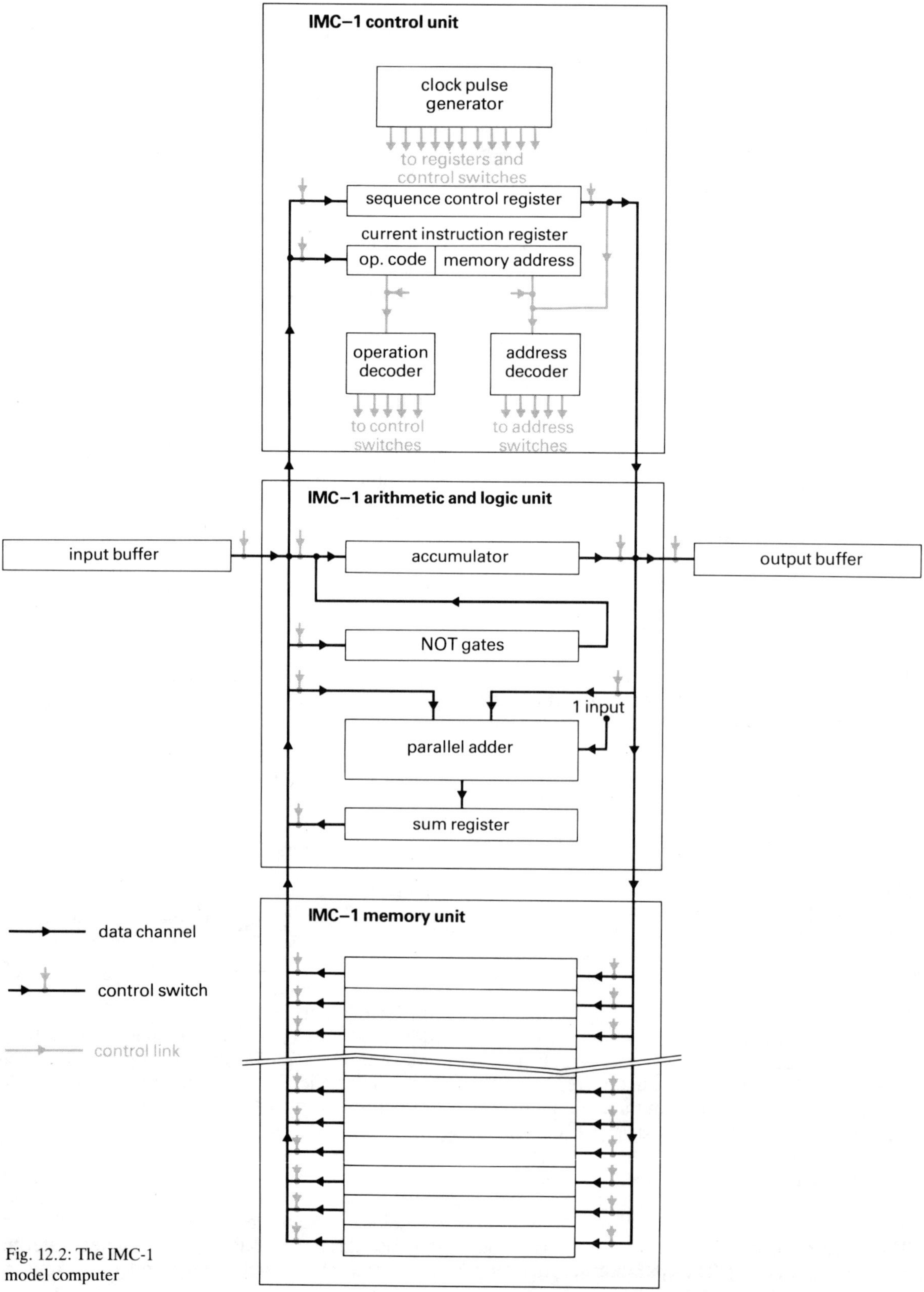

Fig. 12.2: The IMC-1 model computer

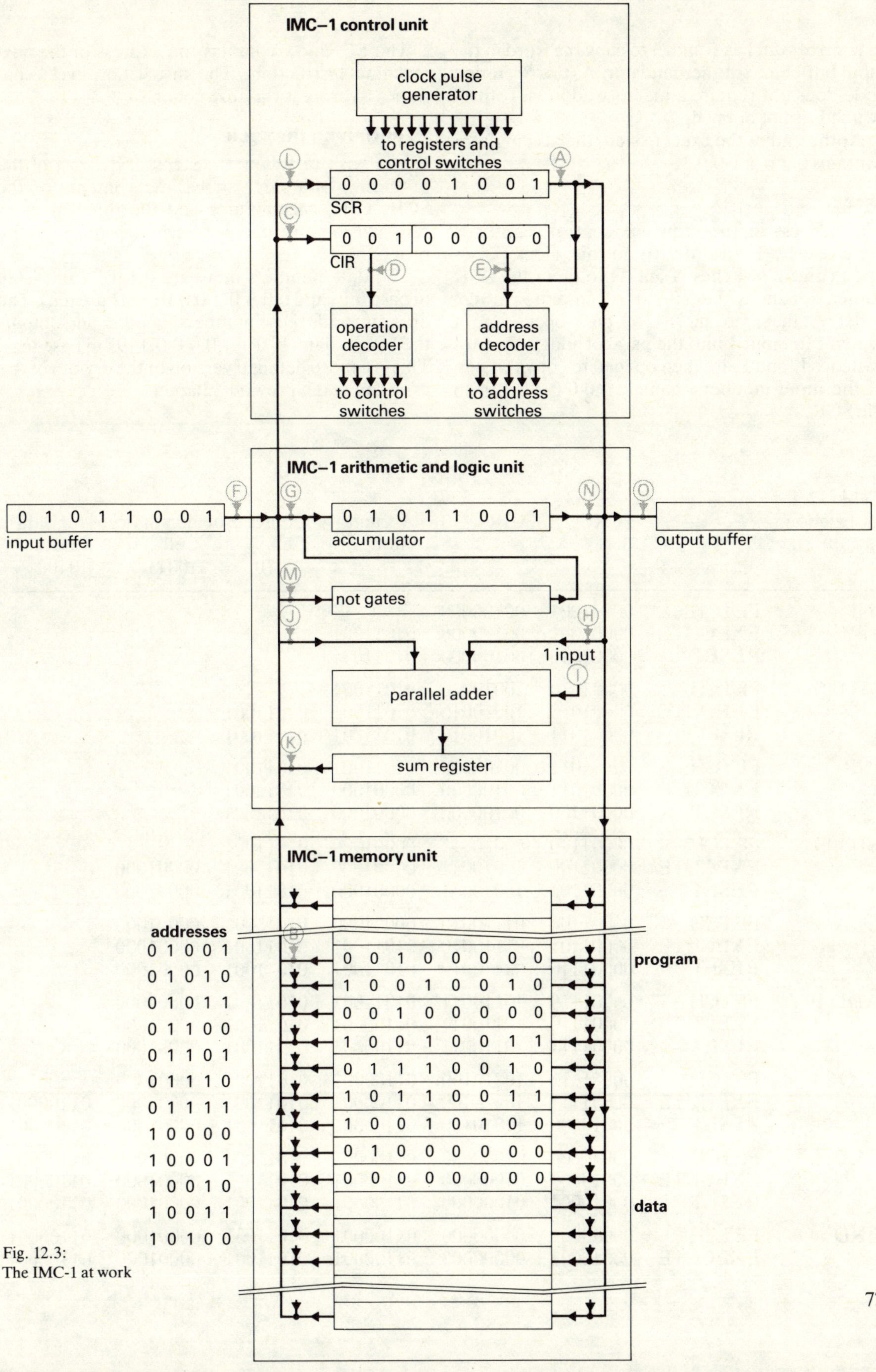

Fig. 12.3:
The IMC-1 at work

to control switches F and G to copy the word in the input buffer into the accumulator. As this operation code does not require a memory address, control switch E is not opened.

At the end of the execute step, the accumulator contains 0 1 0 1 1 0 0 1.

Reset

The address in the sequence control register is increased by 1. In order to do this, clock pulses open control switches A and H to input the SCR contents, namely 0 0 0 0 1 0 0 1, into the parallel adder. At the same time, a clock pulse opens control switch I to input 1 into the parallel adder. Control switches K and L are then opened to copy the sum of the input numbers, namely 0 0 0 0 1 0 1 0, to the SCR.

The SCR now contains the address of the next machine instruction. The instruction cycle continues to process this instruction.

* Continuing the cycle

If you wish to follow the steps of the rest of the program, table 12.1 shows the contents of the SCR, CIR, accumulator and the three memory cells which store data, at each step of the entire program.

The data numbers input are 0 1 0 1 1 0 0 1 (89 in base ten) and 0 0 0 0 1 0 0 0 (8 in base ten). The program adds these numbers together and outputs the result, namely 0 1 1 0 0 0 0 1 (97 in base ten). This is a more detailed version of the dry run of this program in the previous chapter.

Table 12.1

Instruction		SCR	CIR	Accumulator	Contents of memory cells for data Cell 10010	Cell 10011	Cell 10100
INP	FETCH	00001001	00100000				
	EXECUTE	00001001	00100000	01011001			
	RESET	00001010	00100000	01011001			
STO 18	FETCH	00001010	10010010	01011001			
	EXECUTE	00001010	10010010	01011001	01011001		
	RESET	00001011	10010010	01011001	01011001		
INP	FETCH	00001011	00100000	01011001	01011001		
	EXECUTE	00001011	00100000	00001000	01011001		
	RESET	00001100	00100000	00001000	01011001		
STO 19	FETCH	00001100	10010011	00001000	01011001		
	EXECUTE	00001100	10010011	00001000	01011001	00001000	
	RESET	00001101	10010011	00001000	01011001	00001000	
LOA 18	FETCH	00001101	01110010	00001000	01011001	00001000	
	EXECUTE	00001101	01110010	01011001	01011001	00001000	
	RESET	00001110	01110010	01011001	01011001	00001000	
ADD 19	FETCH	00001110	10110011	01011001	01011001	00001000	
	EXECUTE	00001110	10110011	01100001	01011001	00001000	
	RESET	00001111	10110011	01100001	01011001	00001000	
STO 20	FETCH	00001111	10010100	01100001	01011001	00001000	
	EXECUTE	00001111	10010100	01100001	01011001	00001000	01100001
	RESET	00010000	10010100	01100001	01011001	00001000	01100001
OUP	FETCH	00010000	01000000	01100001	01011001	00001000	01100001
	EXECUTE	00010000	01000000	01100001	01011001	00001000	01100001
	RESET	00010001	01000000	01100001	01011001	00001000	01100001
END	FETCH	00010001	00000000	01100001	01011001	00001000	01100001
	EXECUTE	00010001	00000000	01100001	01011001	00001000	01100001

Timing

The timing of each step of the instruction cycle is controlled by the clock pulse generator in the control unit of the CPU. The time for a complete instruction cycle is called the **cycle time** of the computer.

The speed of processing of most computers is very high. A million clock pulses per second, or more, are common. Some units of time often used in this connection are: **millisecond** (thousandth of a second), **microsecond** (millionth of a second) and **nanosecond** (thousand millionth of a second). Typical cycle times are one microsecond or less.

* Some further aspects of processing a program

The instruction cycles of most computers have several features not found on the IMC-1. These features include **micro-instructions** and **macro-instructions, subprogram linkage** and **interrupts.** These are now briefly discussed.

* Micro-instructions and macro-instructions

As you will have realized from the first part of this chapter, it takes several steps to carry out one machine instruction. At each step, control switches at various points in the computer are opened or closed. One way of controlling the opening and closing of these switches in the correct sequence is to use **micro-instructions.** A set of micro-instructions together forms a **microprogram** which carries out the steps of a machine instruction.

A **macro-instruction** is a machine language instruction which calls up a set of other machine language instructions, to perform some task. For instance, if a computer cannot do multiplication directly by hardware, it requires a number of machine language instructions to perform the necessary shifts and additions. It is convenient to store these instructions ready for use, and access them by a single macro-instruction whenever they are required. This considerably reduces the length of machine language programs.

Other uses of microprograms or macro-instructions include controlling the detailed steps of input and output, and transfer of data to or from backing store.

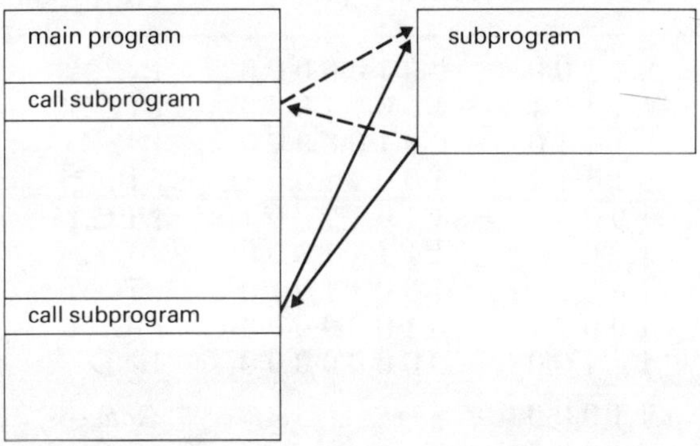

Fig. 12.4: Subprogram linkage

* Subprogram linkage

If some instructions are needed more than once in a program, it is most convenient to write them as a **subprogram.** The subprogram may be accessed from any number of points in the rest of the program, which is called the **main program.** After the subprogram, control returns to the place in the main program from which the subprogram was accessed. See Figure 12.4.

One way of linking the main program and the subprogram in this manner is as follows:

There is a machine language instruction to store the contents of the sequence control register (the address of the current main program instruction) in the memory. The subprogram is then accessed. In this way, the computer 'remembers' its place in the main program while it is processing the subprogram. After the subprogram, this address is once again placed in the SCR, by another machine instruction. Processing of the main program then continues.

* Interrupts

In most computers, it is necessary from time to time to interrupt the processing of a program. An **interrupt** is a signal which causes a break in the execution of the current program. An interrupt can occur for several reasons, the most common being for the input or output of data. This is because peripheral units work much more slowly than the CPU.

When an interrupt occurs, the contents of the sequence control register, (the address of the machine instruction currently being processed), and other important registers, are stored in the memory, and control is transferred to another program. In this way the computer 'remembers' its place in the program. It returns to this place after the interrupt.

Summary

In this chapter, some of the steps involved in processing a machine language program have been

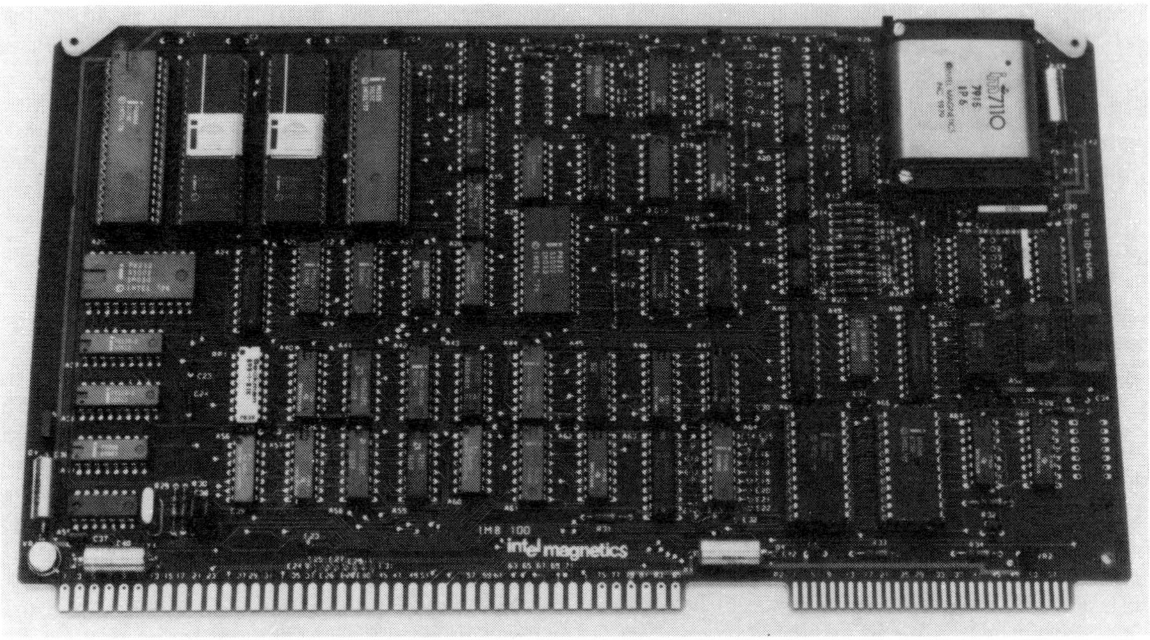

An Intel magnetic bubble memory system

introduced. You will now realize that the step-by-step working of a computer is very complex. Even a simple operation, such as adding two numbers, takes a large number of steps to do on a computer. It is only the very high speed of each step which enables the whole operation to be done so quickly.

This chapter concludes the detailed description of the central processing unit of a computer. The next few chapters show how computers are made to perform useful work, and how they can be used by people who do not have expert knowledge of the structure and functioning of computers.

Exercise 12

1 Write down the meanings of the following words or phrases:
clock pulse generator;
sequence control register;
current instruction register;
operation decoder; data highway;
instruction cycle; cycle time; subprogram;
interrupt; micro-instruction;
macro-instruction.

2 (a) At the start of an instruction cycle, a sequence control register contains 0 0 1 0 0 1 0 1. What will its contents be at the start of the next instruction cycle?
(b) A program consists of ten machine language instructions, starting at address 0 0 1 0 1. What is the contents of the SCR (8 bits), at the start of the last instruction cycle of the program?

***3** Table 1 is a machine language program which subtracts two numbers by finding the complement and adding. It is the second example program in Chapter 11.

Table 12.2

Address	Machine instruction	Decoded instruction
0 1 1 0 0	0 0 1 0 0 0 0 0	INP
0 1 1 0 1	1 0 0 1 1 0 0 0	STO 24
0 1 1 1 0	0 0 1 0 0 0 0 0	INP
0 1 1 1 1	1 0 0 1 1 0 0 1	STO 25
1 0 0 0 0	1 1 0 1 1 0 0 1	NEG 25
1 0 0 0 1	1 1 1 1 1 0 0 0	ADI 24
1 0 0 1 0	1 0 0 1 1 0 1 0	STO 26
1 0 0 1 1	0 1 0 0 0 0 0 0	OUP
1 0 1 0 0	0 0 0 0 0 0 0 0	END
1 1 0 0 0		*Data*
1 1 0 0 1		
1 1 0 1 0		

(a) Using the information in Table 12.2 copy and complete Table 12.3. It shows the contents of the SCR, CIR, accumulator and the three memory cells which store data, at each step of the entire program.

(b) What (binary) number is output?

4 A computer has a card reader which reads a card in 100 milliseconds, and a CPU with a cycle time of 10 microseconds. How many instruction cycles take place while a card is being read?

5 The transfer rate of data from a magnetic disc is one byte every 2 microseconds. If this interrupts every twentieth instruction cycle, what is the cycle time of the CPU?

6 Does the display register on a pocket calculator correspond to the sequence control register, current instruction register or accumulator on a computer?

7 A computer has a cycle time of 100 nanoseconds. Is it true to say that it can add two numbers in this time? If not, how long would it take to add two numbers?

Table 12.3

Instruction		SCR	CIR	Accumulator	Contents of memory cells for data		
					Cell 11000	Cell 11001	Cell 11010
INP	FETCH	00001100	00100000				
	EXECUTE	00001100	00100000	01000010			
	RESET	00001101	00100000	01000010			
STO 24	FETCH	00001101	10011000	01000010			
	EXECUTE	00001101	10011000	01000010	01000010		
	RESET	00001110	10011000	01000010	01000010		
INP	FETCH	00001110	00100000	01000010	01000010		
	EXECUTE	00001110	00100000	00001100	01000010		
	RESET	00001111	00100000	00001100	01000010		
STO 25	FETCH	00001111	10011001	00001100	01000010		
	EXECUTE	00001111	10011001	00001100	01000010	00001100	
	RESET	00010000	10011001	00001100	01000010	00001100	

13

Assembly language

Section A

In this chapter, a type of computer language called **assembly language** is introduced. The intention of introducing this type of language is not to solve complicated problems, nor to teach computer programming, but to give further insight into the step-by-step working of a computer.

The development of assembly language

The earliest computers were programmed in machine language. Each instruction was written in its binary code, and each cell in the memory allocated for a specific purpose. This made programming a slow and difficult task. A single error often meant rewriting large portions of a program.

To speed up this process, **assembly languages,** often called **low level languages,** were introduced.

Features of assembly languages

In an assembly language, each machine instruction is replaced by an instruction using a short English word for the operation code (like IN, ADD, OUT etc.) and, in most cases, a letter, or series of letters, for the memory address. Numbers are in base ten.

It must be emphasized that one assembly language instruction replaces one machine language instruction. Thus an assembly language program still illustrates the step-by-step working of a computer while it is being processed. For example:

Machine language	**Assembly language**
1 0 1 1 1 0 0 1	ADD SALES 3

Assemblers

Programs are not processed in assembly language. Each computer has a program called an **assembler,** usually kept on backing store ready for use. The assembler converts each instruction of an assembly language program into the equivalent machine language instruction. The machine language program is then run.

The flow diagram in Figure 13.1 shows the steps of running a program in assembly language.

An example of an assembly language: CESIL

CESIL is the name of a low level language which has been specially written for introductory computing courses. It can be run on many computers. However CESIL is not used for data processing in industry or commerce, nor does it actually correspond to the machine language of any computer.

Some of the words for operations in CESIL are:

IN	Input next data number to accumulator.
OUT	Output contents of accumulator.
LOAD	Copy from memory to accumulator.
STORE	Copy from accumulator to memory.
ADD	Add number in memory to number in accumulator.
SUBTRACT	Subtract number in memory from number in accumulator.
MULTIPLY	Multiply number in memory by number in accumulator.
DIVIDE	Divide number in accumulator by number in memory.
HALT	End of program.

The memory address in a CESIL instruction is indicated by a letter, or by a string of up to six letters or numbers, starting with a letter. Some examples of complete CESIL instructions are:

LOAD A	Copy from memory cell A to accumulator.
ADD TOTAL	Add number in memory cell TOTAL to number in accumulator.

Compare these instructions with the machine language instructions.

Only whole numbers may be used as data for

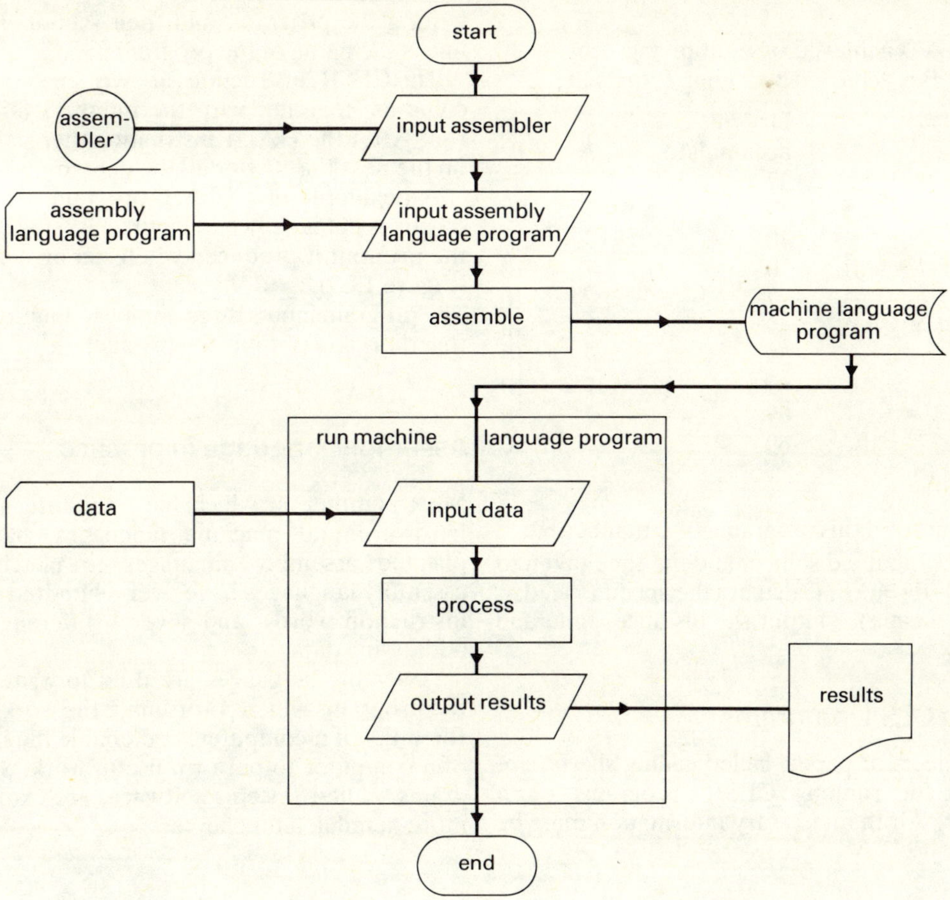

Fig. 13.1: Running an assembly language program

CESIL programs. The numbers may be positive or negative. The DIVIDE instruction gives the whole number part of the answer. (For example 15 DIVIDEd by 4 = 3.)

Some examples of CESIL programs

Some simple CESIL programs are shown in the following three examples. Next to each instruction you will notice some numbers, in columns. There is one column for the accumulator, and another for each memory cell used in the program. Each CESIL instruction is carried out by hand, and the numbers which result are written in the appropriate columns. This process is called a **dry run** of the program. A dry run follows the steps which a computer carries out while processing a program.

Example 1 Input two numbers and add them together. Output their sum.

Only one memory cell is needed, to store the first number.

Program		Dry run Accumulator	**N**
IN		13	
STORE	N	13	13
IN		9	13
ADD	N	22	13
OUT		**22**	13
HALT		22	13

Data 13 9

The output from this program is the number 22.

Compare this program with the machine language program on page 66.

Example 2 Input numbers A and B. Output the value of $A^2 + 2B$.

Squaring A is achieved by multiplying A by itself. Doubling B is achieved by adding B to itself.

Program		Dry run accumulator	**A**	**B**
IN		7		
STORE	A	7	7	
IN		10	7	
STORE	B	10	7	10
LOAD	A	7	7	10
MULTIPLY	A	49	7	10
ADD	B	59	7	10
ADD	B	69	7	10
OUT		**69**	7	10
HALT		69	7	10

Data 7 10

The output from this program is the number 69.

Example 3 Input a distance, and the time taken to travel that distance. Calculate the speed (speed = distance ÷ time). Output the distance, time and speed.

Running CESIL programs

Special sheets of paper, called **coding sheets,** are available for running CESIL programs on a computer. All the necessary information must be written neatly in the correct places.

The first two lines identify the name of the person writing the program, and their school. The third line is the name of the program.

The CESIL instructions are written in the correct columns, together with the numbers for the dry run. After the HALT instruction there is a % sign on the next line. After all the data there is a *.

An example of a CESIL program written on a coding sheet is shown in Figure 13.2, together with the printout it produced when run on a computer (Figure 13.3).

The program inputs three numbers, multiplies them together, and outputs the product.

Assembly language in practice

Most computers, which have sophisticated CPU hardware and machine languages, have complicated assembly languages to match. Many assembly languages have over a hundred different instruction words, and several different ways of addressing data.

Assembly languages are used to write most of the programs which co-ordinate the working of all the units of a computer, and enable the hardware of a computer to perform useful work. Such programs, called **systems software,** are explained in more detail in later chapters.

Example 3

Program		Dry run accumulator	DIST	TIME	SPEED
IN		512			
STORE	DIST	512	512		
IN		16	512		
STORE	TIME	16	512	16	
LOAD	DIST	512	512	16	
DIVIDE	TIME	32	512	16	
STORE	SPEED	32	512	16	32
LOAD	DIST	512	512	16	32
OUT		**512**	512	16	32
LOAD	TIME	16	512	16	32
OUT		**16**	512	16	32
LOAD	SPEED	32	512	16	32
OUT		**32**	512	16	32
HALT		32	512	16	32

Data 512 16

The output from this program is the numbers 512, 16 and 32.

FILL IN THESE BOXES ONLY ON SHEET ONE

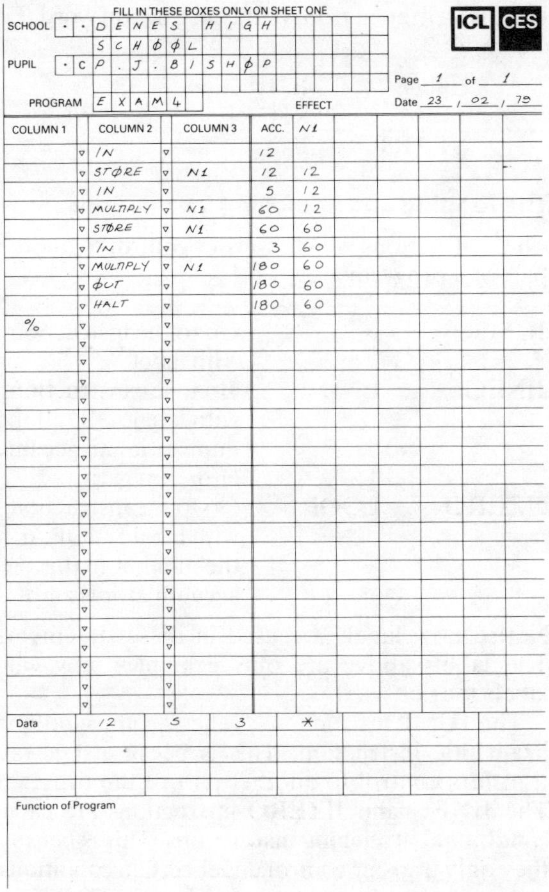
SCHOOL ..DENES HIGH SCHØØL
PUPIL .CP.J.BISHØP
PROGRAM EXAM4 EFFECT
Page 1 of 1
Date 23/02/79

COLUMN 1	COLUMN 2	COLUMN 3	ACC.	N1
	IN		12	
	STØRE	N1	12	12
	IN		5	12
	MULTIPLY	N1	60	12
	STØRE	N1	60	60
	IN		3	60
	MULTIPLY	N1	180	60
	ØUT		180	60
	HALT		180	60
%				

Data 12 5 3 *

Function of Program

FORM 4/3618(8.70) CESIL CODING SHEET © HOSKYNS GROUP LIMITED 1969

Fig. 13.2

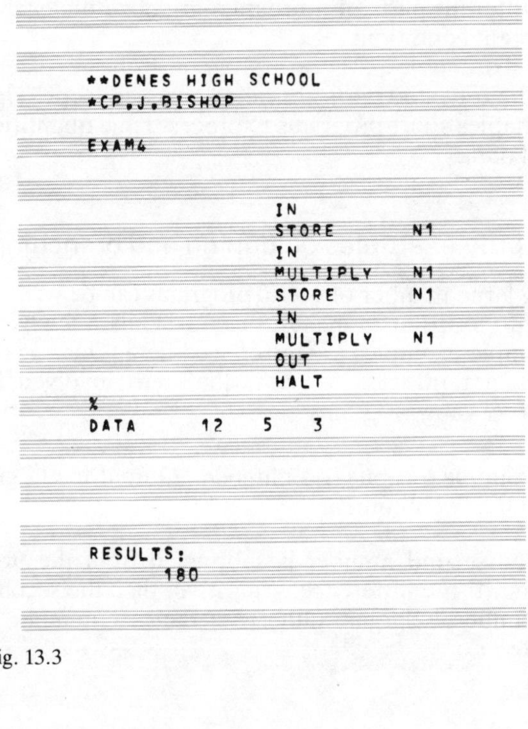

```
**DENES HIGH SCHOOL
*CP.J.BISHOP

EXAM4

             IN
             STORE      N1
             IN
             MULTIPLY   N1
             STORE      N1
             IN
             MULTIPLY   N1
             OUT
             HALT
%
DATA      12    5    3

RESULTS:
          180
```

Fig. 13.3

Another area of use of assembly languages is in programming microcomputers. A number of microcomputers can only be programmed in their assembly language.

Some applications programs are written in assembly languages, though the majority are written in high level languages, which are introduced in the next chapter.

Exercise 13a

1 Write down the meanings of the following words or phrases:
assembler; dry run; low level language.

2 (a) Copy this CESIL program, and complete the dry run:

Program		Dry run accumulator	A	B
IN		7		
STORE	A	7	7	
MULTIPLY	A	49	7	
STORE	A	49	49	
IN				
STORE	B			
MULTIPLY	B			
ADD	A			
OUT				
HALT				
Data 7 3				

(b) What has this program calculated?

Choosing your own data numbers, write CESIL programs for questions **3–6.** Dry run the programs, and run them on a computer if possible.

3 Input four numbers and output their total. Use one memory cell only to store the running total.

4 Input numbers P and Q. Output the values of PQ and 3PQ.

***5** Input four numbers and calculate the sum of their squares. Use as few memory cells as you can.

6 Input the length and breadth of a rectangle. Calculate its area (area = length × breadth). Output the length, breadth and area.

At this stage you should be able to make up simple CESIL programs of your own.

Section 13b: Further CESIL programs

In this section, three more CESIL instructions are introduced. They enable programs to be written which include decisions, or parts of programs which are run repeatedly, called **loops.** The use of constants in CESIL programs is also introduced.

Constants

Instead of referring to a variable number stored in the computer memory, CESIL instructions can refer to a fixed number, called a **constant.** Constants in CESIL must be whole numbers, but may be positive or negative. For example:

LOAD	+ 10	means load the number 10 into the accumulator.
DIVIDE	− 160	means divide the number in the accumulator by − 160.

Notice that constants must have a + or − sign in front.

The following is an example of a program which uses a constant:

Example 5 Input three numbers. Calculate and output their total and average.

The numbers are input and added up. The total is output, then divided by 3 to give the average. The average is output. Only one memory cell is needed, for the total.

Program		Dry run accumulator	TOTAL
IN		10	
STORE	TOTAL	10	10
IN		18	10
ADD	TOTAL	28	10
STORE	TOTAL	28	28
IN		8	28
ADD	TOTAL	36	28
OUT		**36**	28
DIVIDE	+3	12	28
OUT		**12**	28
HALT		12	28

Data 10 18 8

The output is 36 (total) and 12 (average)

Looping and branching

CESIL instructions are usually processed in the order in which they are written in the program. However there are three instructions which transfer control to some other part of the program.

Labels

A CESIL instruction may be identified by a **label.** A label consists of a single letter, or a string of up to six letters or numbers, starting with a letter. The label is written in front of the instruction word. For example:

Label	Instruction	
J	STORE	SUM
START	IN	

The looping and branching instructions

The instructions which transfer control to another part of a program are:

JUMP	X	Go to the instruction with label X
JINEG	END	Go to the instruction with label END, if the number in the accumulator is negative
JIZERO	LOOP	Go to the instruction with label LOOP, if the number in the accumulator is zero

Notice how labels are used in these statements. The labels above are only examples, any valid labels may be used.

The JUMP instruction is called an **unconditional branching** instruction. This is because it always transfers control to another part of the program. The JINEG and JIZERO instructions are called **conditional branching** instructions. This is because they only transfer control under certain conditions.

There are two main uses for these instructions:

1 To enable a computer to make decisions. Different parts of a program are done under different conditions.

2 To enable parts of a program to be repeated. The repeated parts are called program **loops.** This enables short programs to process large quantities of data.

Some examples of looping and branching

A large number of useful programs can be written with loops or branches, or both. Only a few very simple examples are introduced here. Once again the intention is to show the steps involved in processing programs.

Example 6 Input two numbers. Output the larger of the two numbers.

The second number is subtracted from the first one. If the difference is negative, then the second number is larger. Otherwise the first number is larger.

Example 7 Input a set of numbers, and output each number together with its square. The set may be of any length. The end of the set is marked with the number 0, (which is not a number of the set).
This program illustrates the use of an **end-of-data marker,** sometimes called **terminator** or **rogue value,** to control a loop. It is a very common way of processing variable amounts of data.

Example 8 Input a set of four numbers. Calculate their total and average, and output these quantities.

A loop is used to input the numbers and add up the total. The number of repetition of the loop is controlled by a **counter.** The counter starts at 4, and is reduced by 1 for each input number. When the counter becomes zero, the loop is finished.

The total starts at zero, and each input number is added on.

Example 6

	Program		Dry run accumulator	A	B
	IN		17		
	STORE	A	17	17	
	IN		23	17	
	STORE	B	23	17	23
	LOAD	A	17	17	23
	SUBTRACT	B	−6	17	23
	JINEG	X	−6	17	23
	LOAD	A	These instructions are not used with this data		
	OUT				
	JUMP	END			
X	LOAD	B	123	17	23
	OUT		23	17	23
END	HALT		23	17	23

Data 17 23

Note: The JINEG instruction transfers control to the instruction with label X. The output from the program is the number 23, the larger input number.

Example 7

	Program		Dry runs first acc	X	second acc	X	third acc	X
START	IN		5		7	25	0	49
	JIZERO	END	5		7	25	0	49
	OUT		**5**		**7**	25		
	STORE	X	5	5	7	7		
	MULTIPLY	X	25	5	49	7		
	OUT		**25**	5	**49**	7		
	JUMP	START	25	5	49	7		
END	HALT						0	49

Data 5 7 0

Notice that there is a dry run for each repetition of the program. The output consists of the numbers 5, 25, 7 and 49.

Example 8

	Program		Dry runs first			second			third			fourth		
	LOAD	+0	0											
	STORE	TOTAL	0	0										
	LOAD	+4	4	0										
NEXT	STORE	COUNT	4	0	4	3	7	3	2	12	2	1	23	1
	IN		7	0	4	5	7	3	11	12	2	13	23	1
	ADD	TOTAL	7	0	4	12	7	3	23	12	2	36	23	1
	STORE	TOTAL	7	7	4	12	12	3	23	23	2	36	36	1
	LOAD	COUNT	4	7	4	3	12	3	2	23	2	1	36	1
	SUBTRACT	+1	3	7	4	2	12	3	1	23	2	0	36	1
	JIZERO	END	3	7	4	2	12	3	1	23	2	0	36	1
	JUMP	NEXT	3	7	4	2	12	3	1	23	2			
END	LOAD	TOTAL										36	36	1
	OUT											**36**	36	1
	DIVIDE	+4										9	36	1
	OUT											**9**	36	1
	HALT											9	36	1

Data 7 5 11 13

acc TOTAL COUNT acc TOTAL COUNT

acc TOTAL COUNT acc TOTAL COUNT

Note: The total and the counter change their values several times during the running of the program. The output consists of the numbers 36 and 9, and total and average respectively of the input numbers.

Exercise 13b

1 Write down the meanings of the following words or phrases:
constant; end-of-data marker; counter.

2 Study the following CESIL program, and then answer the questions about it:

```
        IN
        STORE       N
        SUBTRACT    +100
        JINEG       END
        LOAD        N
        OUT
END     HALT
```

(a) What does the program do?
(b) Dry run the program using the data number 150.
(c) Dry run the program using the data number 99.

Choosing your own data numbers, write CESIL programs for questions **3** to **8.** Dry run the programs, and run them on a computer if possible.

3 Input two numbers and output the smaller one.

4 Input a set of positive numbers, with the end marker by −1. Output each number together with its cube. (The cube of a number A is $A^3 = A \times A \times A$.)

5 Input a set of ten numbers. Calculate and output their total and average. Dry run the program for the first, second and tenth numbers only.

6 Input a set of numbers, with the end marked by zero. Output only those numbers greater than 100.

***7** Using the constants 1 and 10 only, output the squares of all the whole numbers from 1 to 10. Dry run the program for the first, second ninth and tenth numbers only.

***8** Input the length and breadth of six rectangles. Calculate and output the area of each (area = length × breadth).

14

High level language

Section A

Although assembly languages are a considerable improvement over machine languages, they have two major disadvantages:

1 Even simple assembly language programs are quite long. Consequently, it is difficult to locate and correct errors.

2 Writing assembly language programs requires considerable knowledge of the workings of computers.

Both these disadvantages arise from the fact that there is one assembly language instruction for every machine language instruction.

To overcome these disadvantages, **high level languages** have been developed. High level languages do not follow the pattern of machine code instructions. Detailed knowledge of the workings of computers is not required when writing high level language programs.

This chapter describes some of the features of high level languages, and compares them to low level languages. However, this chapter does not attempt to teach programming in any high level language.

Features of high level languages

A program in a high level language consists of a number of **statements.** A statement may contain several instructions, and is usually equivalent to more than one machine language instruction.

Most high level languages use English words and base ten numbers. Calculation statements usually resemble ordinary algebra.

Each type of computer has its own machine code and assembly language. Most high level languages, however, can be used on many different types of computers.

Assembly languages have to follow the machine code of the particular computer, but high level languages are **problem oriented.** Different high level languages are used for different computer applications.

Compilation and interpretation

Computers cannot process high level language statements directly. The machine code instructions corresponding to the high level language statements must first be produced. There are two ways of doing this – **compilation** and **interpretation.**

Compilation

Compilation is carried out by a program called a **compiler.** A compiler inputs a **source program,** in a high level language, and produces an **object program,** in machine language. Most statements in the source program become several machine code instructions in the object program.

The flow diagram in Figure 14.1 shows the stages of compiling and running a high level language program.

Interpretation

Interpretation is carried out by a program called an **interpreter.** An interpreter inputs a source program one statement at a time. It produces the machine code instructions equivalent to each statement, and supervises the running of these machine code instructions, before it accepts the next source program statement.

Figure 14.2 shows the stages of interpreting and running a high level language program.

Translating a program from high level language to machine language is a slow process. If a program has to be run frequently, it is common for a machine language copy of the program to be kept on backing store.

Some high level languages

Quite a number of high level languages are now in existence. Attempts have been made to agree on a small number of standard ones, but these have not been successful.

The first high level languages to be developed were FORTRAN, ALGOL and COBOL. FORTRAN (the letters standing for **for**mula **tran**slation) is for scientific, engineering and math-

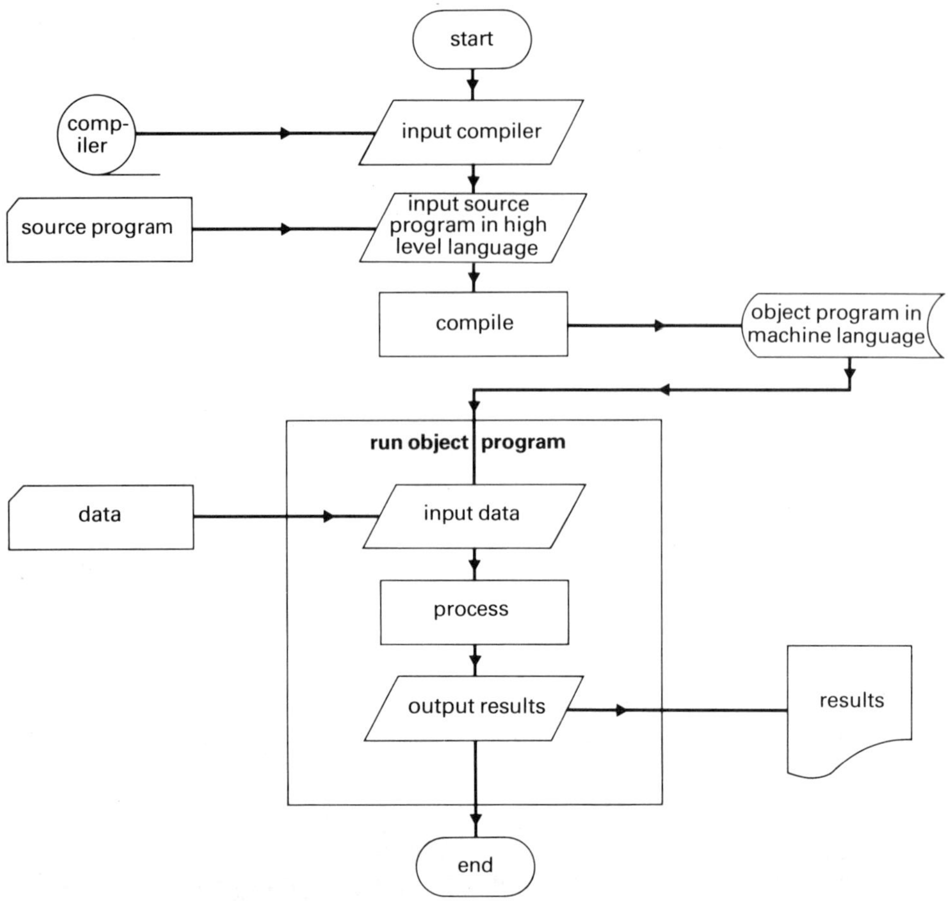

Fig. 14.1: Compiling and running a high level language program

ematical problems, as is ALGOL 60 (**algo**rithmic **l**anguage – an algorithm is a set of instructions for carrying out a task or solving a problem). COBOL (**co**mmon **b**usiness **o**riented **l**anguage) is for commercial work.

Although these are still the most widely used high level languages, several others have been developed. BASIC is a student's language, designed to be as simple as possible. BASIC is also used in some commercial and industrial applications of computers, and is the language of most microcomputers. RPG is for commercial work, PL1 is a sophisticated general purpose language, and APL is a scientific language.

Program structure

Most commercial and scientific programs are of considerable length, often several thousand statements. They are written in a number of parts, called **modules.** Each module performs a specific task.

Some modules must be used several times during the running of a program. They are written as subprograms, as described in Chapter 12.

Utility routines

Some programming tasks are very common, such as sorting a set of data in order. Subprograms to carry out these tasks are permanently stored on many computers, in their **program library.** These subprograms are called **utility routines,** or **library subprograms.** They can be used by any program run on the computer.

Applications packages

An **applications package** is a complete program, or set of programs, to carry out a task such as stock control or wage calculations. Some firms employ their own programmers to write applications packages, others buy them, often together with their computers.

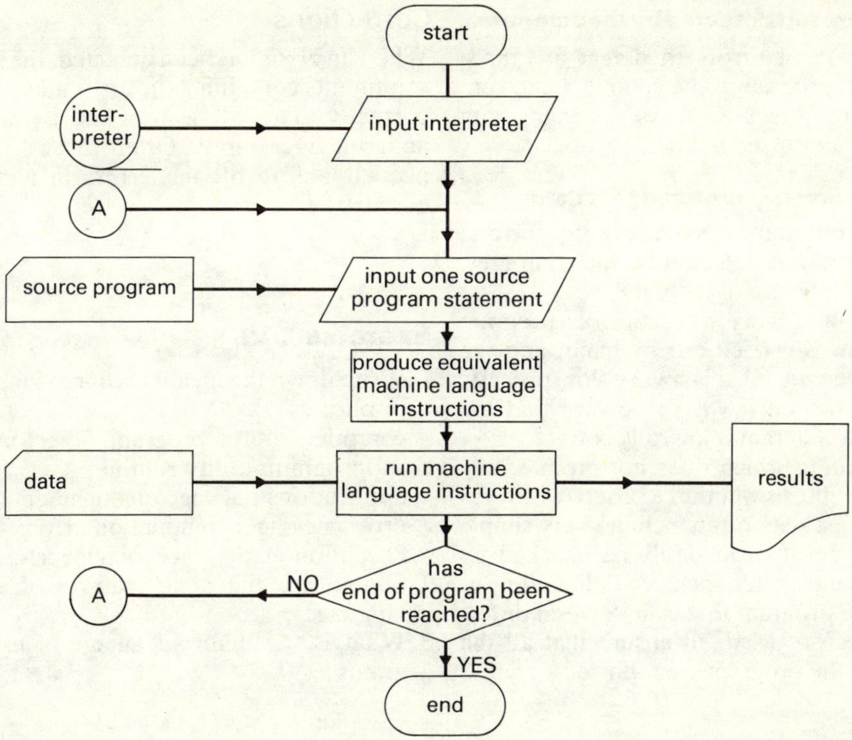

Fig. 14.2: Interpreting and running a high level language program

Errors

This section describes some of the types of errors which can occur in programs, and how they are detected and corrected.

A computer program will not produce correct results unless it is completely free of errors. Some errors are detected by the computer running the program, others are not. Correcting the errors in a program is called **debugging.**

Some errors are detected while a program is being compiled or interpreted, others while it is being run, while others are not detected by the computer, but cause wrong results.

Errors detected by the compiler or interpreter

Every high level language has rules for the construction of statements. Any statement which does not follow these rules, cannot be translated into machine language by the compiler or interpreter.

For example, statements in some high level languages must start with a statement number. If this is missing, then an error occurs.

This kind of error is called a **compilation error.** Programs with compilation errors cannot be run.

Errors occurring during the running of a program

A computer will halt the running of a program if it cannot carry out one of the instructions.

This type of error occurs, for example, if the computer is instructed to divide a number by zero, or if it runs out of input data, or if numbers are produced which are too large or too small to store (called overflow and underflow respectively).

Errors of this type are called **execution errors** or **run-time errors.** Running of a program stops if an execution error occurs.

Diagnostics

Most computers make an attempt to trace the source of a compilation or run-time error. If an error has occurred, a **diagnostic error message** is printed. This usually identifies the statement which contains the error, and indicates the type of error.

Some high level languages have the facility of **tracing** programs, or parts of programs. If a program is being traced, the contents of certain storage locations are output at various times during the execution of the program. This sometimes makes it easier to identify errors.

Errors which are not detected by the computer

The hardest type of errors to detect are those which allow the program to be compiled and run, but produce wrong results. Ways of dealing with these errors are discussed below.

Preventing errors: dry runs and test data

The two most common ways of preventing errors, or locating errors not detected by the computer, are **dry runs** and the use of **test data.**

A dry run is when every instruction of a program or flow diagram is carried out by hand, and the results written down. This is a very slow process, but it is often the only way to be sure that the program or flow diagram is logically correct.

Test data is data which does not produce any useful results, but tests whether a program is working properly. Test data often includes very simple figures so that results can easily be checked by hand. Wrong data is often included deliberately to be sure that the program rejects it. Several different sets of data are used, to ensure that all the logical paths in the program are followed.

Corrections

When an error has been detected, the statement or statements containing the error must be re-written correctly. The whole program is then compiled and run once more. Often several attempts are needed before all the errors in a program are eliminated.

Exercise 14a

1 Write down the meanings of the following words or phrases:
compiler; source program; object program; subprogram; utility routine; applications package; debugging; error message; compilation error; execution error; trace; diagnostics.
2 Summarize the main features of a high level language.
3 What is the main advantage of using subprograms?

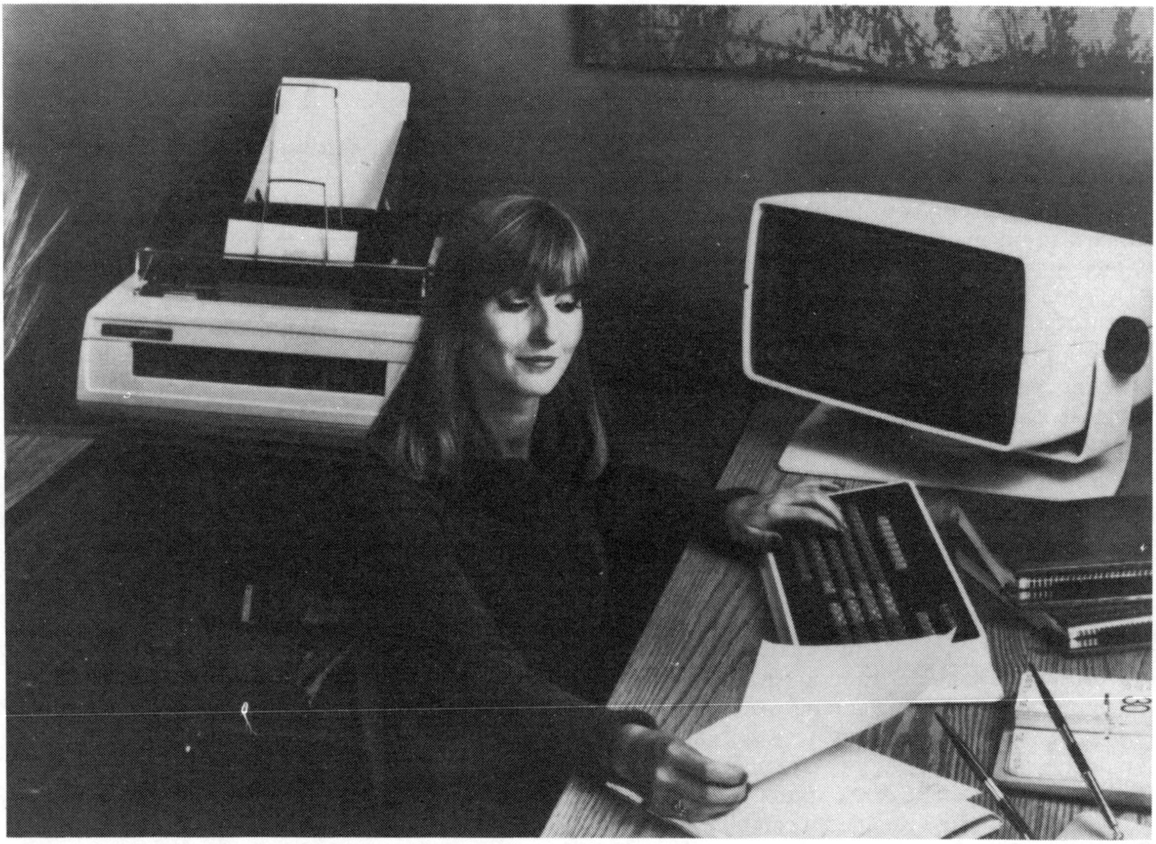

A Data General word processing system

4 A program which has run correctly using test data later produces wrong results. Suggest a possible reason for this.
5 What are the main differences between high level and low level languages?
6 (a) What is the input to a compiler program?
(b) What is the output from a compiler program?
(AEB 78 specimen)

Section B: Comparing high level languages with assembly languages

This section gives some idea how programs in a high level language are compiled or interpreted and run. The same programs are written in the high level language BASIC and in the low level language CESIL. The low level language version of the program is dry run.

This illustrates the function of a compiler or interpreter, with the BASIC program as the source program, and the CESIL program corresponding to the machine language object program.

BASIC language

A BASIC language program consists of a set of statements. Each statement starts with a statement number. Then there is a word for the operation, such as READ, PRINT, LET, etc. Finally there is a list of letters for memory locations, or a formula for a calculation.

Below is a complete program in BASIC language, with an explanation of each statement. The program inputs three numbers and stores them in memory cells A, B and C. The value of A × B ÷ C is calculated, and stored in memory cell D. Finally the contents of cells A, B, C and D are output.

Statement	Explanation
5 READ A, B, C	input numbers into memory cells A, B and C
10 LET D = A * B/C	calculate A × B ÷ C, store result in D
15 PRINT A, B, C, D	output contents of memory cells A, B, C and D
20 STOP	stop processing
25 DATA 3, 7, 15	supplies numbers for the READ statement
30 END	end of program

Notice that the symbols for calculations are not quite the same as those in ordinary algebra. The complete set of symbols is as follows:

Algebra		BASIC
+	stays	+
−	stays	−
×	becomes	*
÷	becomes	/

BASIC and CESIL

Here are some examples of the same program written in BASIC and in CESIL. Notice how most BASIC statements are replaced by several CESIL instructions.

Example 1 Input two numbers and output their difference. See program below.

Memory cells A and B are used for the numbers. Memory cell D stores the difference.

Example 1

BASIC	CESIL			Dry run acc	A	B	D
5 READ A, B		IN		15			
		STORE	A	15	15		
		IN		7	15	7	
		STORE	B	7	15	7	
10 LET D = A–B		LOAD	A	15	15	7	
		SUBTRACT	B	8	15	7	
		STORE	D	8	15	7	8
15 PRINT D		LOAD	D	8	15	7	8
		OUT		8	15	7	8
20 STOP		HALT		8	15	7	8
	%						
23 DATA 15, 7		15 7	*				
30 END							

Example 2

BASIC	CESIL			Dry run acc	P	Q	R	S	T
5 READ P, Q, R, S		IN		4					
		STORE	P	4	4				
		IN		6	4				
		STORE	Q	6	4	6			
		IN		3	4	6			
		STORE	R	3	4	6	3		
		IN		5	4	6	3		
		STORE	S	5	4	6	3	5	
10 LET T = P * Q + R * S		LOAD	P	4	4	6	3	5	
		MULTIPLY	Q	24	4	6	3	5	
		STORE	T	24	4	6	3	5	24
		LOAD	R	3	4	6	3	5	24
		MULTIPLY	S	15	4	6	3	5	24
		ADD	T	39	4	6	3	5	24
		STORE	T	39	4	6	3	5	39
15 PRINT T		LOAD	T	39	4	6	3	5	39
		OUT		39	4	6	3	5	39
20 STOP		HALT		39	4	6	3	5	39
	%								
25 DATA 4, 6, 3, 5		4 6 3 5 *							
30 END									

Example 2 Input numbers into stores P, Q, R and S. Calculate T where T = P × Q + R × S. Output T. See program above.

You will notice, in examples 1 and 2, that the CESIL instructions have been written to match the BASIC statements exactly. However, looking at the CESIL programs on their own, you will realize that some instructions are unnecessary. For instance, the instructions STORE T and LOAD T in Example 2 are not needed.

Many compilers take steps to avoid producing unnecessary object code instructions. The object code they produce is as condensed as possible. Interpreters do not have this facility.

Exercise 14b

In questions **1** to **4**, write CESIL programs to do the same calculations as these BASIC programs. Dry run the CESIL programs.

1 Input two numbers. Divide one into the other and output the quotient.
5 READ A, B 10 LET C = A/B
15 PRINT C 20 STOP 25 DATA 45, 9
30 END

2 Input the length, breadth and height of a box. Calculate and output its volume.
5 READ L, B, H 10 LET V = L * B * H
15 PRINT V 20 STOP 25 DATA 8, 3, 5
30 END

3 Input the radius of a circle. Calculate and output its area.

Formula: $a = \pi r^2$, *a:* area, *r:* radius.
Use $\frac{22}{7}$ for π.

5 READ R 10 LET A = 22/7 * R * R
15 PRINT A 20 STOP 25 DATA 14 30 END

***4** Two BASIC statements which transfer control to another part of the program have the instruction words IF . . . THEN and GO TO. Here are examples of how they are used:
25 IF B = 0 THEN 40
Go to statement 40 if B = 0
30 GO TO 50
Go to statement 50

The following program inputs a set of lengths in feet. It multiplies each length by 12 to convert it to inches. The feet and inches are output. The end of the set of lengths is marked by a zero.
5 READ F 10 IF F = 0 THEN 30
15 LET I = 12 * F 20 PRINT F, I
25 GO TO 5 30 STOP 35 DATA 4, 9, 0
40 END

5 Write BASIC programs for some of the CESIL programs from the previous chapter.

6 Illustrate the difference between LOW-LEVEL and HIGH-LEVEL languages, using suitable examples for
(a) input instructions, (b) decisions,
(c) arithmetic.
Name the languages you have used. (WJEC (CSE)78)

7 Translate each of the BASIC statements in Figure 14.3 into the corresponding CESIL instructions.

If you need a label, make it up by using LIN followed by the BASIC line number. (Line 30 has been translated as an example.)

If these instructions form a CESIL program some of these instructions may be unnecessary. In the final column write 'unnecessary' on the lines where this occurs. (MREB 78)

BASIC	CESIL Col 1	Col 2	Col 3	
10 LET P=1				
20 LET C=1				
30 READ A	LIN 30	IN		
		STORE	A	
40 IF A<0 THEN 60				
50 LET P=P+1				
60 LET C=C+1				
70 IF C≤6 THEN 30				
80 LET N=C−P				
90 PRINT N,P				
100 END		HALT		

Fig. 14.3

15

Operating systems

As you will probably have realized by now, a computer is a complex assembly of different components. The components include logic elements, registers, memory cells, input and output devices, and magnetic backing store devices. They have different functions, and all work at very different speeds.

For a computer as a whole to work efficiently, the operation of all the components must be carefully co-ordinated. Fast devices like the CPU must not stand idle for long periods of time waiting for slow devices like card readers.

The **operating system,** sometimes called the **executive** or **supervisor program,** has the task of co-ordinating all the components of a computer, and providing communication between the computer and the person operating it. Its purpose is to allow the computer to be used in the most efficient manner possible.

An operating system is a program, or a set of programs, written in a low level language. It is permanently stored, either on the computer memory, or on backing store. It takes over control of the computer at the following times:

- ☐ between programs
- ☐ between the compiling and running of a program
- ☐ sometimes when data is input or output
- ☐ sometimes when data is transferred to or from backing store
- ☐ when an error has occurred
- ☐ in response to an instruction from the person operating the computer.

The operating system allocates memory space to programs, and shares CPU time among them. It also schedules the use of backing store, and input/output devices.

Types of operating systems

There are several types of operating system, depending on the size of the computer, and the type of work it does. Some operating systems are very simple, others are extremely complex. The operating systems described in this chapter are **single program operation, batch processing, multiprogramming, remote job entry** and **multi-access.**

Single program operation

Many small computers and most microcomputers can only process one program at a time. The operating system supervises the input, compilation, running and output of each program, and reports any errors.

Batch processing

The operating systems of most medium and large computers enable them to do **batch processing.** A number of programs are batched together, and then run as a group. Although the programs, are actually processed one at a time, the input stage of one program can sometimes overlap with the output stage from the previous program. Similarly, input and output from the same program can sometimes be done at the same time. (Note that the phrase 'batch processing' also applies to batches of data. This is explained in Chapter 17.)

Multiprogramming

Most fairly large computers have **multiprogramming,** or **multitasking,** operating systems. To avoid wasting CPU time waiting for slow input or output devices, a multiprogramming operating system can switch the CPU from one program to another during processing.

At any time there are several programs in the computer memory. Parts of each program are processed in turn, according to their input and output requirements. Programs can have a priority rating to determine which is done first. In addition, the computer operator can intervene to change the order of processing.

Remote job entry

Some computers have card readers, line printers or other peripheral devices connected from distant sites. Programs and data are input and output at these sites, and processed by the computer. A batch processing or multiprogramming operating system is most commonly used.

Multi-access

Computers with terminals generally work in such a

way that each person using a terminal appears to have the whole computer at his or her disposal. A multi-access operating system enables this to be done.

The terminals are connected to the computer via a device called a **multiplexer** (Figure 15.1). The multiplexer enables the operating system to allocate short intervals of CPU time to each terminal in turn. During these time intervals, data is passed to or from the CPU, and any processing required by the terminal is carried out. Because the CPU works so much faster than a terminal, each terminal appears to be working continuously, when in fact it is not. The operating system also controls the memory and backing store allocated to each terminal. Magnetic disc backing store is almost always used.

Combining operating systems

Many large computers combine a multiprogramming and a multi-access operating system. The resulting operating system is extremely complex. It has the task of co-ordinating all the different hardware and software resources of the computer in the most efficient manner possible.

Some examples of operating systems

Most operating systems have unusual, often amusing names. Here are some examples:

MAXIMOP: Used on ICL 1900 series computers, it is a multi-access operating system.

GEORGE 3: Also used on ICL 1900 computers, it is both multiprogramming and multi-access.

DOS VS: The letters stand for Disc Operating System, Virtual Storage. It is a multiprogramming operating system, used by IBM 360 and 370 computers. It enables the disc backing store of the computer to be used as if it is the actual computer memory. The computer appears to have a much larger memory capacity than it actually has.

Very large computers

In very large computers, processing is often done at more than one place simultaneously. Ways of doing this include **parallel central processors, distributed processing** and **distributed array processing.**

Parallel central processors

Two or more large CPU's work side by side (in parallel, or in tandem), sharing all the peripherals between them. There is often a smaller, separate CPU called a **front-end processor,** which controls the flow of data to the other CPU's.

The operating system of this sort of computer usually allows both multiprogramming and multi-access. Each program is allocated memory space and processing time in one of the CPU's, and access to various peripherals as required.

Distributed processing

The terminals used by some computers are capable of doing a certain amount of processing on their own. These are called **intelligent terminals.** On

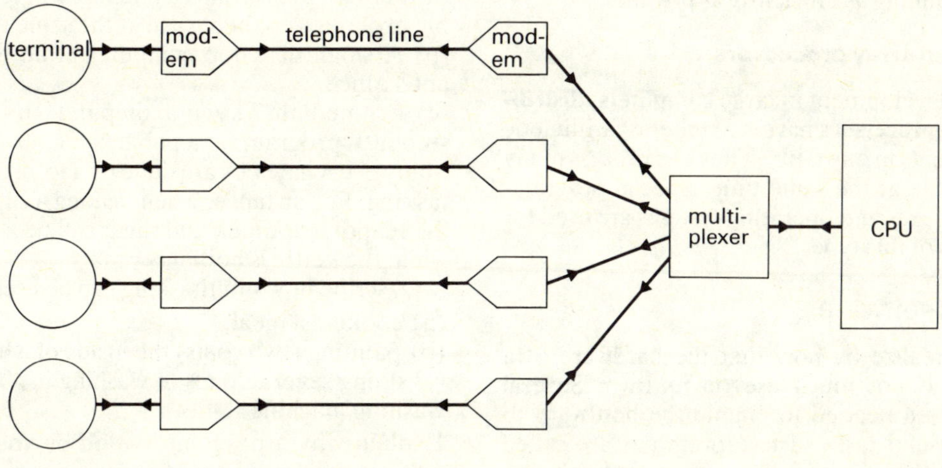

Fig. 15.1: A multiplexer

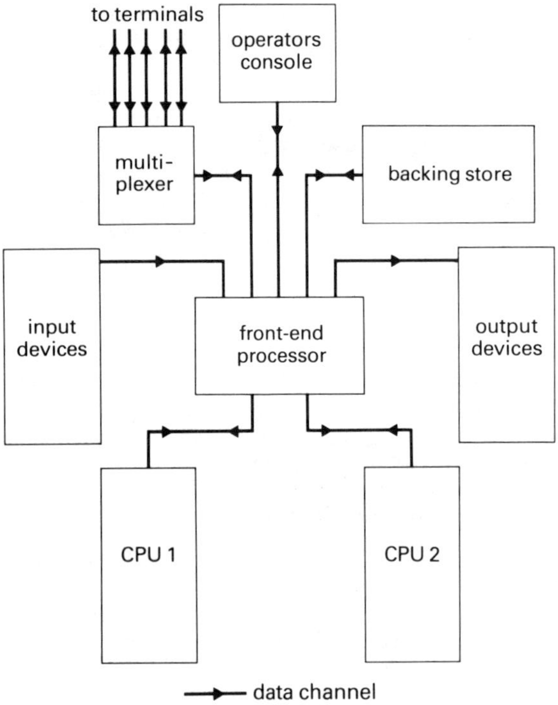

Fig. 15.2: A large computer, with parallel central processors

these computers, the processing is shared between the CPU and the terminals.

A few very large computer systems have more than one CPU at different sites. These central processers are linked by telephone lines or radio channels. Processing is shared by all the CPU's in the network.

The task of the operating system is to share the work between the different CPU's and intelligent terminals, in order to keep the whole computer network running as efficiently as possible.

Distributed array processors

A recent development in large computers, **distributed array processors** have a number of arithmetic and logic units in one CPU. They can process many items of data at the same time. Special programming languages and operating systems are used for computers of this type.

Systems software

You will realize by now that the hardware of a computer is not much use on its own. Several programs are needed to enable the hardware to perform useful tasks. These programs are called **systems software,** and include operating systems, assemblers and compilers.

The work of the computer takes the form of **user programs,** written in an assembly language or a high level language. See Figure 15.3.

The capability of a computer is determined not only by its hardware, but also by its systems software.

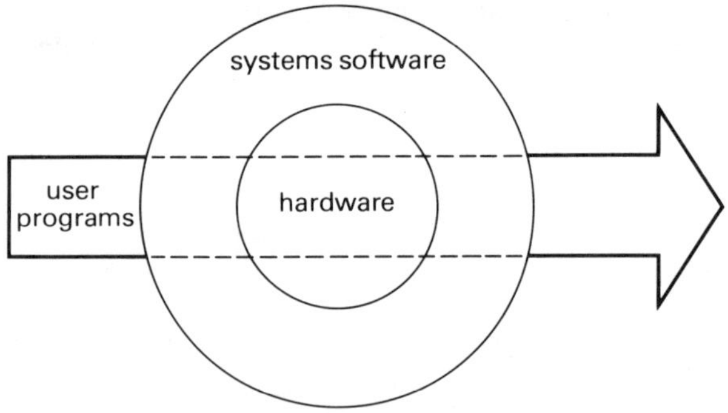

Fig. 15.3: The relationship between user programs, systems software and hardware.

Exercise 15

1 Write down the meanings of the following words or phrases:
batch processing; multitasking; multi-access; multiplexer; systems software; user programs; front end processor; distributed processing.

2 Find out what type of operating system is used by the computer on which your programs are run.

3 MAXIMOP, GEORGE 3 and DOS VS are the names of three operating systems mentioned in the text. Find out the names of other operating systems, and what types they are.

4 What type of operating system would be most likely to be used on the following computers:
(a) At a large insurance company where several big programs are being run at the same time.
(b) A small desk-top computer at an accountant's office.
(c) A medium sized computer processing students' programs at a polytechnic.

5 Many everyday jobs are done by a form of multitasking. For instance, when making a cup of tea, the teapot, cup, milk and sugar can be got ready while the kettle is boiling.
Describe how multitasking can be used in
(a) cooking a meal,
(b) painting (two coats) the inside of a house,
(c) doing several loads of washing in a twin-tub washing machine.

6 Explain why a program written by you *cannot* occupy the entire main store of a computer. (AEB 78 specimen)

16

The people who work with computers

The widespread use of computers has created many jobs. Some of the jobs are highly skilled, most of them are well paid. There are two main areas of work: the manufacture of computers, and the application of computers. This chapter describes the work done by people in jobs related to computers.

Computer manufacture

Most large computers are made by large companies. The various stages of computer design and manufacture are usually carried out by teams. These stages are shown in Figure 16.1.

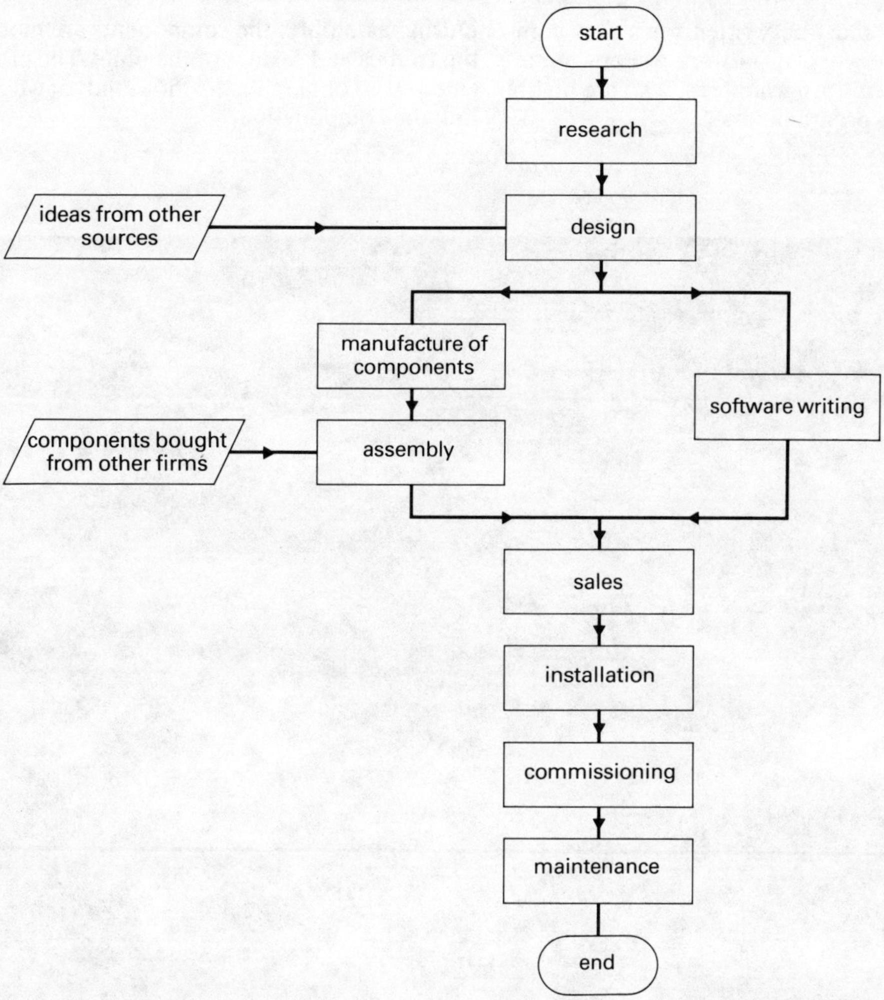

Fig. 16.1: The work of a computer manufacturing company

Research

Computer manufacturers spend large sums of money on research. People working in this field include **research engineers** and technicians. They invent and test new devices to make computers faster, smaller, more efficient and cheaper. Other researchers investigate new possible uses of computers.

Design

Computers are designed by **computer architects.** They take many factors into consideration in designing a computer. Ideas and devices come from the research teams, and from outside sources, particularly universities. The market of a new computer is carefully studied. This determines the size and cost of the machine.

Systems software – operating systems, assemblers and compilers – must be written for a new computer. This is the work of **software writers,** sometimes called **systems programmers,** who are highly skilled computer programmers.

Construction

There are two main stages in the construction of computers: making the components and assembling the units.

Making the components

A computer manufacturer usually makes some of the components, and buys others from outside firms. All solid state components must be made extremely carefully. Working conditions are often similar to those in an operating theatre. The air is free of dust, and the temperature precisely controlled. Microscopes and test circuits are used to examine finished components, which are rejected if there are any defects.

Assembling the units

During assembly, the components are mounted in the frames and casings of the units. The most intricate job is connecting the thousands of wires which link the components.

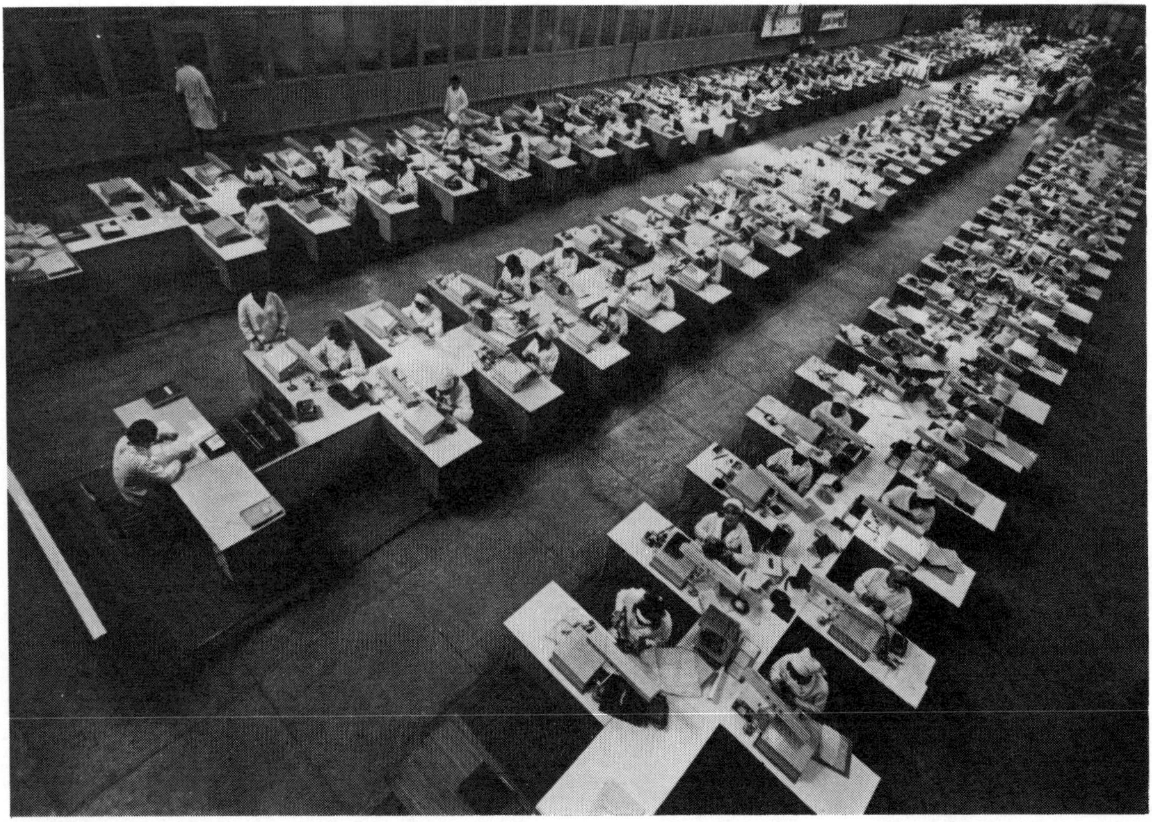

Manufacture of computer components in the USSR

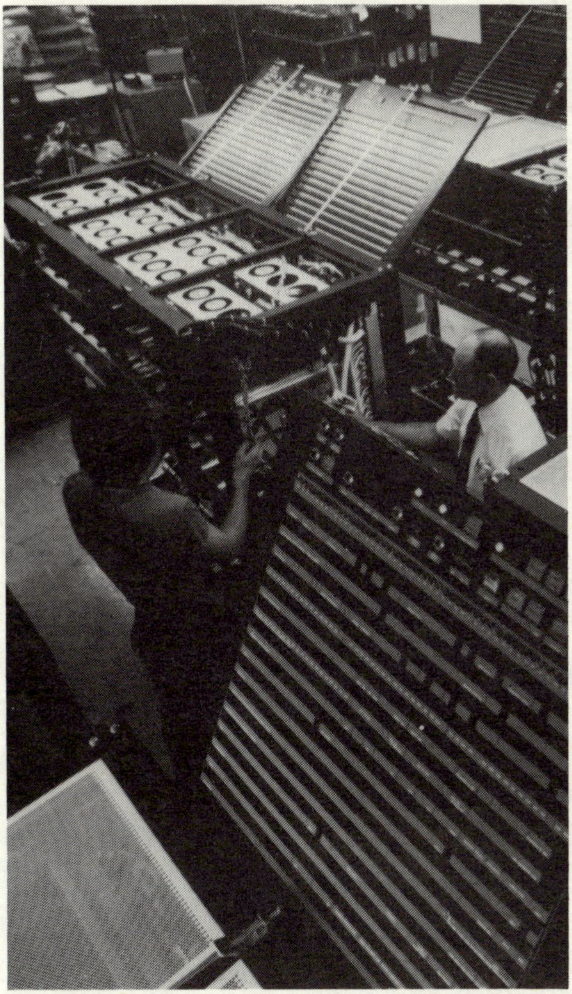

The central processing units of large Burroughs computers being assembled

Sales

Computer salesmen have the job of matching a computer system (both hardware and software) to the needs of each customer. Salesmen arrange demonstrations of computers, and provide printed material describing the computers and their advantages. Selling a large computer is a long and complex process.

Computers are either bought or loaned by customers. A sale or a loan usually contains an arrangement for the maintenance of the computer.

Installation

Installation is supervised by **installation engineers.** A suitable room, with air conditioning and security arrangements, is prepared. The units of the computer are transported to the site, and connected together.

The computer is then started and tested. This is done by **commissioning engineers.** First the hardware is tested, and then the systems software (operating system, compilers and assemblers) is loaded. Special programs are used to test the systems software. If the whole computer system is satisfactory, then the computer is handed over to the customer. The first user programs are run.

If an existing computer is enlarged by the addition of new units, then the new units are installed and commissioned by a similar way.

Maintenance

Maintenance engineers from the computer manufacturer visit installations to inspect and repair the computers. Maintenance is done on a regular basis (as often as once a week in many cases) and whenever there is a breakdown.

Some computer manufacturers

International Business Machines (IBM) is the world's largest computer manufacturer. Based in the U.S.A., it has a number of factories and research centres in North America and Europe. IBM computers are sold and serviced in many countries.

International Computers Limited (ICL) is the largest British computer manufacturer. Partly government owned, it has several research laboratories and factories throughout the U.K.

Digital Equipment Corporation (DEC) is an American company specializing in small and medium sized computers. Its best known machines are the PDP 8 and the PDP 11.

Other prominent American manufacturers are Sperry Univac, Burroughs Corporation, National Cash Register (NCR), Texas Instruments, Honeywell, Control Data Corporation and Hewlett-Packard.

A newcomer to computer manufacturing is the Amdahl Corporation, an American firm which makes large computers, competing with IBM.

Putting computers to work

The use of computers has created even more jobs than the manufacture of computers. A computer needs a number of people to operate it, program it and supply it with data.

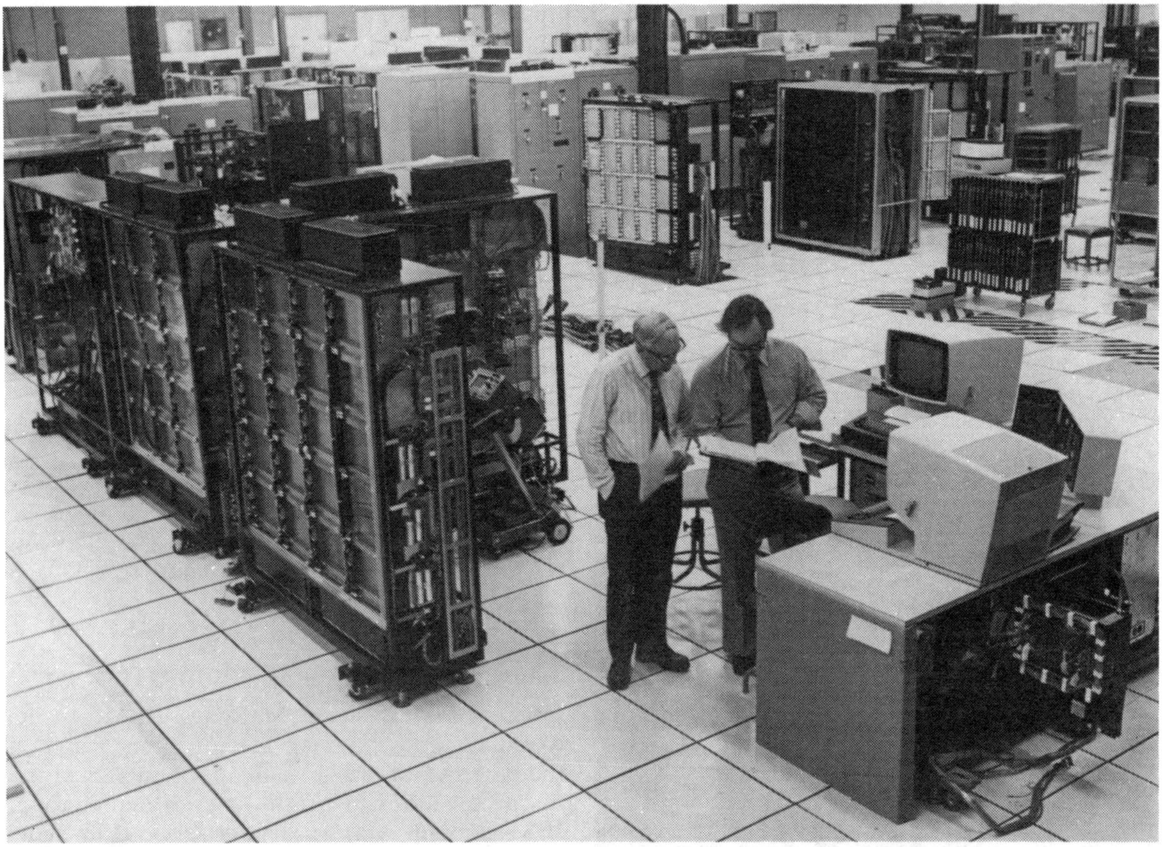

An IBM central processing unit being assembled in Havant, UK

Data processing departments

In most commercial or industrial companies which have computers, the people who work directly with the computer work together in the **data processing department.** Very often a large number of staff have access to the computer via terminals.

Most data processing departments employ people in the jobs shown in Figure 16.2.

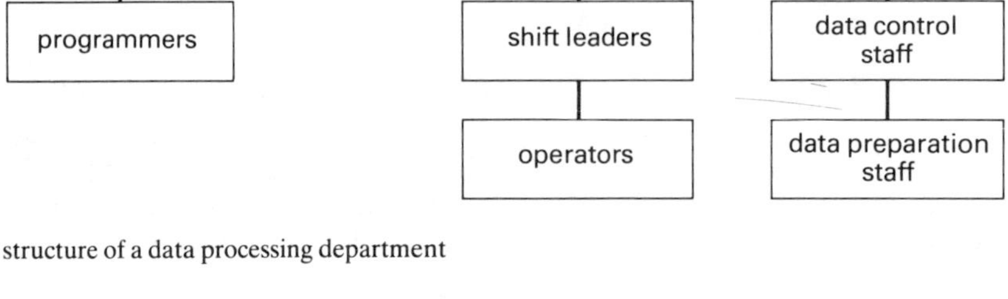

Fig. 16.2: The job structure of a data processing department

Data processing manager

The **data processing manager** is responsible for the overall running of the department. It is his (or her) responsibility to see that the data processing department co-ordinates with the rest of the company. The data processing manager has a say in the appointment of other members of the data processing department.

Systems analysts

Systems analysts are concerned with planning how work is done on the computer. They consult with the people in the firm, called the **users,** whose work is to be computerized, and study the operation in detail. Each step of the operation, both on and off the computer, is precisely described. The description often takes the form of a **systems flow diagram.** The plan may have to be modified before agreement is reached with the users. (The next chapter describes some techniques of data processing in more detail.)

Programmers

Computer **programmers** write programs according to the requirements of the system flow diagrams. Large programs are written in separate parts, or **modules.** Each module is usually written by a different programmer. The modules are tested very carefully until all the errors have been removed. The complete program is then put together, and again tested. The checking process is called **debugging.**

An important task of a programmer is **documentation.** This is writing a detailed explanation of how a program works, so that other people can understand it, and change it if necessary. Detailed instructions are also written for the people who are going to use the program. These instructions are called **user documentation.**

Once in use, programs must be altered from time to time in the light of experience or changing requirements. This is another job for a computer programmer, called **program maintenance.**

Computer programmers doing the work described here are sometimes called **applications programmers,** to distinguish them from systems programmers who write systems software.

Operations manager

The **operations manager** is in charge of allocating computer time to different programs, and arranging for the maintenance and repair of the computer when necessary. The operations manager allocates work to the computer operators and data preparation staff, and supervises the ordering of stationery and other supplies.

Computer operators

Computer operators keep the computer running. They often work in shifts if the computer works 24 hours per day. They use the keyboard on the operator's console to type instructions to the computer. They change magnetic discs and tapes, load card readers with cards, and supply line printers with paper.

The operator's console produces the **computer log.** This is a record of the names of all the programs run, with their starting and finishing times, and any errors which have occurred. The log also records instructions by the operator and messages from the computer.

Data preparation staff

Data preparation staff punch and verify cards or paper tape, which inputs both programs and data into the computer. On newer computers, they operate the key-to-disc input devices.

If there are several computer operators or data preparation staff working in shifts, there are **shift leaders** to supervise them. Data processing departments with large numbers of magnetic tapes or discs have **file librarians** to look after them. Large companies have **data control staff** whose job it is to ensure that all the data for a program reaches the computer at the right time.

Data processing departments

The flow diagram in Figure 16.3 shows all the stages of developing, writing and running a program in a large data processing department. These job descriptions vary somewhat amongst different firms. In smaller companies, the same person may do more than one job, such as systems analyst and programmer. In large firms, teams of people work on each job.

The current tendency is away from separate data processing departments. The computer and the data processing staff are integrated into the other departments of the firm.

Computer bureaus

Many firms which use computers do not have their own data processing department. All computer work is sent to a **computer bureau.** This is an independent company, doing data processing for others. The bureau usually has its own computer, and a staff structure like that of a data processing

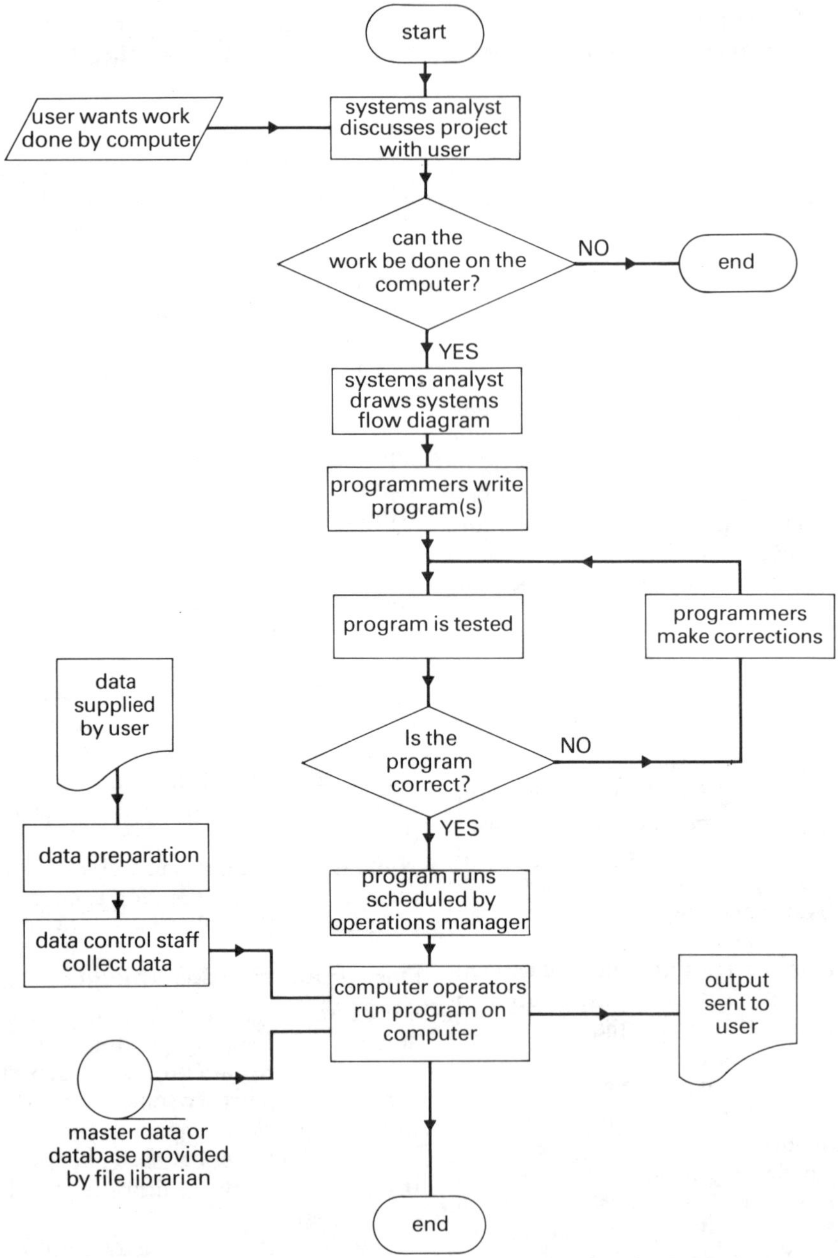

Fig. 16.3: The development, writing and running of a program in a large data processing department

department. Some bureaus provide programs for other firms to run on their own computers.

Most bureaus use up-to-date, efficient computers, and can often provide a better service to a small (or even medium sized) firm than its own data processing department. Many growing firms use bureaus to try out computerized methods for a few years before they buy their own computer and set up their own data processing department.

Exercise 16

1 Write down the meanings of the following words or phrases:
program maintenance; computer log;
data processing department;
commissioning a new computer;
documentation.

2 From the job descriptions, decide which person would do the following tasks:

(a) Connect together the units of a new computer.
(b) Persuade a data processing manager to buy a new computer.
(c) Decide what kind of memory circuits to use in a new computer.
(d) Write a detailed description of how a program works.
(e) Start up a new computer and check that it works properly.
(f) In a commercial firm, decide not to computerize part of their accounting system.
(g) Correct a program that has produced wrong results.
(h) Decide what information must be supplied for a program.
(i) Decide whether or not to buy a new magnetic tape drive.
(j) Deal with a complaint that the computer was not being used properly.
(k) Verify a set of punched cards.
(l) Invent a new kind of line printer.
(m) Supply more paper for a line printer.
(n) Decide when a program will be run.
(o) Write a compiler for a new computer.

3 A school leaver is thinking of applying for his or her first job in a computer establishment and has asked you for advice.

Write suitable notes which will explain the types of opportunities which are available and what each will demand. Bearing in mind the background and training needed, discuss the areas for which he or she should apply to make best use of particular aptitudes. You should give advice on computing as a future career, including any doubts or reservations which should be pointed out to someone whose working life will extend well into the next century. (JMB 78)

4 The job titles of some of the persons associated with a computer system, from its concept to its use by the customer, are given below:

Commissioning Engineer; Customer's Systems Analyst; Software Writer; Installation Engineer; Sales Engineer; Key-punch Operator; Manufacturer's Research Engineer; Data Processing Manager.

(a) Show clearly which job titles are associated with the customer's organization and which with the computer manufacturer. By means of a diagram, or otherwise, show the order in which the tasks performed by all these people, in their association with the computer system, are carried out.

(b) State, briefly, what is involved in *each* of *four* jobs mentioned above. (AEB 78 specimen)

5 (a) A firm already possesses a computer. Explain briefly what the following three people would do if they all worked for this firm which wanted to computerize some part of its work that had not been computerized before:
Systems Analyst; Programmer; Data Processing Manager.
(b) The firm could have chosen (i) to write their own programs, (ii) to buy an already written piece of software, (iii) to commission a specialist company to write the programs for them.
Give the advantages of each of these methods. (MREB 77)

17

Data processing

Although a large number of computers are used for scientific and engineering purposes, and at universities, the majority of computers are used in commerce and industry. Here they assist in paying wages, keeping accounts, keeping records of stock levels, storing information for rapid access, and many other activities. All these activities involve **data processing.** The purpose of this chapter is to describe how some of these data processing operations are done.

As mentioned previously, data processing does not necessarily involve computers. If a computer is used, the process is more correctly called *electronic data processing*. However, in this chapter the phrase 'data processing' is used whether or not computers are involved.

Data processing systems

Data processing generally involves setting up a **system** to carry out all the stages of the work, on a regular basis. A data processing system includes all the people involved in various stages of the work, and (if one is used) a computer. Some of the people work directly with the computer, others do not. The various jobs involved are described in the previous chapter.

Figure 17.1 shows the composition of an electronic data processing system. As mentioned previously, the planning of a data processing system is the responsibility of a systems analyst.

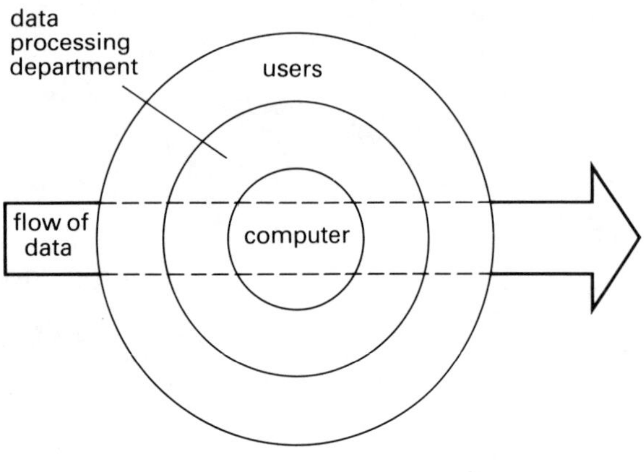

Fig. 17.1: An electronic data processing system

Files

Most data processing systems handle very large quantities of data. This data is usually collected together in **files.** Several examples of files are given in this chapter, and a more detailed discussion of them follows in the next chapter.

The data processing questions

In planning how a data processing operation is to be done, either with or without the aid of a computer, it is useful to start by asking some questions. The questions used in this chapter include those used in Chapter 1. They are:

1 What is the purpose of the system?
2 What input data is required?
3 How is the data captured and stored?

Note: The word 'capture' is commonly used for the process of obtaining information.

The remaining questions are:

4 What processing is done?
5 What is the output?
6 What computer hardware is used?
7 How well does the system work?

For systems which have not been tried out yet, question **7** becomes:

How well is the system likely to work?

Having answered the data processing questions, the steps of the operation can be described in more detail.

Systems flow diagrams

A convenient way of describing the steps of a data processing operation is to use a **systems flow diagram.** In many ways, systems flow diagrams resemble the ordinary flow diagrams introduced in Chapter 1. A systems flow diagram has a box for each step, and arrows to show how the steps fit

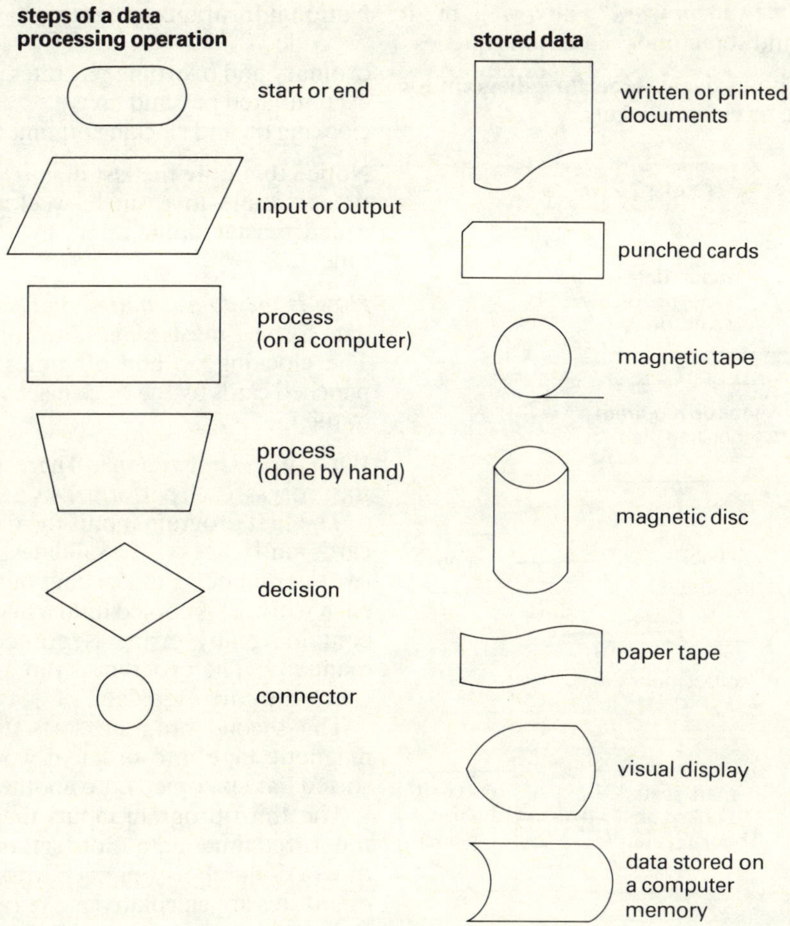

Fig. 17.2: Systems flow diagram symbols

together. There are also symbols for data stored in various ways.

The systems flow diagram symbols used in this book are shown in Figure 17.2. They are a compromise between the various sets of 'standard' symbols in current use, all of which they resemble fairly closely.

Some examples of data processing

A few examples of data processing systems are included here. They illustrate a systematic approach to data processing, by answering the data processing questions, and drawing systems flow diagrams.

The first example is of a system which does not make use of a computer.

Example 1: Booking theatre or cinema tickets.
What is the purpose of the system? To enable people to reserve seats to see a play or a film.

What input data is required? The date and time of the show, the number of seats required, and sometimes their position and/or price.

How is the data captured and stored? The input data is spoken to the person doing the booking, either directly or over the telephone. The seats which have already been booked are recorded on a booking plan. The tickets are written or printed.

What processing is done? The booking plan for the required performance is located. If seats are available, they are marked on the booking plan, the tickets are issued, and the money is collected. If no suitable seats can be found, then no booking is made.

The booking plan now contains new information. In computer language, it has been **updated.**

What is the output? The tickets

What computer hardware is used? None

How well does the system work? Fairly well, but it is rather slow, and sometimes causes long queues.

Figure 17.3 shows the systems flow diagram for booking theatre or cinema tickets.

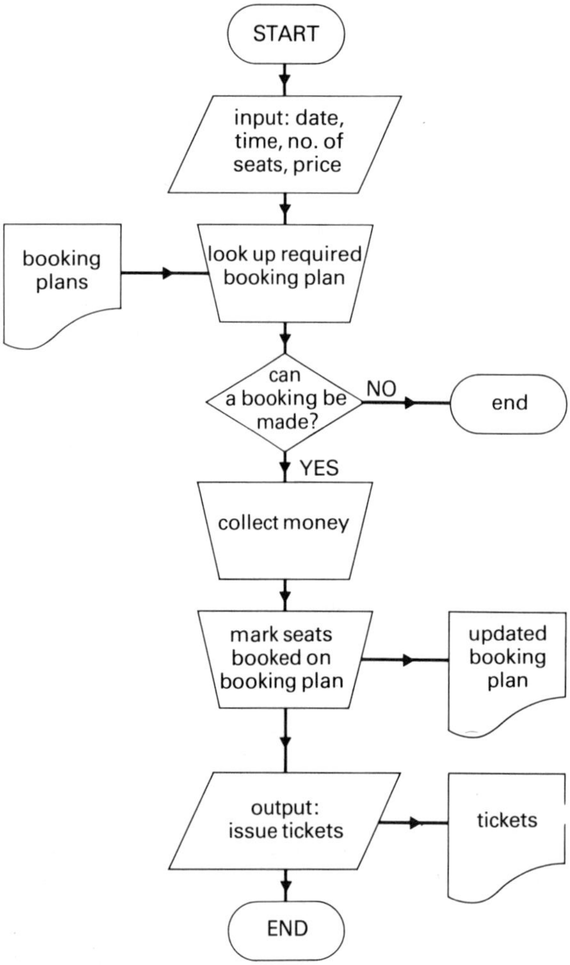

Fig. 17.3: Booking theatre or cinema tickets

Example 2 Calculating Weekly Wages. A payroll system of this sort is used in many factories and shops for their weekly wages.

What is the purpose of the system? To produce weekly wage slips for all workers who are paid at an hourly rate. These slips show the hours worked, pay rate, gross wage, income tax, National Insurance contribution, etc. and nett wage, after all the deductions have been made.

What input data is required? For each worker:
works number;
name;
National Insurance number;
tax code;
ordinary and overtime pay rates per hour;
accumulated pay and tax;
clocking on and clocking off times during the week.

Notice that only the last item (clocking on and off times) refers to a single week. The other data, called **master data,** refers to a longer period of time.

How is the data captured and stored? The master data forms a **master file,** stored on a magnetic tape. The clocking on and off times are captured on punched cards by the clock machines at the entrance to the factory.

What processing is done? There are three stages to the process, each performed by a separate program.

The first program inputs the data from the clock cards and checks, or **validates,** it. Correct data (works number and clocking on and off times for each worker) is copied onto a magnetic tape. Data containing any errors is printed, and corrected manually. The program is run again to input and check the corrected data.

The second program sorts the data from the magnetic tape into order of works number. The sorted data is copied onto another magnetic tape.

The third program inputs the master data and the sorted times data. Both sets of data are in order of works number. For each worker, the following quantities are calculated:
ordinary hours and overtime hours worked;
ordinary pay; overtime pay and gross pay;
income tax; National Insurance contributions;
graduated pension contributions and
other deductions; nett pay;
accumulated gross pay; tax and nett pay.

What is the output? Payslips are printed, showing the works number, name and above data for each worker. A new version of the master file is created, containing updated accumulated pay and tax. The payslips are printed on wage slip forms by the computer's line printer.

What computer hardware is used? A small or medium sized computer, with 8 K to 32 K of main store, including a special reader for the clock cards, at least two magnetic tape units and a line printer.

How well does the system work? Very well in most cases. The master data needs to be updated from time to time as pay rates change, and workers arrive and leave.

Figure 17.4 shows the systems flow diagram for calculating weekly wages.

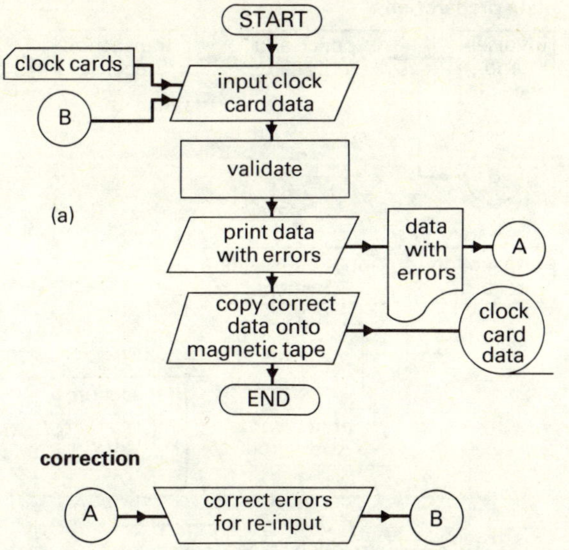

Fig. 17.4: Calculating weekly wages (a) Program 1: input/validation

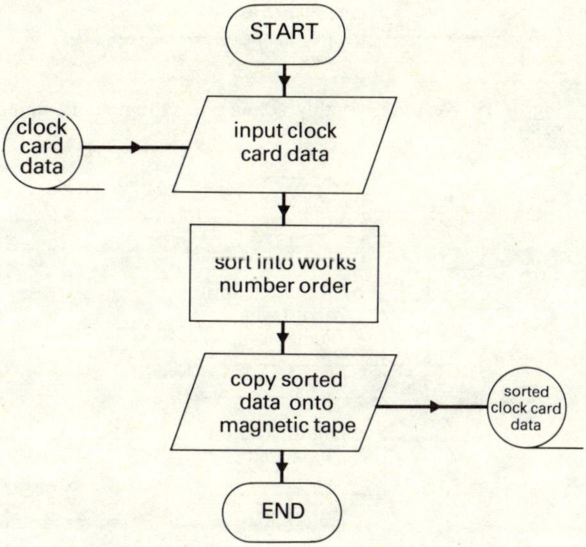

(b) Program 2: sorting

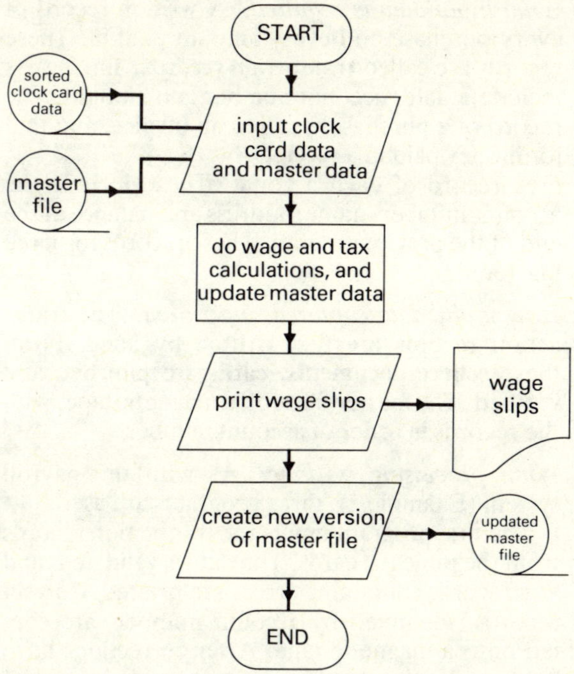

(c) Program 3: calculating wages, printing wage slips and updating master file

Example 3 Keeping monthly accounts. A system of the type described below is used by many shops and businesses with customers who have monthly accounts.

What is the purpose of the system? To keep a record of all purchases and amounts of money received.

To produce a monthly **statement** for each account, showing all the purchases and payments for that account for that month, together with the amount owing at the end of the month, called the **balance.**

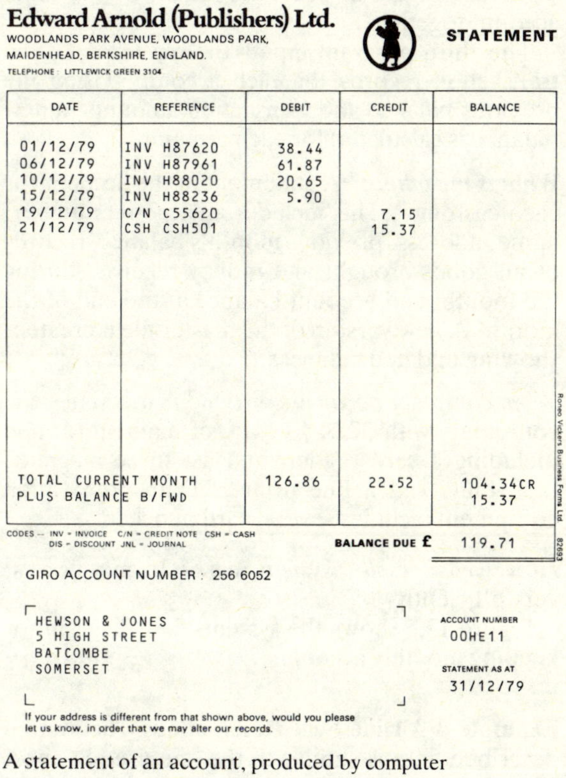

Edward Arnold (Publishers) Ltd.
WOODLANDS PARK AVENUE, WOODLANDS PARK,
MAIDENHEAD, BERKSHIRE, ENGLAND.
TELEPHONE: LITTLEWICK GREEN 3104

STATEMENT

DATE	REFERENCE	DEBIT	CREDIT	BALANCE
01/12/79	INV H87620	38.44		
06/12/79	INV H87961	61.87		
10/12/79	INV H88020	20.65		
15/12/79	INV H88236	5.90		
19/12/79	C/N C55620		7.15	
21/12/79	CSH CSH501		15.37	
TOTAL CURRENT MONTH		126.86	22.52	104.34CR
PLUS BALANCE B/FWD				15.37

CODES — INV = INVOICE C/N = CREDIT NOTE CSH = CASH
DIS = DISCOUNT JNL = JOURNAL

BALANCE DUE £ 119.71

Roneo Vickers Business Forms Ltd 82693

GIRO ACCOUNT NUMBER : 256 6052

HEWSON & JONES
5 HIGH STREET
BATCOMBE
SOMERSET

ACCOUNT NUMBER
00HE11

STATEMENT AS AT
31/12/79

If your address is different from that shown above, would you please let us know, in order that we may alter our records.

A statement of an account, produced by computer

What input data is required? A written record of every purchase and every amount paid in. These records are called **transaction records,** and always include a date, account number and amount. The record of a purchase is called an **invoice,** and that for money paid in a **receipt.**

A record of each account. These include the account number, name, address and balance at the end of the previous month. These records form the master file.

How is the data captured and stored? The transaction records are first written by hand. From these **source documents,** cards are punched and verified. The master file is on a magnetic tape, with the records in order of account number.

What processing is done? As with the payroll system (Example 2), three programs are used.

The first program inputs the transaction records from the punched cards. The data is validated, and any records containing errors are printed. Correct records, identified by account number, are copied onto a magnetic tape. After corrections have been made, the program is run again to input and validate the corrected transaction records.

The second program sorts the transaction records into order of account number. The sorted records are copied onto another magnetic tape. The sorting process puts all the transactions of the same account together.

The third program inputs the master data and transaction records for each account. Using the previous balance and transaction amounts, a new balance is calculated for each account.

What is the output? A statement of the account for each customer. This includes an account number, name, address, previous month's balance, records of all goods brought and money received during the month, and account balance at the end of the month. A new version of the master file is created, showing updated balances.

What computer hardware is used? A medium sized computer, with 32 K to 64 K of main store, and including a card reader, at least three magnetic tape units and a line printer. Data preparation equipment includes several card punches.

How well does the system work? In most cases, very efficiently.

Figure 17.5 shows the systems flow diagram for keeping monthly accounts.

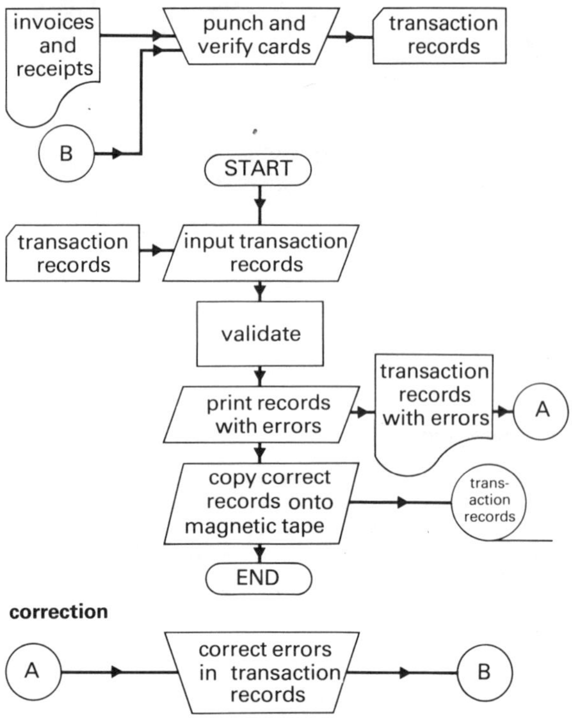

Fig. 17.5: Keeping monthly accounts (a) Program 1: input/validation

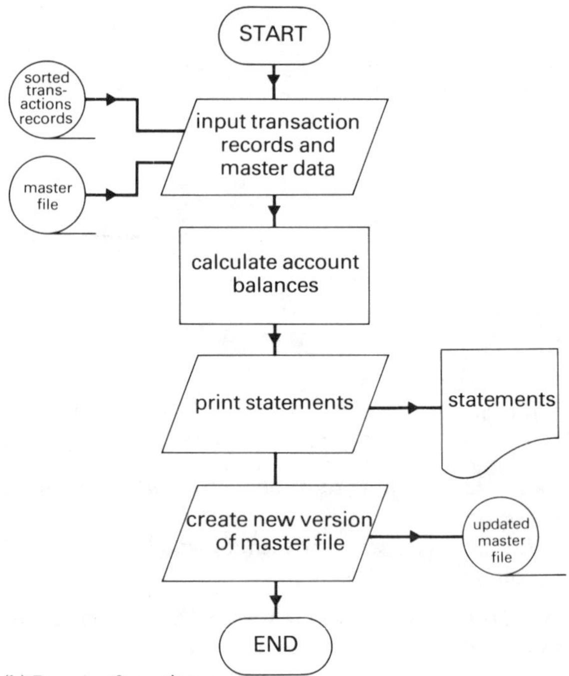

(b) Program 2: sorting

Example 4 Airline Seat Reservations The system described here is similar to the one used by most airlines to reserve seats on their flights. The computer, at an office of the airline, is accessed by a

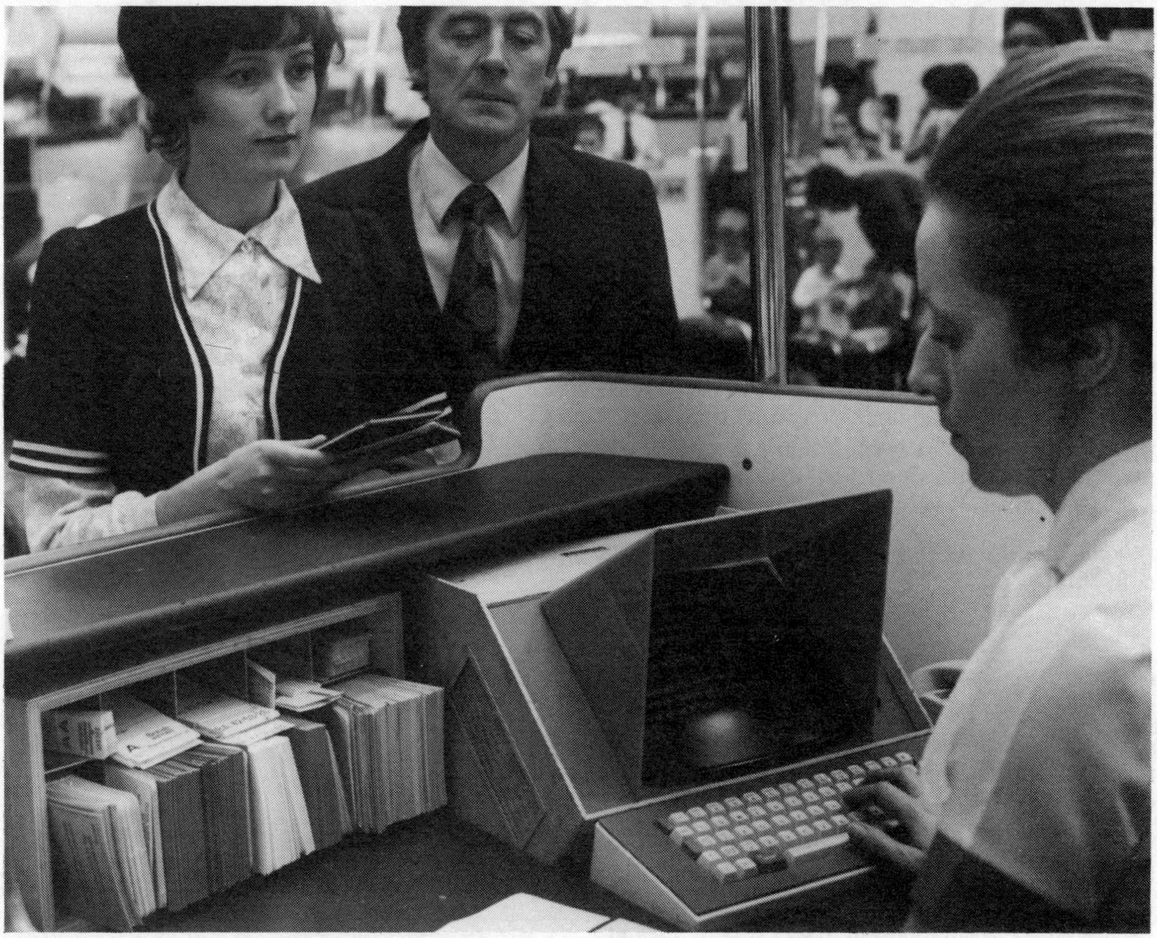

A visual display unit at an airport. Passenger reservations are being checked prior to departure

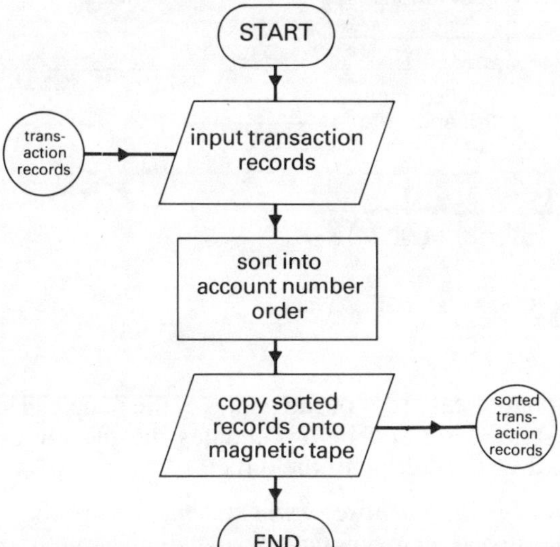

(c) Program 3: calculating account balances, printing statements and updating master file

large number of remote access visual display units. The VDU's are at travel agents and airports. Computers belonging to different airlines are connected together by an international communication network called SITA (Societé Internationále de Telecommunication Aeronautiques).

What is the purpose of the system? To enable passengers to reserve seats on any forthcoming flight from any travel agent who has a VDU connected to the computer.

What input data is required? The flight number, date, number of seats required, name(s) of passenger(s).

How is the data captured and stored? The input data is typed on a VDU keyboard and displayed.

A file containing records of all forthcoming flights is stored on magnetic discs. A flight record includes the flight number, date, airports of call, a list of the names of the passengers who have already booked seats, and the number of vacant seats. As this file is also used for other purposes, such as checking in passengers at airports, it is called a **database.**

What processing is done? There are two steps in the process of reserving a seat. These are:

1 Finding out if there are sufficient vacant seats on the required flight.

2 Making reservations if so.

The first step is called **accessing** the database, and the second is called **updating** the database.

To make a reservation, the flight record is accessed, and the number of vacant seats is displayed on the VDU screen. If a reservation can be made, the new names are added to the flight record, and the number of vacant seats is reduced.

What is the output? A message on the VDU screen confirming that the booking has been made. The tickets are then written by hand, and the money is collected.

What computer hardware is used? A fairly large (64 K to 256 K of memory), fast computer, with several magnetic disc drives and a number of VDU terminals, linked via a multiplexer. The airline seat reservation program is available at all times.

How well does the system work? The computer-based system replaced a manual one where each travel agent was allocated a fixed quota of seats on each flight. The manual system was very inefficient, as some travel agents had to turn away passengers because their quota of seats were all booked, while others did not fill their quotas.

The computerized booking system is a considerable improvement. However, in recent years, many airlines have begun to offer various fare reduction schemes, including standby systems. These schemes made the reservation process more complicated. There has been confusion and delay at airports during busy times.

Figure 17.6 shows a systems flow diagram for making airline seat reservations.

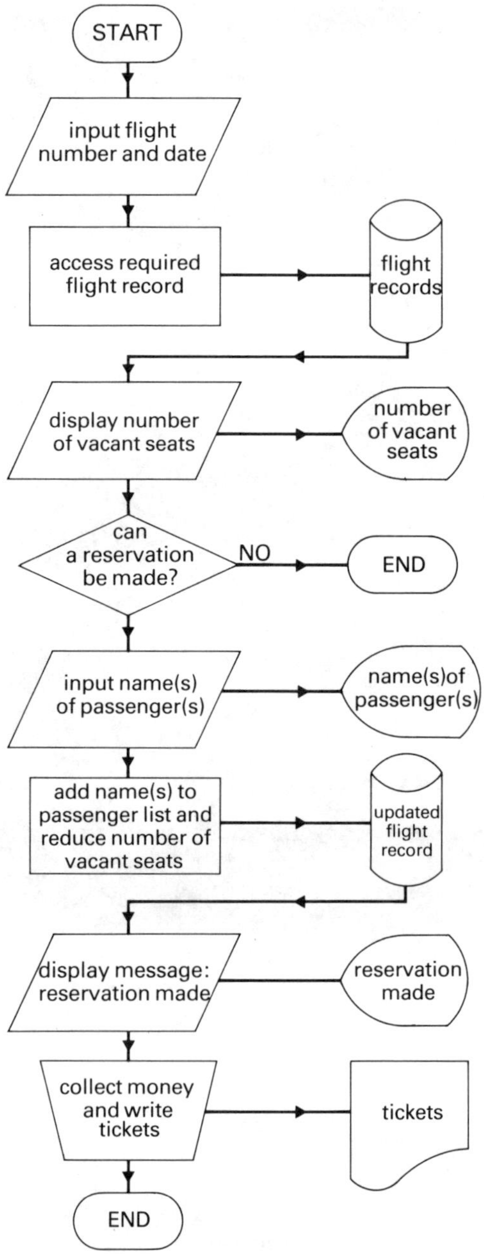

Fig. 17.6: Airline seat reservations

Example 5 Updating a telephone directory.
Computers can be used to assemble and store the information for a telephone directory, and update this information for the new edition of the directory each year.

The first time that a computer is used, the data is input from an existing directory, and copied into a file, on a magnetic tape, or tapes. The file is in alphabetical order of the names of the people. The system described below updates the file for the next year's edition of the directory.

What is the purpose of the system? To produce a file, stored on magnetic tape, containing up-to-date information for the next edition of a telephone directory. The directory is then printed from the magnetic tape.

What input data is required? The information from the previous year's edition of the directory.

A list of all the changes in the directory: names to be added or removed, new addresses and telephone numbers.

How is the data captured and stored? The information for the changes and new entries is filled in on various forms. It is then typed by direct data entry onto a magnetic tape.

Information from the previous year's directory is already on a magnetic tape.

What processing is done? Three separate computer programs are used.

The first program inputs the changes and new entries data from the magnetic tape. The data is validated, and any data with errors is printed for correction manually. The correct data is copied onto another magnetic tape. When the corrections have been made, the program is run again to input and validate the corrected data.

The second program inputs the validated data, and sorts it into alphabetical order of names. The sorted data is copied onto another magnetic tape.

The third program combines the changes and new entries data with the data from the previous edition. Both sets of data are in alphabetical order. Two processes are actually involved. Existing entries may be altered or deleted. This is called updating. New entries are inserted into their correct positions on the updated tape. This process is called **merging.** Merging is combining data from two (or more) sources, each of which is in order. The combined data is also in order.

What is the output? An up-to-date file, on a magnetic tape, containing information for the next edition of the telephone directory.

What computer hardware is used? A medium sized computer, with 16 K to 64 K of main store, including at least three magnetic tape units, and at least one visual display unit for direct data entry to magnetic tape.

How well is the system likely to work? Fairly well. The slowest part of the job is typing all the data. On the computerized system, this only needs to be done once, as opposed to two or three times on the manual system.

Figure 17.7 shows a systems flow diagram for updating a telephone directory.

Types of data processing systems

There are several types of data processing systems, depending on the type of communication between

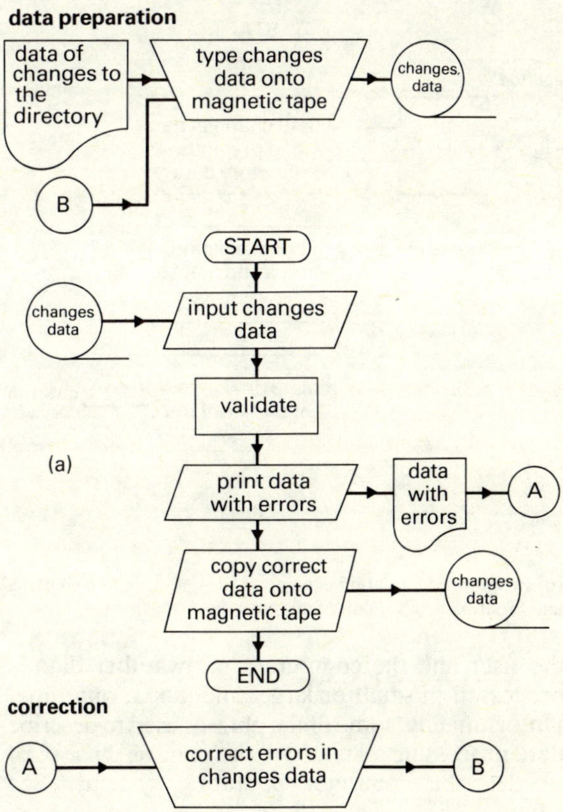

Fig. 17.7: Updating a telephone directory (a) Program 1: input/validation

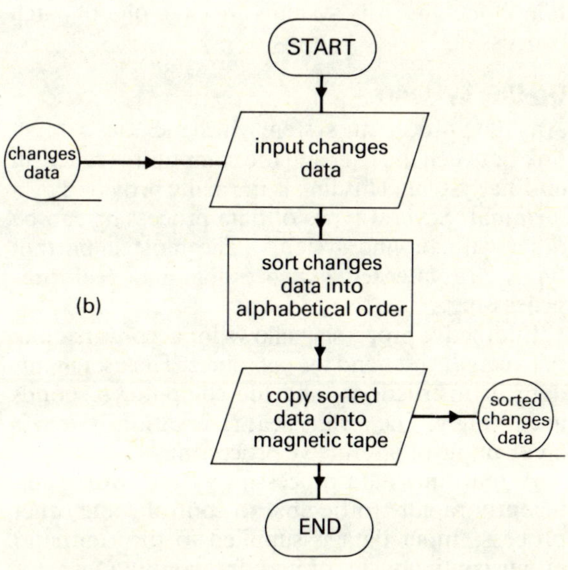

(b) Program 2: Sorting

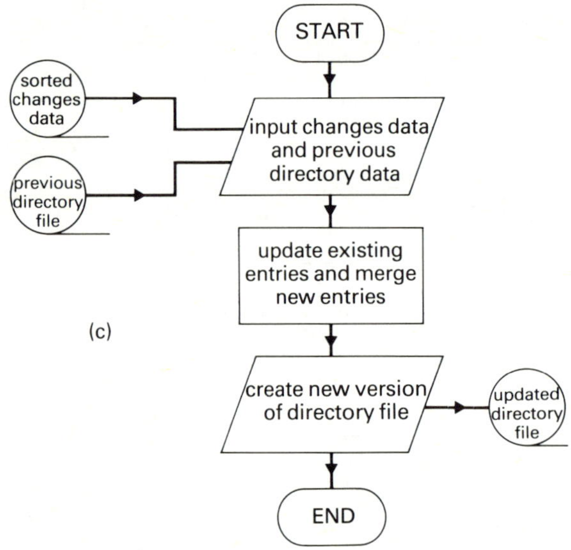

(c) Program 3: Updating existing entries, merging new entries and creating new version of directory file

the user and the computer, and whether data is processed in small or large amounts at one time. Unfortunately, some of the phrases used to describe data processing systems are the same as those used to describe computer operating systems (See Chapter 15).

Batch processing systems

Batch processing systems are those which process data, not in single items, but in batches, at one time. The weekly wages, monthly accounts and telephone directory systems are examples of batch processing.

On-line systems

Any data processing system which includes a direct link between the user and the computer is called an **on-line** system. This link is normally provided by a terminal. Several types of data processing can be done with on-line systems. The most important types are **interactive processing** and **real time processing.**

Interactive processing allows for a 'conversation' between the user and the computer. The user inputs data or instructions, and the computer responds accordingly. The airline seat reservation system is an example of interactive processing.

A real time data processing system works sufficiently rapidly to be able to control some other process. Input data is supplied to the computer either continuously, or very frequently. Output is available almost immediately.

An example of a real time processing system is controlling spacecraft. Data concerning the course of the spacecraft is continuously input into the computer. The computer outputs control instructions in response to the data, rapidly enough to keep the spacecraft on course.

Backing store: Discs or tape?

As you will have noticed in the examples, some data processing systems use magnetic tape backing store, while others use magnetic discs. A few systems, not described here, use both.

Batch processing systems are generally suited to magnetic tape. Processing is usually done in the order in which data occurs on the tape. This takes advantage of the serial access property of magnetic tape. Some of the data may have to be sorted into the correct order before processing. If so, the sorting operation is usually the slowest part of the whole process.

On-line data processing systems generally use magnetic disc backing store. On these systems, requests for data occur in a random fashion. With random access magnetic discs, all requests can be dealt with in approximately the same time.

Conclusion

This chapter has introduced the idea of a data processing system, and outlined some common examples of them. Methods of organizing data, and several important techniques of data processing have been mentioned. They are discussed in more detail in the next chapter.

In conclusion, one important feature of electronic data processing is worth emphasizing: it involves the close co-ordination of work done by people, and work done by computers. Both the people and the computers are essential if the system is to work properly.

Exercise 17

1 Write down the meanings of the following words or phrases:
master data; validate; source document;
balance (of an account); invoice; receipt;
transaction record;
statement (of an account); database;
accessing; updating; on-line processing;
data capture; merging; real-time processing;
interactive processing.

2 Parts (a) to (g) are brief descriptions of some common data processing operations. For each

operation, answer the data processing question on page 106, and draw a systems flow diagram.

The descriptions contain most of the information required to answer the data processing questions. Supply any additional information needed yourself, based on the way the data processing examples are done.

(a) Goods are received by and despatched from a warehouse. Whenever goods arrive, or are sent out, a note is written, showing the item number and the quantity. At the end of each day, a computer uses this data, and the previous day's stock levels, to calculate the current stock levels of all the items in the warehouse.

The previous day's stock levels are stored on a magnetic tape. A new magnetic tape is created, showing the current stock levels.

(b) Whenever money is paid into or withdrawn from a bank, a slip is written, with a date, account number, person's name and amount. These slips, called deposit and withdrawal slips respectively, are the transaction records for the system. Every night, the bank's computer runs a program to input this data and calculate the amount of money (the balance) in each account. A magnetic tape inputs the balances from the previous night.

A list of account number, names and balances is printed. The new balances are stored on another magnetic tape.

(c) Another bank has a terminal at each cashier's desk. Whenever money is paid in or withdrawn, the date, account number and amount are typed on the terminal. The computer accesses the account, which is stored on a magnetic disc. A record of the transaction is stored, and the balance increased or decreased by the amount paid in or withdrawn.

The date, the amount paid in or withdrawn and the new balance are printed in the person's bank book by a special device attached to the terminal.

(d) A reference library has an index of its books stored on a magnetic disc. A person may use a terminal to find out whether or not the library has a particular book. Either the author's name or the title is input on the terminal. The index is then accessed.

If the book is found, its entire reference is displayed: author, title and subject code number. If the book is not in the library, a message is displayed.

This is an example of an **information retrieval** system.

(e) A computer is used to store and process the data for a dictionary. The data consists of a number of words, in alphabetical order, each with its meaning. The data is stored on a magnetic tape.

From time to time, a new edition of the dictionary is produced. New words are inserted, a few words are deleted, and the meanings of many of the words are revised.

A magnetic tape is produced of the data for the revised edition of the dictionary.

(f) The information for a telephone directory is stored on a magnetic disc and accessed from VDU terminals. A name is input, and the address and telephone number are displayed, or there is a message to say that the name is not in the directory.

(g) Use any other system with which you are familiar.

3 A firm which publishes magazines keeps records of its subscribers on cards in a file. The information is either handwritten or typed onto the cards. When anything has to be posted to the subscribers a clerk selects the appropriate cards and copies the names and addresses onto envelopes. The envelopes are then sent to the dispatch department for filling and posting.

(a) The file may need to be updated by (i) an insertion, (ii) an amendment (iii) a deletion. Suggest what each of these could be caused by.

(b) Explain how the clerk would update the file in the event of these cases: (i) Inserting a record, (ii) amending a record, (iii) deleting a record.

The firm is thinking of using its computer to replace this manual system. The file will be stored on magnetic tape, the labels will be printed on the line-printer and the information will be input on punched cards.

(c) The magnetic tape file will be updated only once a week whereas the manual file could be updated at any time. Explain why the magnetic tape file would be updated only once a week.

(d) If someone phones the clerk and asks for details of a particular subscriber, why would the clerk find it difficult to give the information from the magnetic tape even if he had the tape on his desk?

(e) To overcome this difficulty a complete list of the file is printed out each time the file is updated. Explain whether the clerk can, or can not, now give accurate up-to-date information.

(f) Draw a system flowchart to show the updating of the file and the printing of the list. (*Hint:* you will need a sort program.)

Explain why you need a sort program.

(g) Draw a systems flowchart to show the printing of the labels.

(h) Question (c), (d) and (e) above seem to suggest that the computerized system will not be as good as the manual card file system. Give *two* advantages that the firm would hope to gain from the computerized system. (MREB 78)

4 Shortly before the motor vehicle licence of each car is due for renewal, the Department of the Environment sends a reminder to the owner of the vehicle. A computer is used to prepare the reminder by printing information on a standard form.

On one section of the reminder are printed (a) particulars regarding ownership and (b) particulars of the vehicle concerned. If these particulars are correctly printed the owner is invited to tear off this section and return it together with the tax due. If the particulars are not correct (e.g the car has been resprayed in another colour) the owner is required to apply for a new licence on a separate form on which the changes can be recorded. New licences are subsequently despatched by post.

Outline, with the aid of a **systems flowchart,** how the computer can be used, in conjunction with the above procedure, to issue licences and to correct the computer's information regarding each vehicle. You should assume that the computer records are held on magnetic tape. (UCLES 78 II)

5 You are carrying out a survey of the types of residence in which the pupils in your school live. The accommodation in your area is made up of semi-detached houses, detached houses, flats and terraced houses.

Describe the procedure that you would follow to carry out this task. Your answer should include your method of data capture, your method of data organization and a flow diagram to show how you would determine the number of pupils living in each type of residence. (YREB 76 II)

6 The theatre booking system (Example 1) is to be computerized. An on-line system is planned, with VDU's at box offices and booking agencies, accessing a central computer with magnetic disc backing store.

Answer the data processing questions and draw a systems flow diagram for the new system.

18

Organizing data

The previous chapter introduced, in broad outline, some methods of data processing. This chapter describes ways of organizing the data which is used, and looks at some of the data processing techniques mentioned previously, in more detail. These techniques are data capture, validation, sorting, accessing and merging. The chapter concludes with a section on the security of data.

Files

Data processing, with or without computers, would be impossible if the data were not organized in some way. As a first step in organizing data, related data is collected together in **files.**

In its most general sense, a file is any collection of data. However, in the vast majority of cases, files contain data referring to a specific topic, and strictly arranged according to some structure.

Computers inherited files from manual systems, mainly commercial systems. Although there are many differences between pieces of paper in a filing cabinet, and magnetized areas on a tape or disc, many of the ideas involved are the same in all three cases.

The next few sections introduce some general ideas of file structure, and then outline how these ideas can be put into practice when files are stored on magnetic tape or magnetic discs.

File structure

The structure of a file depends on the type of data which it stores, particularly how individual data items are related, and how the data is used. A wide variety of file structures are used in practice. Some of the simpler and more common ones are mentioned below.

In most files, individual data items are grouped together in **records.** Each record generally has the same structure, though the length may vary. Data items within the record refer to the same event,

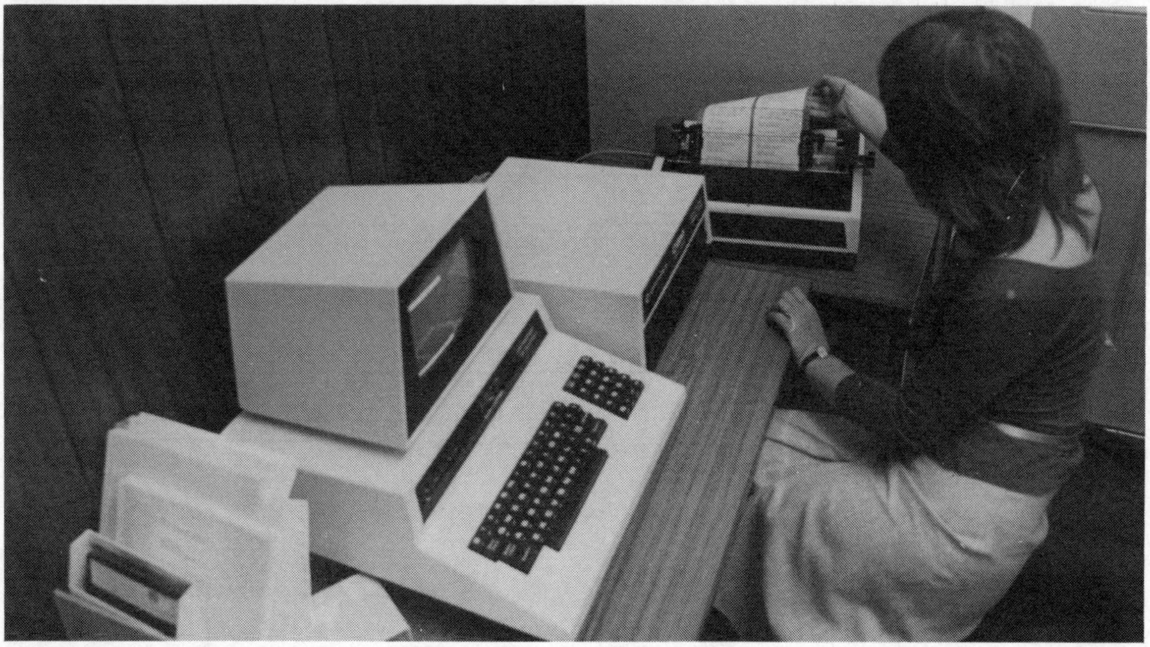

A Commodore Pet in a file processing application

person or object. The area of the storage medium reserved for one data item is called a **field.** A file consists of a set of records, a record consists of a set of fields.

For example, most businesses keep a payroll file. Each record concerns one employee, and includes fields for his or her name, works number, tax code etc.

A few of the records in a file may have special purposes. For example, the first record usually identifies the file. It includes the name of the file, and the date it was created, or last updated. In most cases, the last record simply marks the end of the file.

Keys

There are several ways of arranging the records in a file. In all cases, the records must be identified. One data item in the record, called a **key,** is used for this purpose. The key may already be part of the record, such as the works number in the payroll example, or it may be a special number or code used for identification only. The most important requirement of keys is that no two records have the same key.

Sequential files

A very common file structure is to arrange the records in order of their keys. Such files are called **sequential** files. See Figure 18.1. Accessing records in sequential files is a fairly simple process. It is described later in this chapter. However, if records are added or removed frequently, or if it is important to preserve some relationship between them, then a sequential file is not the best structure.

File directory

One convenient way of describing other arrangements of records is to use a **file directory.** The file directory contains a list of the keys, usually in order, together with a set of numbers which indicate the positions of the records in the file. The file directory is usually stored at the beginning of the file. See Figure 18.2.

Another convenient way of arranging the records in a file is to have a formula, or a specified procedure, for finding the location of the record from its key.

Files stored on magnetic tape

You will recall from a previous chapter that magnetic tape is a serial access medium, and that data stored on magnetic tape is usually in blocks, with gaps between the blocks.

Magnetic tape is best suited to store files where the records are not in any order, or sequential files. A block of tape contains one or more records.

If the records are not of fixed length, a certain character, or group of characters is used as an **end-of-record maker.** Other characters may be used to mark the ends of blocks, and also the end of the whole file.

For example, the master data for the monthly accounts system outlined in the previous chapter is kept on a magnetic tape. The most suitable structure is a sequential file, with each record containing the data for one account, using the account number as the key. Other data in a record includes the customer's name, address, and current balance. A block might contain ten records.

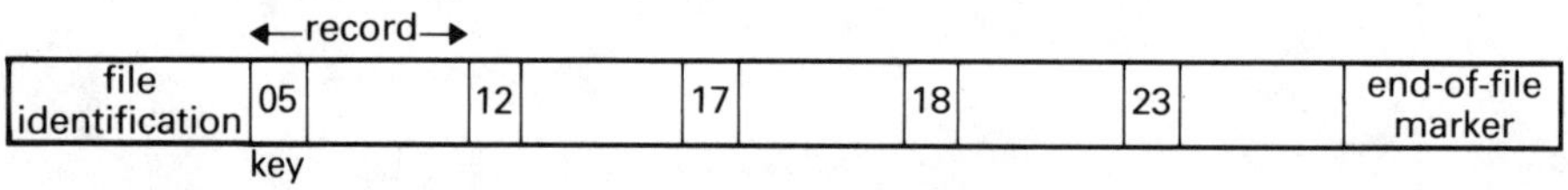

Fig. 18.1: A sequential file

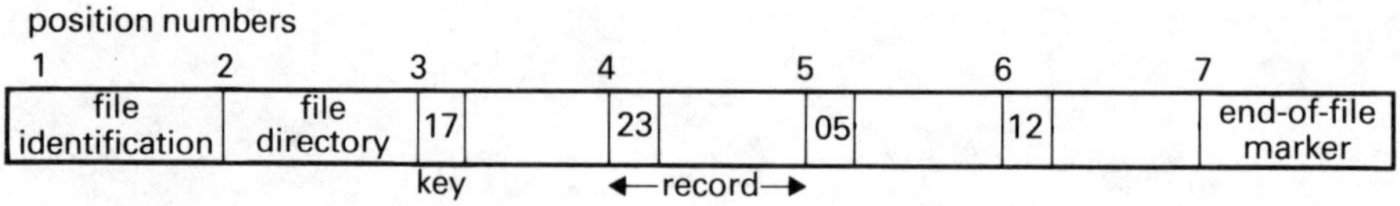

Contents of the file directory:

key	**position**
05	5
12	6
17	3
23	4

Fig. 18.2: The use of a file directory

Files stored on magnetic discs

As mentioned previously, magnetic discs are random access media. Any data item can be accessed more or less equally quickly, regardless of its position on the disc. Each storage area on a disc can be located by means of an address, in a manner somewhat similar to locating a data item in a CPU memory.

Magnetic discs can be used to store non-ordered or sequential files. In the latter case, the order of keys is usually the same as the order of addresses of the records.

Magnetic discs are also suited to storing more complex file structures. If a file directory is used, it contains the keys together with the addresses on the disc of the records to which they refer. While the file is being used, the file directory is usually copied onto the CPU memory. If a file directory is not used, there is some procedure for calculating the magnetic disc address of a record from its key.

For example, the flight records for the airline seat reservation system in the previous chapter form a file, stored on a magnetic disc (or discs). The key for each record is derived from the flight number and the date. A record also includes the times and airports of call, a current passenger list, and the number of vacant seats. The file directory associates each key with the magnetic disc address of the flight record to which it refers.

After a flight has taken place, its record is removed from the file, and the disc space allocated to another flight record. The file directory is updated accordingly.

Types of files

There are several types of files, depending on the nature and purpose of the data they contain. Obviously, master data is stored on **master files.** **Transaction files** store commercial transaction records, as previously mentioned, though the phrase is also used to describe any files which contain data used to update master files.

Database

An important type of file is one which stores data used in more than one application. A file of this type is called a **database.** The structure of a database must take into account all its applications, as well as the procedure for updating the data. In adddition, the file structure must reflect all the interrelationships existing within the data.

Some data processing techniques

The previous few sections have indicated how files contain data strictly organized in some structure. The next few sections describe how such data is collected and checked, and some ways in which data in files is processed. The operations discussed, namely **sorting, accessing** and **merging,** were all introduced in the data processing systems of the previous chapter.

Data capture

Data capture is obtaining the information required by a data processing system. The information must be accurate, relevant and concise, and the method of capture efficient, reliable and designed for possible expansion of the system.

Many methods have been developed to suit these rather exacting requirements. The particular method used in any system depends on the nature and quantity of the data, and how frequently it is collected.

Probably the most common manual method of data capture is filling in a form. This source document is then copied onto some input medium like punched cards, or input directly by optical or magnetic character reading, or by direct data entry onto a magnetic disc or tape. These methods have been discussed in Chapter 5.

In other situations, data is captured by some sensing instrument, changed into digital form, and input as pulses of electricity.

Validation

If any input data is wrong, the output it produces will be wrong (Garbage In, Garbage Out). Wrong input data can also cause a computer program to stop, for example if it instructs the computer to divide by zero.

For these reasons, it is essential that all input data is thoroughly checked by a computer program before it is used. Wrong data cannot usually be corrected by a program. In most cases it is output for correction and re-input.

Input data from punched cards will already have been verified, to ensure that the cards have been punched correctly. Validation, sometimes also called **vetting,** carries out further checks. Common checks are **range checks,** and the use of **hash totals,** **batch totals** and **check digits.**

Range checks

Range checks detect any numbers that are too big or too small. For example, if a shop has account numbers in the range 1 to 10000, then any account number less than 1 or more than 10000 is wrong.

Hash totals

Hash totals are totals of other data numbers. For example, if a person's works number, and ordinary and overtime hours worked are input, they are added up, and the total also input. The program adds up the numbers again, and checks its total against the one which was input. If the totals are different, then one of the input numbers is wrong.

Batch totals

Batch totals are totals of data items from a batch of input data. They are checked in a similar way to hash totals. They are particularly useful with punched cards, as they indicate whether a card has been lost.

Check digits

A check digit is an extra number or letter placed on the end of a data item. The purpose of the check digit is to detect whether an error has been made in copying the data item from one medium to another.

A check digit is first calculated when the data item is created. Each time the data item is copied, the process of obtaining the check digit is repeated, and the results compared. If the check digits are different, then the data item has been copied wrongly.

Most methods for assigning check digits to numbers start by multiplying each digit of the number by a **weighting factor,** and then adding up the products.

For example, using the number 4281 and weighting factors 7, 3, 5, and 9:

number	4	2	8	1
weighting factors	7	3	5	9 ×
products	28 +	6 +	40 +	0 = 8**3**

One method is to use the last digit of the sum as the check digit (**3** in this case). Another method is to divide the sum by a suitable number (which must not be a weighting factor) and use the remainder as the check digit.

If the above number had been copied wrongly, as 4821 for example, the check digit would be as follows:

number	4	8	2	1
weighting factors	7	3	5	9 ×
products	28 +	24 +	10 +	9 = 7**1**

The check digit, using the last digit of the sum, is **1.** Previously, this method produced a check digit of 3.

Another method of obtaining check digits is introduced in the exercise at the end of this chapter.

Sorting

Sorting is a very common data processing technique. It is usually applied to the records of a file, though individual data items may also be sorted into numerical or alphabetical order.

Tag sort

The records in a file are sorted in order of their keys. It is not usual to move entire records during the sort. The keys are sorted separately, and then the records accessed in order, and copied onto another storage medium. This operation is called a **tag sort.**

Bubble sort

Considerable effort has been made to devise efficient procedures for sorting. One of the simpler procedures in common use is called a **bubble sort.** It may be used with numbers, or literal data. For a set of numbers, the steps are as follows:

Each number is compared with the following one. If the first number is larger, the numbers and interchanged. After all the numbers have been compared, the largest number is at the end. For example, sorting the numbers

76 34 11 45 89 21 32

The steps are:

(arrow) numbers compared

76	34	11	45	89	21	32	interchange
34	76	11	45	89	21	32	interchange
34	11	76	45	89	21	32	interchange
34	11	45	76	89	21	32	no interchange
34	11	45	76	89	21	32	interchange
34	11	45	76	21	89	32	interchange
34	11	45	76	21	32	89	

The largest number is now at the end. The process is repeated for the other numbers:

34	11	45	76	21	32	(89)	interchange
11	34	45	76	21	32	(89)	no interchange
11	34	45	76	21	32	(89)	no interchange
11	34	45	76	21	32	(89)	interchange
11	34	45	21	76	32	(89)	interchange
11	34	45	21	32	76	(89)	

The second largest number is now second last. The

process continues for the other numbers. They usually become completely ordered before all the comparisons have been made.

Even this brief example shows that sorting is a fairly slow process.

Merging

Merging is when data from two sources is combined. Before merging, both sets of data are in order. After merging, the data is again in order. For example, if two magnetic tapes have numbers as follows:

Tape A	11	18	23	31	47	58		
Tape B	10	16	17	24	53	56	59	71

after merging, the output magnetic tape has the following numbers:

Tape C	10	11	16	17	18	23	24	31	47
	53	56	58	59	71				

At each step of the merging process, the next numbers on the input tapes are compared. The lower number is copied onto the output tape.

When merging is used with files, the records are merged according to their keys.

Accessing

Accessing involves locating one name out of a large set of names or one number out of a large set of numbers, or one record in a file. It is usually too slow to read for the beginning of the data until the required name, number or record is found.

Binary search

A method frequently used, if the data is in order, is called a *binary search*. It involves moving forwards or backwards in the data, one step at a time. The first step is half the length of the list of data. Each subsequent step is half the length of the previous step. The direction of the step is always towards the required data item.

For example, to find the number 81 from the eight numbers below, the steps are as follows:

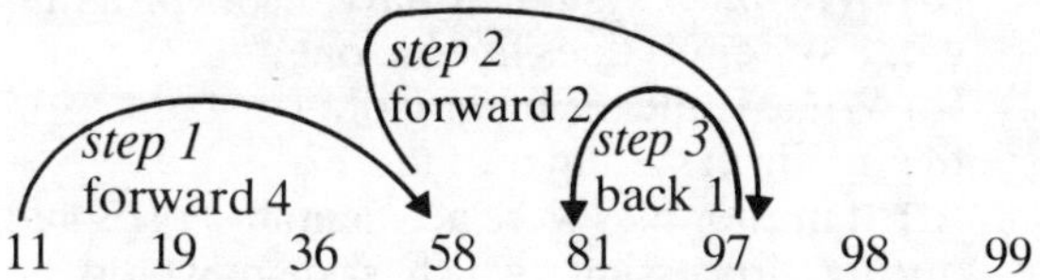

The required number is found fairly quickly.

Applied to files, accessing usually implies locating a certain record, identified by its key. The numbers used in the binary search are the keys of the records in the file.

Security of data

As you will realize from the data processing systems outlined in the previous chapter, large quantities of data are kept on magnetic tapes and discs. This data is often vital to the running of a system. Steps must be taken to prevent the accidental (or deliberate) erasure of the data, and to enable the data to be recovered if this does happen.

The most common security precautions are as follows:

Whenever a magnetic tape file is updated, the up-to-date file is on a new magnetic tape. The previous version of the file is kept, as well as the one from which it was copied. The transaction data which was used to update the files is also kept. Thus there are three **generations** of the file. This is called the **grandfather-father-son** principle.

Files on magnetic discs, which are continuously being updated, are copied onto magnetic tape from time to time. This creates **security copies** of the file. Copies of transaction data are also kept.

To prevent unauthorized access to data, a system of **passwords** is generally used. Each person entitled to use the data is allocated a password, which must be entered whenever that person 'logs in' to the computer. There are generally different levels of security, with some passwords giving wider access to data than others, and only a few passwords permitting the updating of files. The password often acts as a 'signature' on data entered onto a file.

Exercise 18

1 Write down the meanings of the following words or phrases:
file; record; key; sequential file;
file directory; hash total; check digit;
transaction file; tag sort; bubble sort;
generation (of a file);
grandfather-father-son principle.

2 The file of data for the telephone directory (Example 5, Chapter 17) contains the names, addresses and telephone numbers of the people in the directory.
(a) List the contents of a record.
(b) Which item in the record is the key?
(c) What type of file is it?

3 This question refers to the monthly accounts system (Example 3, Chapter 17).
(a) List the contents of a record in the master file.
(b) List the contents of a record in a transaction file.
(c) How many transaction files are there?

(d) Which data item is the key in all the records?
(e) Which data item is likely to have a check digit? Give reasons for this.

4 Four punched cards contain the following data. The last figure is a hash total.

2361	141	17.92	2519.92
3616	247	15.41	———
4117	234	8.63	———
6121	191	27.41	6380.41

(a) Fill in the missing hash totals.
(b) Which card contains an error?
The following card contains the batch totals of the previous cards:

16215 —— 110.37 ——

(c) Copy and complete the missing totals.
(d) Which of the above totals is wrong?
(e) From your answers to parts (b) and (d), identify the data item which is wrong.

5 A shop has accounts numbered 0001 to 5000. One transaction may not exceed £250.00. A transaction record contains a date, transaction type (1: invoice, 2: receipt), account number and amount.
(a) What kind of checks can be used on transaction records?
The following is a set of transaction records:

25/02/78	1	4167	203.75
19/01/78	2	5613	150.75
31/04/78	1	4030	3.74
09/01/78	3	1161	57.23
10/02/78	2	3137	193.62
16/01/78	2	4203	416.62

(b) Identify the errors in these records.

6 Calculate the check digits for each of the following numbers, using the weighting factors 7, 3, 5, 9 and 1, and taking the last digit of the sum of products as the check digit.

60623 31695 72693

7 The last digits of the following numbers are check digits, calculated as in question **6.** Which numbers are incorrect?

41533**6** 65927**5** 31460**8**

8 Another way of calculating the check digit for a number is divide the number by 9 and write the remainder as the check digit. For example, the number 285 has check digit **6,** because 285 ÷ 9 = 31 remainder 6. This method is called a **modulo 9** or **residue 9** check.

(a) Using the above method, complete the check digits on these numbers:

416____, 2125____, 20060____

(b) Which of these check digits is wrong:

512**8,** 275**3,** 4032**0**?

9 Carry out all the stages of a bubble sort on these sets of numbers:

(a) 1 4 3 5 2
(b) 9 8 7 6 5
(c) 1 3 2 4 6
(d) 6 3 4 7 1 9 2 8

***10** What additional decision can be made to prevent unnecessary repetition of the bubble sort process?

11 Two magnetic tapes containing the numbers:

6 9 11 12 19 23 24 and
1 2 3 7 10 17 18 29

Show the numbers on a magnetic tape merged from these two tapes.

12 Show the steps of a binary search to find the number 37 in each of the following sets:

(a) 5 19 37 46 71 85 89 97
(b) 7 9 15 23 24 25 27 28
30 31 32 34 36 37 52 71

***13** Draw a flow diagram to show the steps in the process of merging two sets of ordered data.

14 A hire purchase company keeps records of all its customers' accounts on computer files. The master file contains details of customers' names, addresses, amount owed and monthly payments due. Each week all the details of that week's payments arrive at the computer centre on a magnetic tape, called the transaction file. This tape is processed against the master file. Figure 18.3 shows two possible ways of doing this: system A and system B.

(a) Which system uses a direct access device?
(b) Why *must* system A have a sort program when system B does not use one?
(c) What is meant by grandfather-father-son files? Which system uses these?
(d) If master files were accidentally corrupted during processing, which system would be better at recovering correct files? How could the other system be improved to overcome this difficulty?
(e) Which system could be adapted for real time processing? Explain why. (MREB 77)

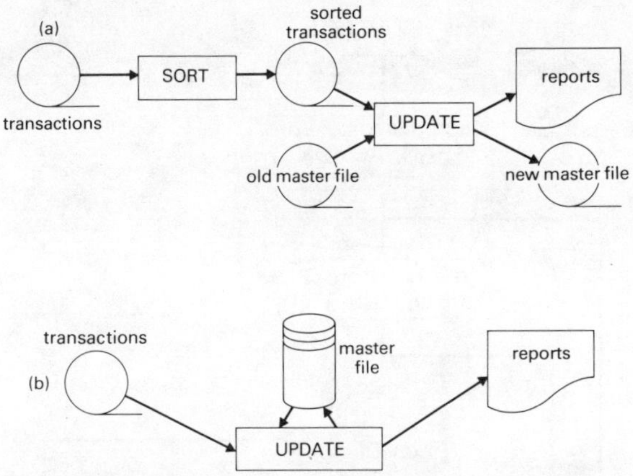

Fig. 18.3: (a) System A, (b) System B

15 When a library in a particular town catalogues a book, details of the title, the author and the catalogue number of the book are recorded on a computer file.

Explain the checks that would be incorporated in a data validation program used in conjunction with the input of these data into the computer file. (JMB 78)

16 A mail order firm receives and despatches orders every day. Describe, preferably by means of a systems flowchart, the steps taken to produce a validated transaction file by the end of the day. (UCLES 76 II)

17 With particular reference to a computer system you have studied, e.g. payroll, stock control, medical records, etc., explain the meaning of the following terms. (Your answer should include the type of information considered in each case.)
(a) master file, (b) updating,
(c) transaction file. (YREB 75 I)

18 The flowchart (Figure 18.4) is designed to insert a new record into a file held on magnetic tape. Each record has a key field and other information. The file is in ascending key order i.e., the smallest key value is at the beginning. The flowchart is incomplete and carefully chosen test data will be used to help complete it. When you dry run the flowchart ignore empty ACTION boxes; follow lines labelled NO at empty decision boxes. In each case (a) to (f) below, write down the keys in NEW MASTER.

(a) Dry run the flowchart with the following test data:

Key of P is 729; Keys in OLD MASTER are 126, 329, 513, 8888.

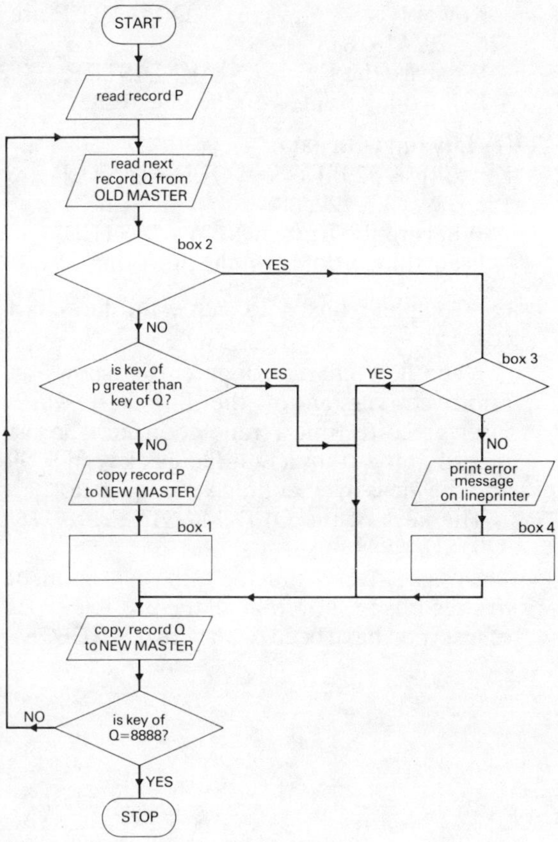

Fig. 18.4

What are the Keys in NEW MASTER?

(b) The first set of data should have worked properly. However, a different choice of data might produce a different result. Dry run the flowchart with the following test data:

Key of P is 86; Key in OLD MASTER are 126, 329, 513, 8888.

What are the Keys in NEW MASTER.

(c) Write in box 1 'set key of P to 8888'. Dry run with the following data:

Key of P is 86; Keys in OLD MASTER are 126, 329, 513, 8888.

What are the Keys in NEW MASTER.

(d) Write 'Key of P = Key of Q?' in box 2. Dry run with data:

Key of P is 86; Keys in OLD MASTER 126, 329, 513, 8888.

What are the Keys in NEW MASTER.

Is anything printed on the line printer?

(e) Write 'Key of P = 8888' in box 3. Dry run with data:

Key of P is 86; Keys in OLD MASTER are 126, 329, 513, 8888.

What are the Keys in NEW MASTER.

In anything printed on the line printer?

(f) Dry run with data:
Key of P is 329; Keys in OLD MASTER are 126, 329, 513, 729, 8888.

What are the Keys in NEW MASTER.

Is anything printed on the line printer?

(g) Complete box 4 to make the flowchart correct.

(h) The flow chart in Figure 18.5 shows an improved version of the flowchart which inserts records from a transaction file. The last record in the transaction file has key of 9999 and the file is in ascending key sequence.

The keys of the OLD MASTER are 126, 329, 513, 8888.

Design a transaction file with a maximum of *five* records to show that all the possible types of insertion have been dealt with. (MREB 78)

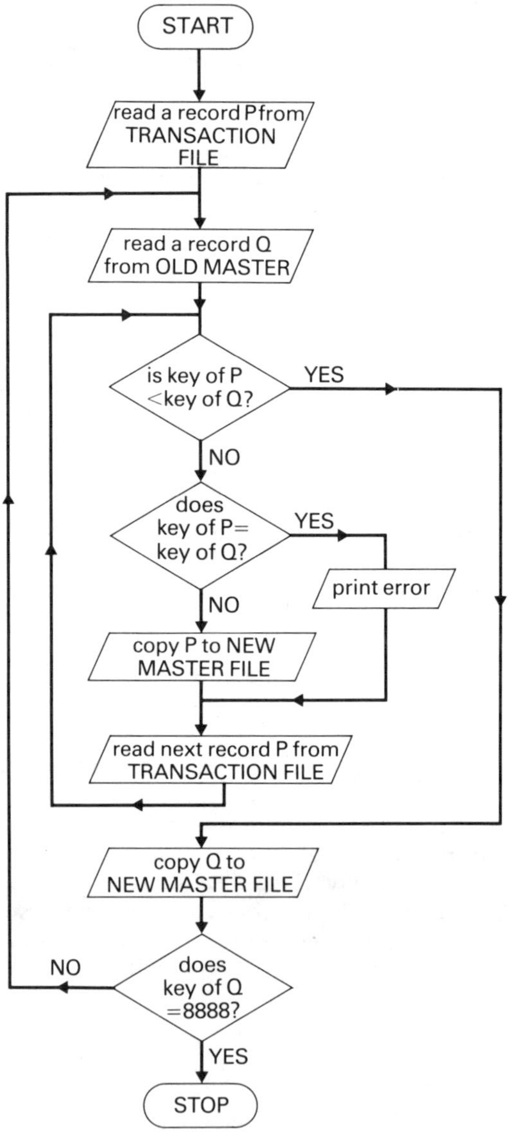

Fig. 18.5

19

Some applications of computers

At present there are over a quarter of a million computers in the world. They are used in many different ways. In some areas of industry and commerce, manual systems are the exception rather than the rule. The first computers were large and complicated, but remote access terminals and microcomputers have brought electronic data processing into many smaller firms.

Cost has been an important factor. In recent years, as wages have risen, computing costs have fallen. In 1952, it cost 57 pence to do one hundred thousand multiplications on a computer. In 1976 the same cost was 0.5 pence. A small computer system can be set up for about £5000, and run for about £80 per week, often doing work that could not be done manually at a comparable cost.

Modern small computer systems are simple, versatile and reliable. Programs are supplied with the hardware, and specialized staff are not needed. Existing staff can be trained in a short time to run the computer.

At the other end of the scale, very large systems with expert staff have made such activities as space research, long range weather forecasting and the co-ordination of multinational corporations a reality. Without computers, none of these would have been possible.

Most computers consist of several units. These units can often be exchanged for other (usually larger) ones, and more units can be added to the system. This enables a computer to grow as the demand for it increases. Many expanding businesses have used computers in this way to help sustain their rate of growth.

The applications described in this chapter give some idea of the many areas in which computers are proving their worth.

Banking

Banks in western countries handle huge amounts of money in many different currencies every day. Without computers, the flow of money would be very much slower.

Cheque processing

One use of computers in banking is to process cheques. A cheque is an instruction to a bank to pay an amount of money to a person or (more commonly) into their bank account. When a cheque is cashed, it must be returned to the bank from where it came for the actual payment to be made.

All the information on a cheque is printed in magnetic ink characters, which enable the sorting of cheques and updating of accounts to be done by computers. An example of the process of clearing a cheque is shown in Figure 19.1.

Computer are used at the central clearing house (in London for British cheques) to sort the cheques according to the bank from where they came. Computers are again used by the individual banks to record the deduction of the amount from one account, and its payment into the other account. British banks handle 6 million cheques per day, on average, by this method.

Bank accounts

In addition to clearing cheques, computers are used by banks to process deposits, withdrawals, standing orders and other transactions. Every night, a program is run which deals with all the transcations from the previous day, and updates the balances in all the accounts. The output from this program, on microfilm in most cases, is distributed to all the branches of the bank ready for the start of business the next day.

Banking of the future: Electronic transfer of funds

Inceasing use is being made of transferring money by a direct link between the computers of the two banks involved. This process is called **Electronic Funds Transfer (EFT).**

Bank accounts are stored on magnetic discs, with input and output on terminals. A switching network links the computers of the two banks. All records of a transaction are made as the transaction takes place.

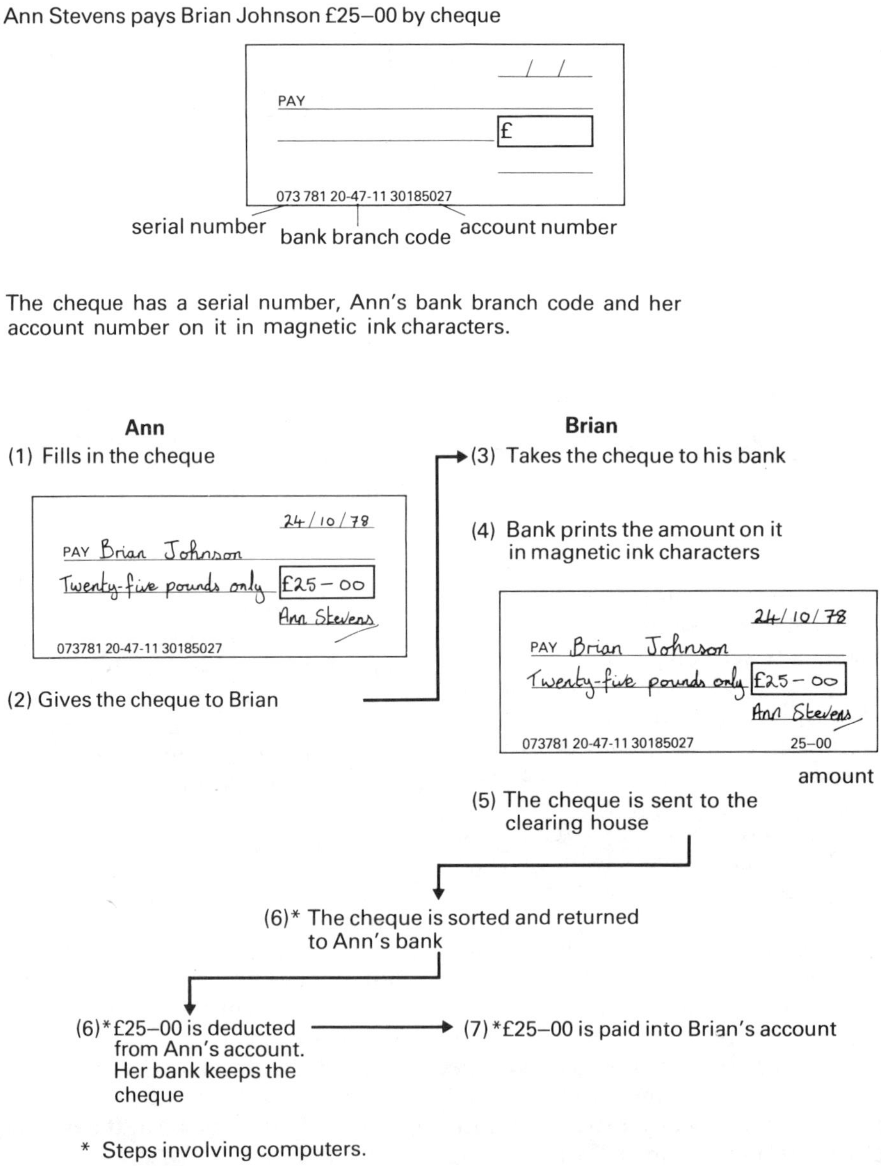

Fig. 19.1: Paying by cheque

A request to transfer money from one account to another (equivalent to writing a cheque) is input on a terminal, either at a bank, or linked to one. The account of the person making the request is accessed to see if the money is available. The switching system then accesses the bank to which the money is to be transferred. When the account is located, the transaction is recorded in both accounts. A message is displayed on the terminal to confirm that the transaction has been recorded. The whole process takes a few seconds. An example of Electronic Funds Transfer is shown in Figure 19.2.

Electronic funds transfer will become generally

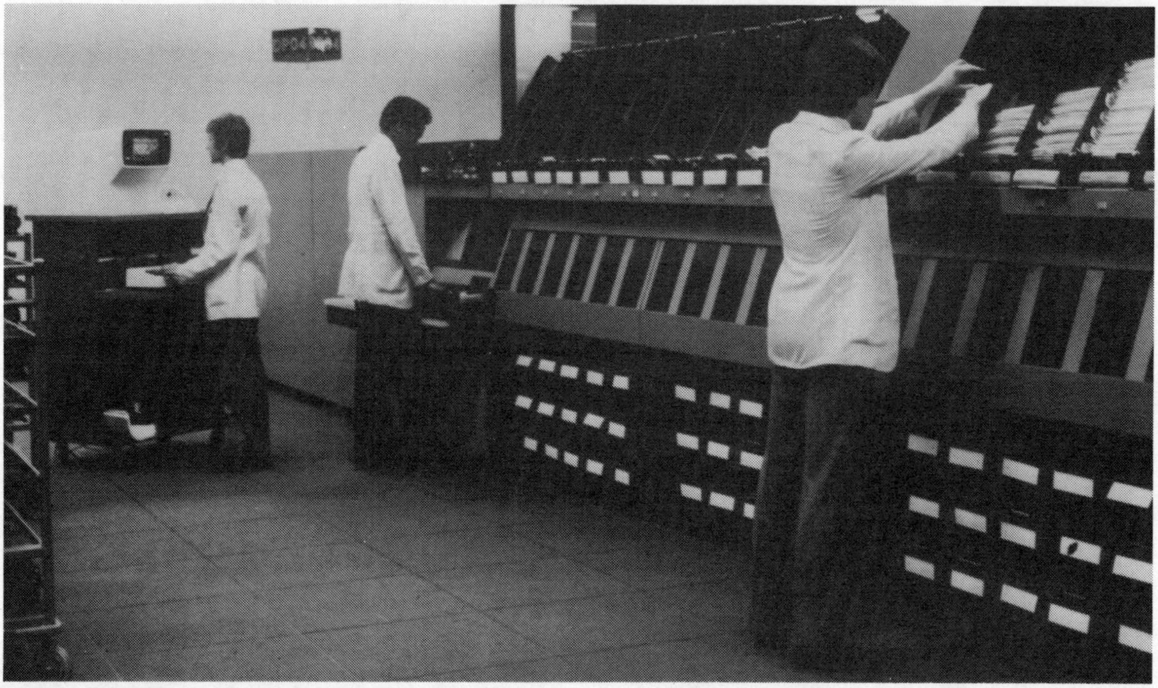

A cheque sorting machine at Lloyds Bank

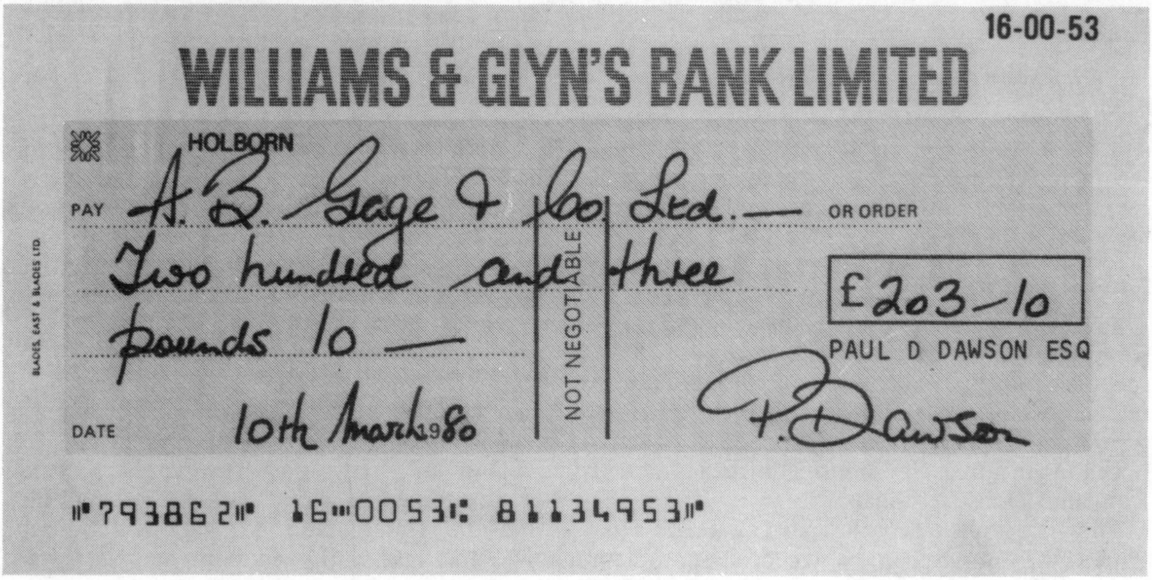

A cheque, showing the characters printed in magnetic ink along the bottom

available as soon as banks have changed their computers to ones using magnetic discs to store accounts, and installed terminals in their branches.

Most major banks will be linked to a worldwide message switching system, centred on two computers operated by the Society for World Interbank Financial Telecommunications (known as SWIFT) in Belgium.

However, not all banks are in favour of EFT, and some are considering alternative systems. It remains to be seen how widely this method of banking will be applied.

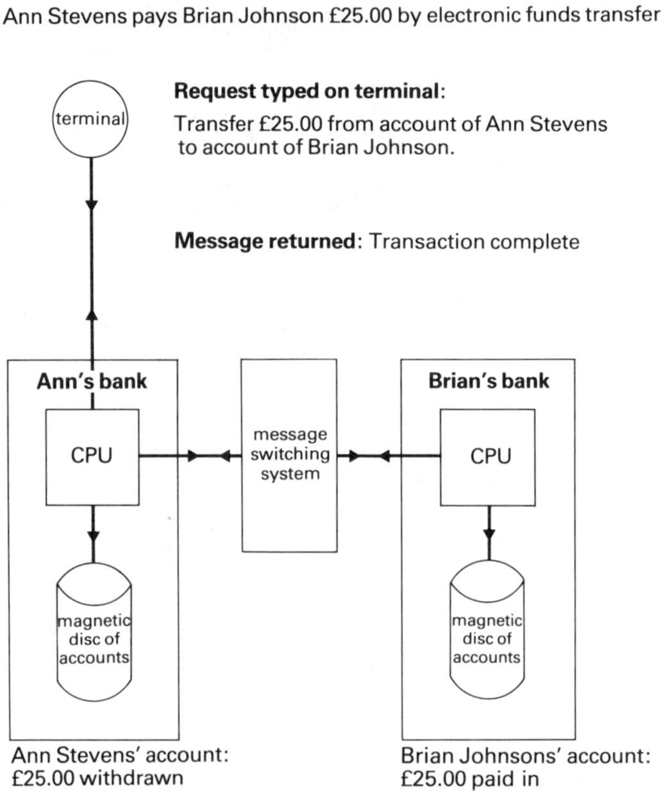

Fig. 19.2: Paying by electronic funds transfer

Medicine

An increasing number of hospitals and medical research establishments have installed computers, for a variety of uses.

Patient records

This is the commonest medical application. Computers are used to file and retrieve medical records of hosptial patients. The records are stored on magnetic tapes or discs, and accessed from terminals in wards, offices, laboratories or even operating theatres. New information can be added from any of these terminals.

The main advantage is the speed of access to the data by the various people who need it. A problem is the confidential nature of the information, fairly easily accessible to unauthorized people.

Blood transfusion service

The British blood transfusion service keeps records of blood stocks and information about all its donors on computerized files. The files can be accessed from a number of places.

Information about donors includes telephone numbers and hours during which they can be used. Records are also kept of appointments and any illnesses of donors.

Up-to-date information on blood stocks is essential because blood can only be kept for about three weeks. The computerized system has the advantages of efficiency and rapid response to an emergency.

Medical research data

Much current medical research involves mathematical modelling of organs such as the lungs, or collection and analysis of large quantities of statistics (on epidemics, etc.). Mathematical modelling is the use of mathematical equations to describe how something works. In both these activities, computers are of valuable assistance.

Assistance with diagnosis

One of a doctor's most important tasks is to diagnose an illness from its symptoms. With the number of known diseases rapidly increasing, and with pressures of time, some doctors believe that an information retrieval system, accessed by a terminal, can be used to assist diagnosis. Such a system is currently being used at a few places.

Intensive care and surgery monitoring

Computers are being used to assist staff in intensive care units, and surgery teams during operations. They continuously monitor the patient's condition. Inputs are temperature, blood pressure, electrocardiograph (heartbeat) pulses and other monitor readings. The program checks that these are within acceptable limits, and alerts the medical staff at the first sign of any irregularity.

Supplies

Hospitals need large quantities of medicines, equipment and other supplies, and shortages could be fatal. Stock records are often kept on computerized files, and orders automatically made out when needed.

The debate: Are computers in medicine a help or a hindrance?

The widespread use of computers in medicine has been opposed by many people. The question is whether computers are making it easier for medical staff to care better for their patients, or making the attitude towards patients even more impersonal.

The question is at present unresolved, but a point to be remembered is that psychological factors (tension, boredom, loneliness, etc.) play a major part in many diseases. Personal relationships established between doctors, nurses and patients are very important.

The Police National Computer

One of the most useful weapons available to police in their fight against crime is rapid access to accurate, up-to-date information. Police forces in Britain are making increasing use of computers to provide this facility. Many forces have their own regional computers, and all forces are linked to the Police National Computer in Hendon, London. The Police National Computer provides immediate access to centralized records from several hundred places throughout Britain.

The computer stores files of four types of information: stolen and suspect vehicles, vehicle owners, names of people with criminal records, and fingerprints.

Stolen and suspect vehicles

The stolen and suspect vehicles file contains registration numbers, chassis/engine numbers and descriptions of all vehicles reported stolen, or otherwise suspect.

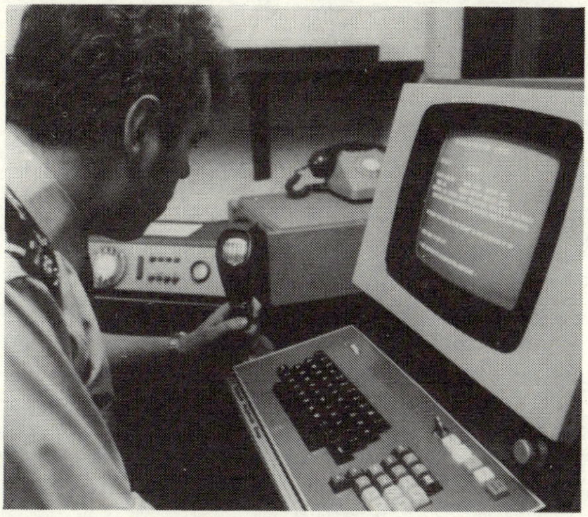

A police officer entering data at a terminal

Vehicle owners' index

The vehicle owners' file contains details, including names and addresses, of all vehicle owners in Britain.

These two files, used in conjunction, make the task of tracing and recovering stolen vehicles much easier. Over 500 cars are stolen in Britain every day, and often driven rapidly over long distances, in the hopes of avoiding detection. Stolen cars are often used in other, more serious crimes.

Names index

This file contains the names of people with criminal records, people wanted by the police or who have been reported missing, disqualified drivers and anyone with a suspended or deferred prison sentence.

Fingerprints index

This file contains a coded index of all the fingerprints in the New Scotland Yard collection.

In addition to providing access to these files, the computer has a broadcast facility, enabling urgent messages to be transmitted from one terminal to others.

Hardware

The hardware of the system is designed for continuous operation, uninterrupted even by the failure of a part of the system. Most essential units are duplicated to ensure this.

There are two Burroughs B6700 central processing units working in parallel. Each CPU has access to a shared 360 K core store. Backing store consists of twenty 100 megabyte magnetic disc drives, and thirteen magnetic tape units. A disc file optimizer ensures most efficient use of the disc storage space.

Three types of hardware device are used to provide a rapid link between the two CPU's and the 300 terminals in the system. There are input/output processors, responsible for passing data between core store and peripherals. Each input/output processor is connected to two data communications processors which control the allocation of CPU time to terminals. Then there are adaptor clusters which act as multiplexers for the low speed (teletype) and medium speed (VDU) communication lines.

Other peripherals include four operator's console displays, four line printers (1100 lines per minute), two card readers (1400 cards per minute), a card punch, two paper tape readers and a paper tape punch. There is a configuration control unit which enables the system to be split into two parts to allow maintenance and development work.

Finally there is a third separate B6700 CPU, with its own peripherals and core store. This computer is used for testing and modifying programs. In this way, the main computer is entirely devoted to operational use.

The development of the system

The Police National Computer Unit was set up in 1968. The equipment at Hendon was installed in 1972, and the communications network by the end of 1973. The first information file (stolen and suspect vehicles) became available in 1974, and work has continued since then adding the other data.

A proposal to extend the names file to contain a large amount of information on people suspected of crimes has not been implemented. Complaints about the dangers of storing such information were made by a number of people, and various organizations, including the National Council for Civil Liberties. There have also been complaints that additional personal information is already being stored on the computer.

However, the Police National Computer has provided a service to police throughout Britain which could not be provided by any manual method. It has helped to increase the chances of a criminal being caught, which is one of the most effective ways of bringing about a reduction in crime.

Traffic control

Most cities are faced with problem of ever-increasing volumes of traffic crowding inadequate

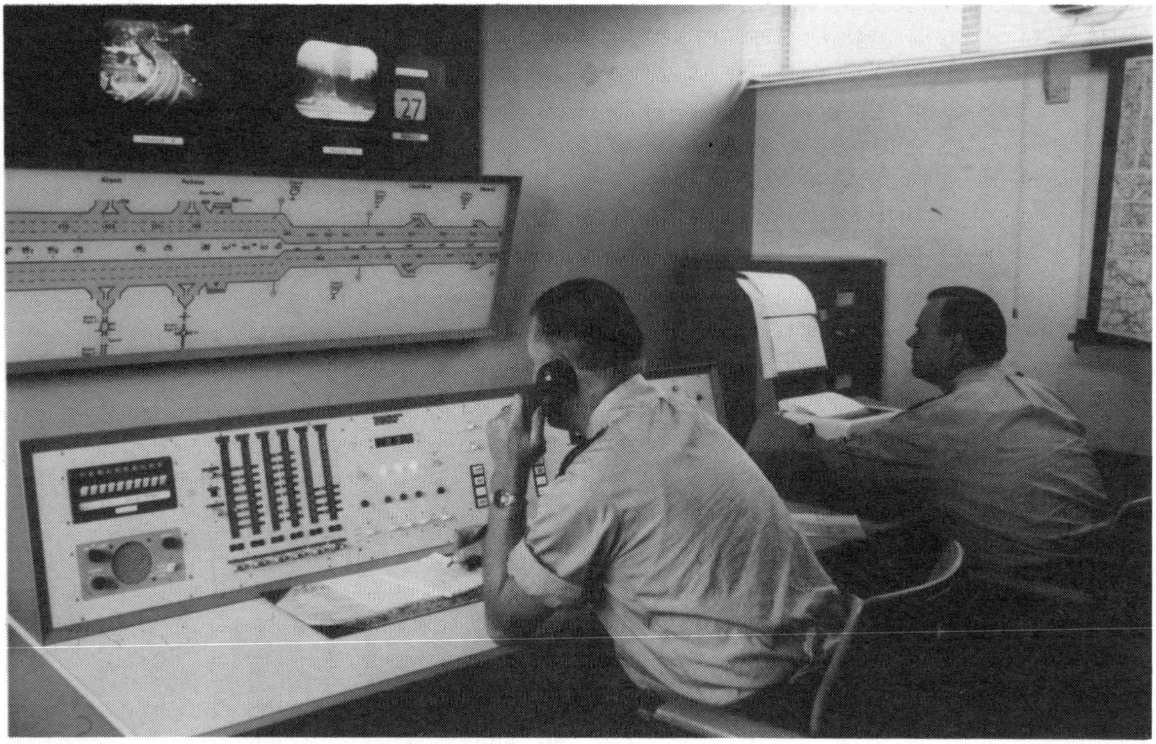

The control room of a computer-assisted traffic control system

road networks. Lack of space, historical buildings that cannot be demolished, and a shortage of money usually prevent major road improvements.

Computers have been used in several attempts to make the best of the existing situation, using integrated traffic control systems which can respond quickly to changing traffic flow patterns. Details vary, but most cities use a combination of computer and manual control.

Data is supplied to the control system by traffic sensors, counting vehicles, and closed circuit television cameras at key intersections. The computer program adjusts the timing of the traffic lights, and displays re-routing messages in response to the data. The intention is to ensure the smoothest possible traffic flow under the current conditions. Obstructions due to road repairs, accidents and vehicle breakdowns are also taken into account.

There is usually a control room with the television screens, and a display board showing the colours of the traffic lights in the area. The operator can override the computer instructions if necessary.

In most cities, computer-assisted traffic control systems have improved conditions, though the extent of the improvement is limited by the roads themselves.

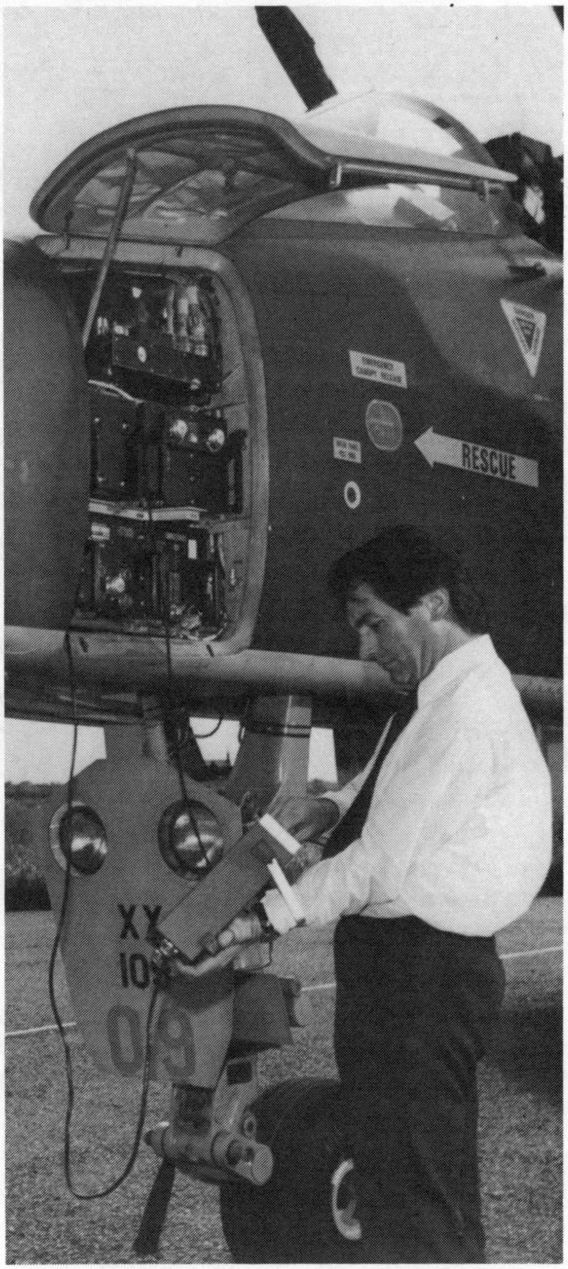

An engineer checks the navigation and weapon aiming computer of a Jaguar fighter plane

Military uses

Much of the development of computers has been for military purposes. Research teams, working in secret, laid the foundations of modern computers during the Second World War. The threat of a third world war has been a major incentive for computer research.

The first use for military computers was to calculate ballistic tables, used in firing shells and dropping bombs. This use has extended to the guidance of missiles, many of which carry on-board computers.

The storage and processing of military information is now done largely by computers. This data can be accessed to aid military decisions and planning.

Modern warships and submarines have on-board computers to assist with navigation, assessment of radar and sonar data, and weapons guidance. The tendency is towards several small computers in different parts of the vessel, to make it more difficult to put the whole system out of action. Small computers are sometimes fitted in tanks and aeroplanes.

Military computers are in constant readiness to assess the significance of a tank buildup along some border, or direct the strike-by-strike progress of an all-out nuclear war.

Space research

Space research and exploration has been one of the most challenging applications of computers, where little would have been achieved without

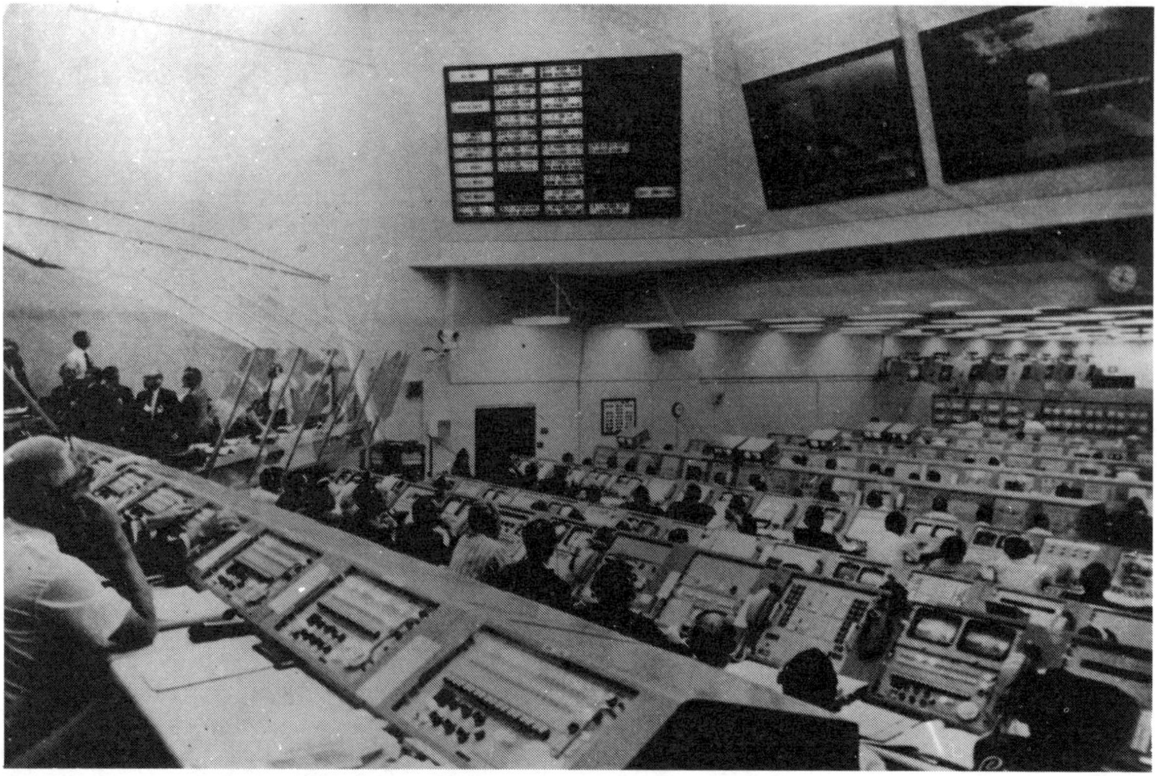

Banks of computerized equipment at the launch control centre of an Apollo moon mission

them. Because of the high standards required, many of the computers and programs developed for space research have found applications elsewhere.

Different types of computers are required for different purposes: The guidance of rockets and satellites in flight requires extremely complex calculations to be done very quickly. The Saturn rockets carrying Apollo spacecraft need twenty five steering instructions per second, provided by an on-board computer in the third stage. The docking of manned space vehicles and the soft landings on the moon and on Mars require very sophisticated computers in the craft. The new generation of manned U.S.A. spacecraft, the orbiting-flying space shuttle (code named Enterprise), has four linked computers on board to assist with control and navigation.

On-board computers are compact, very fast, reliable, and able to withstand the rigours of space. On the other hand they are not very versatile, only being able to carry out a small number of programs. These programs are on permanent storage.

On the ground, very large computers provide the overall control of a space flight and assist with the co-ordination of all the preparatory work. Much of the administration of the projects is done with computers.

At the height of the Apollo space program, there were over one hundred computers in use.

Weather forecasting

A very large computer system at Bracknell in Berkshire processes weather data for much of the northern hemisphere, providing the basis for forecasts.

Twice a day, information such as pressure, temperature, wind speed and direction, amount of rainfall and extent of cloud cover, is supplied by a large number of observation posts in the northern hemisphere, and by weather satellites. The information is sorted, and then used in an extremely complicated program to predict the same figures over the next 24 or 36 hours. In spite of the complexity of the program, weather charts are available two hours after the information has been received.

The staff at the weather centre can make alterations during the running of the program. They use the output as the basis for their forecasts.

A medium range forecasting system is also

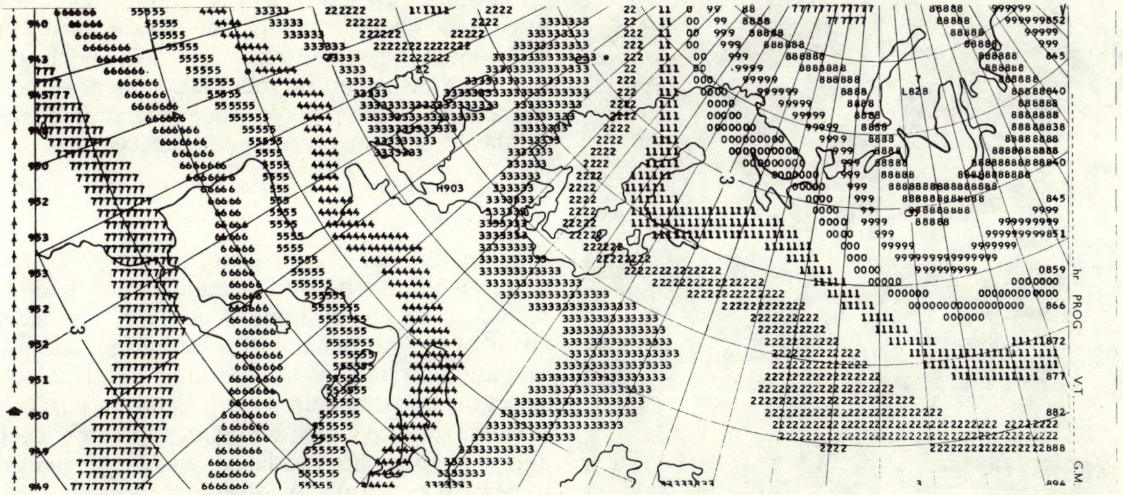

A weather map produced by a computer

planned. It will use two extremely large computers to provide a daily forecast covering four to fifteen days in advance.

Computers have changed weather forecasting from an art to a science. Short term predictions are more reliable (about 75% accurate) and long term predictions (up to weeks ahead) are possible.

Newspaper production

Newspaper production is an example of an application of computers that has been delayed because of the large number of redundancies, and the entire disappearance of some jobs, that it will cause.

The traditional newspaper production process involves the reporter typing the first copy of a story, which is then edited (and often retyped) and sent to be typeset. Advertisements are similarly processed two or three times. Pages are assembled from prints of articles and advertisements.

The computerized system reduces the number of times the information must be typed. Reporters input their news items on a visual display unit, which copies the data onto a magnetic disc.

Editors use another VDU to access the data and amend it. Headings are added, and a program arranges the columns and calculates the space needed.

The page layouts are prepared on another VDU, called a page view terminal. This displays a scaled down image of an entire page. The operator adjusts various combinations of articles to produce the best fit. The final page arrangement is then passed automatically to an on-line printing process.

Changing to a computerized system will involve a large amount of money spent on equipment (estimated at over £50 million for the Fleet Street newspapers), but will bring big savings in running costs. Far fewer staff will be needed, and traditional skills such as typesetting will disappear.

For these reasons, several trade unions have effectively blocked the change to computers in most large British newspapers. For example, one of the reasons for the suspension of publication of the London 'Times' newspaper in November 1978, was the opposition by staff to the introduction of a computerized production process. However it seems that the union action will only delay the change, but not prevent it.

Navigation

Several ships, including Cunard's QE2, have on-board computers to assist with navigation.

The computer receives a radio signal from an orbiting satellite which enables it to calculate the position of the ship very accurately. There are several navigation satellites in very precise orbits passing over the poles. One of these passes within range of the ship every twenty minutes or so.

If it is supplied with additional data about the destination, the positions of any obstacles, and wind and sea conditions, the computer can calculate the course of the ship. It provides a route that will use as little fuel as possible.

An order processing system

This system, used by a modern book publishing company, is a typical example of a commercial

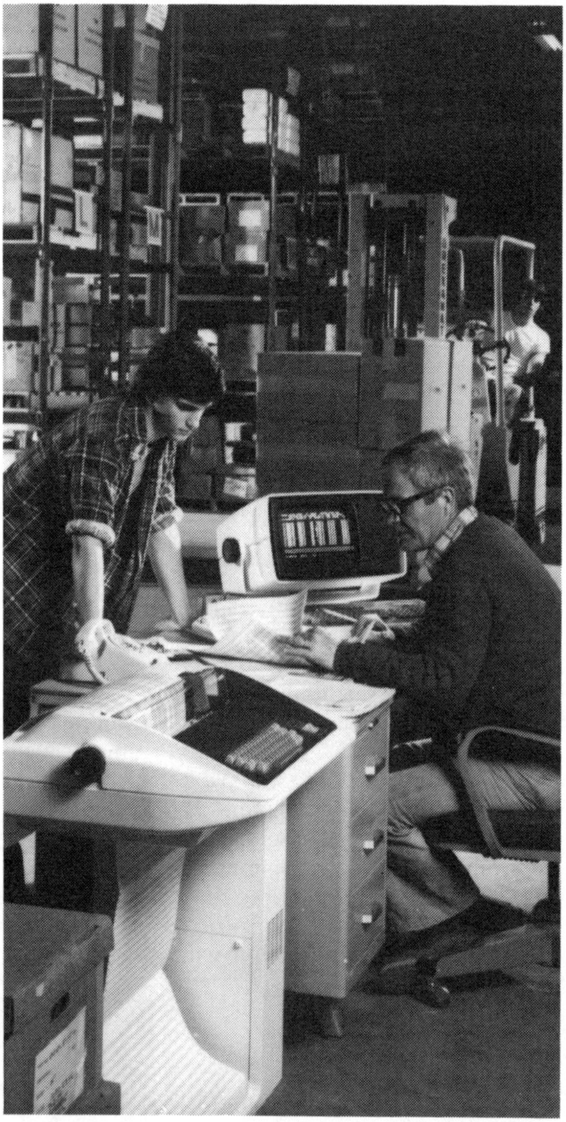

An order processing system, using a Data General minicomputer

application of a small computer. It is described in some detail.

The publishers supply books from their warehouse to booksellers. Several thousand titles are available, and hundreds of orders are received every week from a large number of customers.

The computer includes a visual display unit linked to a central processor, with magnetic disc backing store, and a line printer using special stationery.

For each order received, several items of information are input:

☐ The customer's name and address, which is checked against the file of customers.

☐ The first few letters of the author's name and title of each book ordered. The book is looked up in the index, stored on a magnetic disc, and the full reference displayed on the VDU screen. If there are several possible books, their references are all displayed, and the correct one is selected.

☐ The quantity ordered is entered next to the corresponding book title.

From this data, an invoice, packing note and parcel label are printed. Details of the sale are recorded on the customer's account. The stock levels of the various books are adjusted, and lists prepared for the warehouse staff to be able to select the books required as efficiently as possible.

From time to time, summaries of stock levels and sales totals are produced, enabling managers to be better informed when making decisions.

Word processing

A very promising new development in computers is word processing. Letters, book texts, insurance policies and legal contracts may soon be written, corrected and transmitted by computers, with hardly any paperwork involved at all.

A computer used for word processing includes several visual display units, a line printer and magnetic disc backing store. Systems currently in operation vary considerably in size.

The text is typed and displayed on the VDU screen. Corrections are made by backspacing and overtyping. Various editing facilities enable words, sentences or paragraphs to be inserted or removed, or the order of material to be changed. The final form of the text can be stored, printed or transmitted to another computer.

Smaller systems use modified typewriters connected to cassette tape recorders or floppy disc stores, and visual display screens. As a letter is typed, it is displayed on the screen and recorded magnetically. It can be altered at any stage, and the final, correct version is then printed. Text can be recalled from the store for reprinting or altering.

Links between the word processing computers of different companies may soon provide and electronic mail service.

Information access from your armchair: Ceefax, Oracle and Prestel

The first major use of computers in the home has been information access systems using television sets. In Britain there are two systems, one provided by the television companies (Ceefax from B.B.C. and Oracle from I.T.V.), and the other by the Post

Office (the viewdata system, marketed under the name Prestel).

Ceefax and Oracle

In both of these systems, information stored on computers is braodcast by television transmitters. Each system provides 200 'pages' of up-to-date information (one 'page' occupies the screen of a T.V. set) on such topics as news, weather and sport. A modified T.V. set is needed, with a special dial to select the required page.

Prestel

The Prestel system stores information on a linked network of computers which are accessed by telephone. The information is supplied by a number of information providers, and there is virtually no limit to the number of pages which can be stored. The system started with 50000 pages, and updating and addition of new information is taking place all the time.

The user enters the system by dialling the number of the nearest Prestel computer, and connecting the telephone to the specially adapted television set. Each page of information displayed includes simple instructions on how to access other pages. A Prestel directory is also provided to assist with this. Instructions are given by pressing buttons on a simple, hand-held keypad.

Each Prestel user has a user number, which is also his account number. Apart from the cost of the telephone call, some pages of information cost a few pence to access. Prestel accounts are sent out quarterly. Information providers pay a subscription fee to join, and then a fixed amount per page of information stored.

The range of information stored is enormous. In addition to news, weather and sport, there is information on gardening, forthcoming events, train times, educational courses (including a simple maths test), horoscopes and much else. In addition, users can store simple messages of their own, and send messages ('happy birthday', etc.) to other users.

The Prestel system is part of an international information network, linked by the world telephone system.

Applications in brief

☐ Holiday Inns, the worldwide chain of hotels, use a satellite-linked, computerized communications network for reservations. A reservation can be made at any one of their hotels, anywhere in the world, in a matter of seconds.

☐ The U.S.A.'s nuclear-armed cruise missile carries an on-board computer coupled to a ground scanning radar. The computer guides the missile almost at treetop height to within a few hundred feet of its target, which may be 1500 miles from its launching site.

☐ In California, computers are used to analyse weekly data on soil conditions and crop development. They predict precisely how much moisture the crops need during the next sixty days. This has helped farmers economize on water, and withstand two consecutive years of drought.

☐ A winning idea in the 1978 Rolex Awards for Enterprise competition combines computer technology with surgery. People who have been paralysed by spine injuries will have electrodes inplanted in their leg muscles. Controlled by a tiny computer, these electrodes will transmit control signals to the leg muscles, replacing the signal which have been blocked by the damage to the spine. This could enable many disabled people to walk once again.

☐ Computers are used in the control of Japan's high-speed 'bullet' trains.

☐ A minicomputer has been mounted in a racing car to monitor its performance. It enables the car to be adjusted better to suit the driver and the track.

☐ In an effort to conserve energy, some computer installations in the U.S.A. are using heat generated by their computers to help heat their entire buildings.

Exercise 19

1 Write down the meanings of the following words or phrases:
cheque; EFT; SWIFT;
mathematical modelling; electrocardiograph;
page view terminal; word processing.

2 Find out about other applications of computers, particularly in the following areas:
the Stock Exchange;
controlling production processes in industry;
parliament; education; fire services;
local government;
air traffic control and automatic landing systems;
flight simulators; telephone exchanges.

*__3__ In your opinion, which applications of computers have contributed most to the development of new ideas in computing? Give reasons for your answer.

4 Which applications of computers combine them with other advanced technologies such as radar, satellites, etc.?

5 Suggest some new applications of computers.

6 Try to find an application of computers which has been discontinued, and the computer replaced by a manual system. Write a brief report on the situation.

7 The types of data processing system introduced in Chapter 17 are batch processing, interactive processing and real time processing.

From their descriptions in Chapter 17, classify each of the following applications as one of the three types above:
(a) Cheque clearing
(b) Electronic funds transfer
(c) Traffic control (d) Rocket guidance
(e) Weather forecasting
(f) Newspaper production
(g) Order processing (not all systems are the same type as the one in the text)
(h) Word processing (i) Prestel

8 A chain of supermarkets uses a central supply depot. When a supermarket is running out of goods it places an order for more stock with the central depot.

The central depot collects orders from all the supermarkets in the chain and places orders for large quantities of stock with the suppliers. When the stock arrives at the depot it is distributed to those individual supermarkets that placed the original orders.

The central depot plans to install a computer. Explain how it could be used to help with

(a) the assembly of orders for new stock from the supermarkets,
(b) the placing of orders with the suppliers,
(c) the distribution of stock to the supermarkets.

What additional computing equipment might be installed in individual supermarkets? (WMEB 77 I)

9 Describe, in detail, a computer application with which you are familiar. Include details of data collection, input and output devices used, details of the central processor relevant to the application chosen, storage devices and any important human elements of the system. (AEB 78 specimen)

20

Analogue computers

As mentioned in Chapter 1, there are two types of electronic computers: **digital computers** and **analogue computers.** All the other chapters in the book have been concerned with digital computers. This chapter gives a brief introduction to analogue computers.

In the past, there have been a number of successful mechanical analogue computers. However, virtually all present day analogue computer are electrical. This chapter is mainly concerned with electrical analogue computers.

Representing numbers by electricity

Electricity may be used to represent numbers in one of two ways. One way is to send a series of pulses of current to represent the digits of the number in a binary code. The other way is to have a steady current, where the strength of the current is proportional to the size of the number represented. The first method is used by digital computers, the second by analogue computers. See Figure 20.1.

A further point to be made in connection with Figure 20.1 is this: The presence or absence of two digital pulses can be made to represent the numbers 0, 1, 2, or 3. No numbers between these values can be represented. The digital method is a **discrete** way of representing data.

On the other hand, the steady, analogue current can represent any value in the range 0 to 3. The analogue method is a **continuous** way of representing data.

Time variation

If a quantity varies with time, an analogue representation of the quantity has several advantages

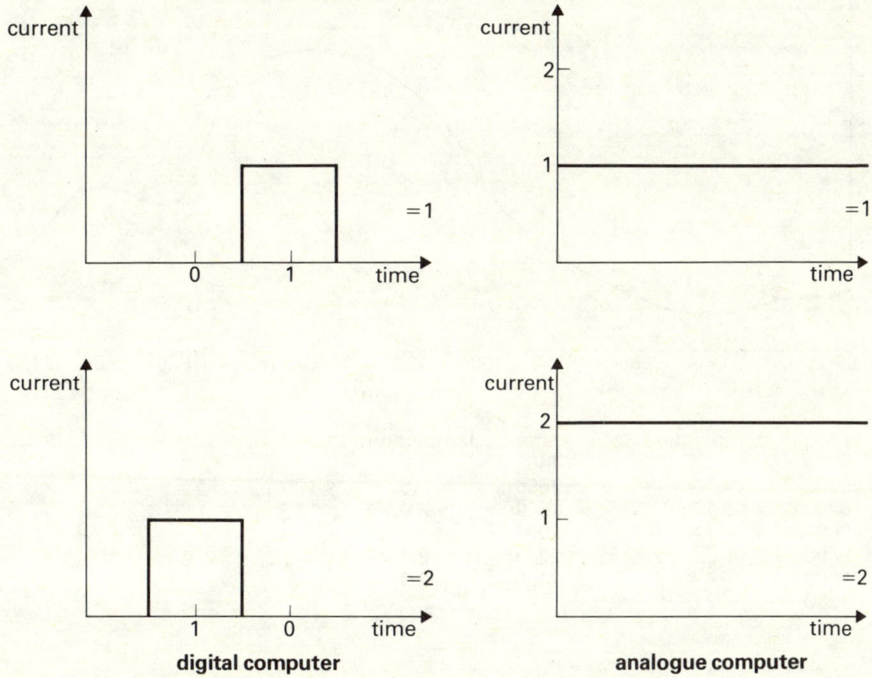

Fig. 20.1: Analogue and digital methods of representing data by electricity

over a digital representation. For example, consider the variation of temperature at a particular place over a period of 24 hours.

An analogue representation of this data could be a graph, drawn directly by a special type of thermometer, showing the precise temperature at any time. A digital representation of this data could be a set of temperatures, accurate to (say) 0.1°C, taken at regular intervals (say 2 hourly). See Figure 20.2.

In a similar way, analogue currents can be made to vary with time to represent a changing physical quantity.

Features of analogue computers

Electrical analogue computers are based on the fact that electric circuits can be set up to behave in a way similar to physical systems. For example, a circuit may be set up to behave like water flowing in a pipe. See Figure 20.3.

The flow of current in the wire is proportional to the flow of water in the pipe.

Analogue computers consist of a large number of electrical components such as resitors, sources of voltage, switches, etc. They are programmed by connecting these components to form circuits. The circuits behave in a similar way to the system which the computer represents.

Data is input by setting the voltages, resistances, etc. at appropriate levels. Meters are connected at suitable points in the circuit to provide output. It is rather difficult to store information in electrical analogue form. Analogue computers do not usually have any form of backing store.

Hybrid computers

Analogue and digital units are sometimes combined in a single computer. The combination is called a **hybrid** computer. A common combination is digital input, output and backing store, and analogue processing.

The link, or interface, between the analogue and the digital units is provided by an **analogue-to-digital converter** (ADC). It converts a digital input signal to an analogue output signal, and vice versa. See Figure 20.4.

(a)

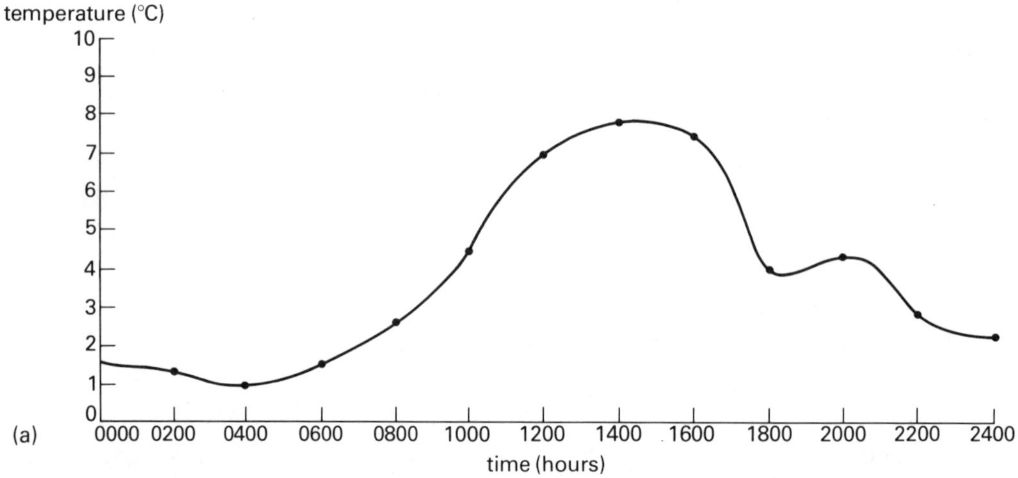

(b)

time	temperature	time	temperature
0000	1.6	1400	7.9
0200	1.2	1600	7.5
0400	1.0	1800	4.0
0600	1.4	2000	4.3
0800	2.6	2200	2.7
1000	4.4	2400	2.2
1200	7.0		

Fig. 20.2: (a) Analogue representation of time-varying data, (b) Digital representation of time-vary data

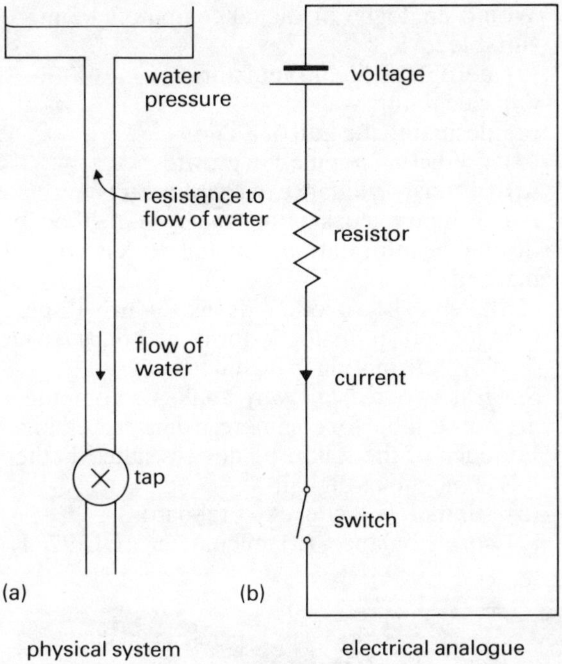

Fig. 20.3: An electrical analogue of a physical system (a) Physical system, (b) Electrical analogue

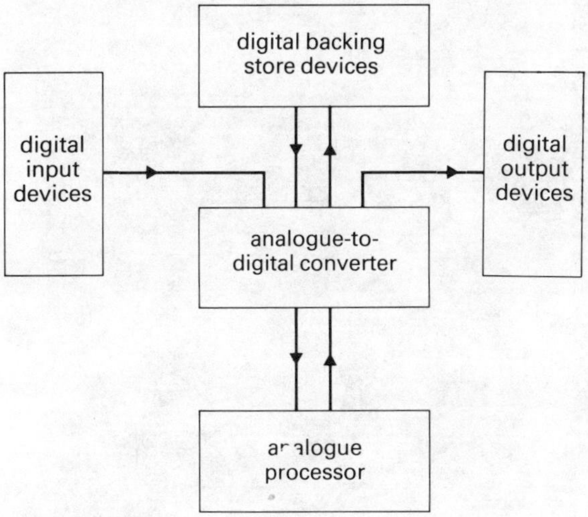

Fig. 20.4: A hybrid computer

Applications

Analogue computers are mainly used for scientific and engineering purposes. They have no commercial applications.

Uses of analogue or hybrid computers include aeroplane design and flight simulators, monitoring and controlling chemical processes (see Figure 20.5) and steelmaking, design and testing of hydraulic systems, heat flow problems, and military uses such as anti-aircraft gun aiming. However digital computers, because of their lower costs, are replacing analogue computers in many applications.

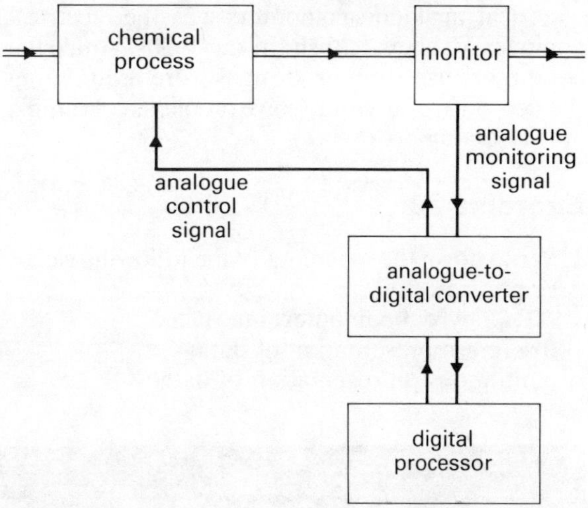

Fig. 20.5: A hybrid computer monitoring and controlling a chemical process

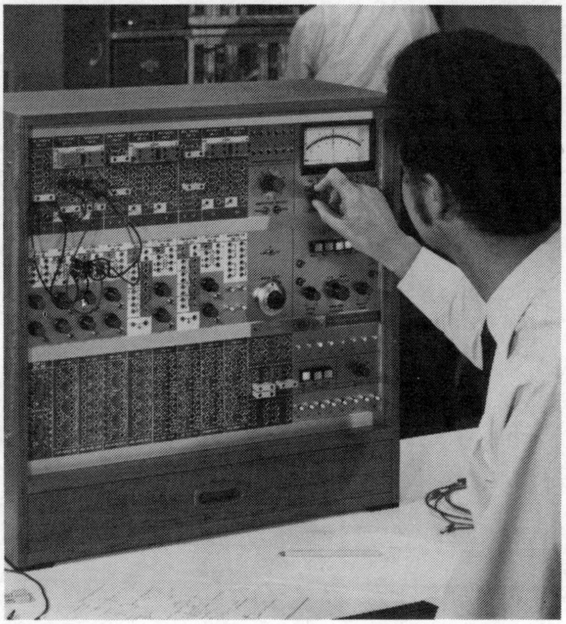

A desk-top analogue computer made by Electronic Associates

History

One of the first analogue calculating devices was the slide rule, invented by William Oughtred in 1620.

The first analogue computers were mechanical, using trains of gears for their working. A well-known model used Meccano parts. An early mechanical analogue computer was the tide simulator, made by Lord Kelvin in 1872.

A major contributor to the development of electrical analogue computers was the electrical engineer Vannevar Bush, in the 1930s. Analogue computers based on his designs were used during the Second World War to solve problems concerning anti-aircraft guns.

Exercise 20

1 Write down the meanings of the following words or phrases:
ADC; hybrid computer; interface;
discrete representation of data;
continuous representation of data.

2 Would analogue or digital computers be more suitable for:
(a) aeroplane flight simulators,
(b) calculating wages,
(c) designing the hull of a ship,
(d) predicting population growth,
(e) on-board guidance of space rockets.

3 An ordinary clock is an analogue method of displaying information, a digital clock is a digital method.

Make a list of other devices which display information in analogue form, and ones which display information in digital form.

4 Suggest two reasons why analogue computers are not suitable for commercial data processing.

5 For each of the following devices state whether it is analogue or digital:
(a) sundial, (b) cricket scoreboard,
(c) spring balance, (d) mileometer. (OLE 76 I)

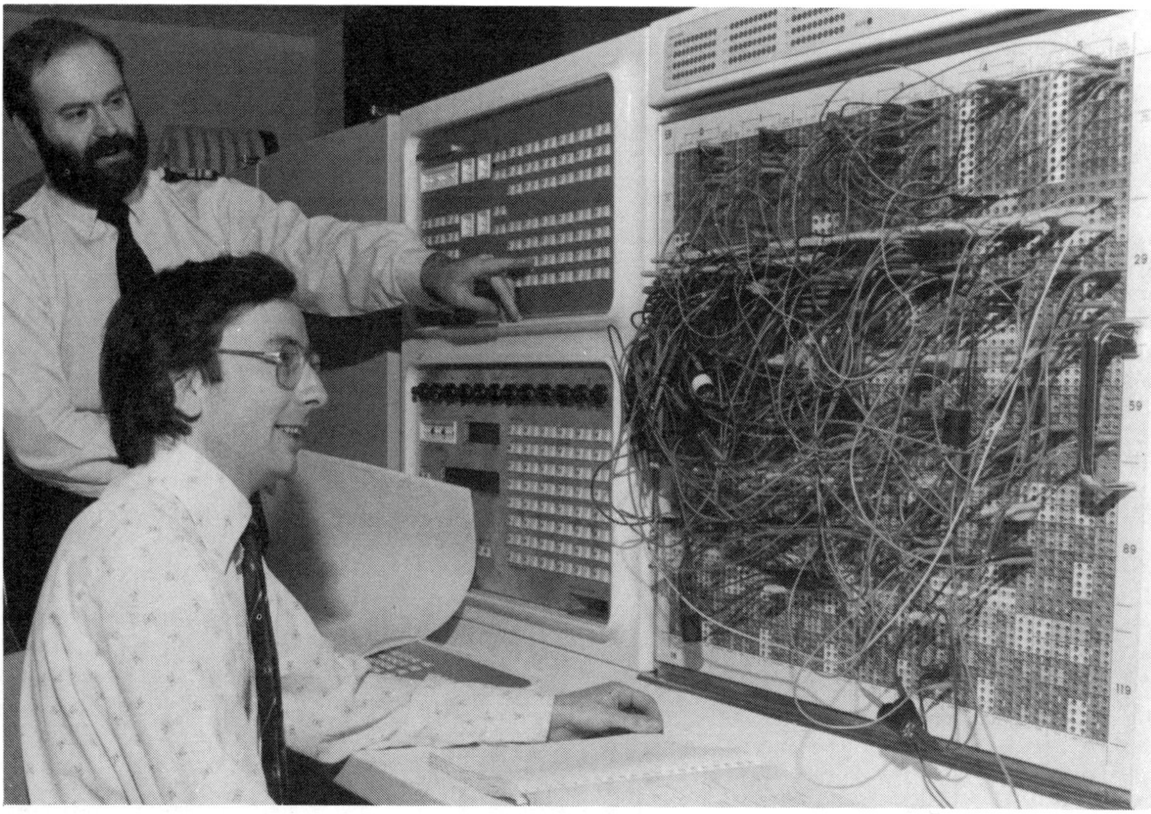

A hybrid computer in use at the Royal Naval College, London

21

The history of computers

Although most of the work on electronic computers has been done in the last thirty years, their origins can be traced in ideas and inventions over several centuries. There have been three phases in the development of computers – the early work on mechanical calculating devices by such men as Napier, Pascal and Leibnitz, the work of Jacquard, Babbage, Hollerith and others to establish the principles of information processing, and the extremely rapid progress of electronic machines during and after the Second World War.

The first phase: Mechanical calculators

The first calculating aid was undoubtedly the fingers. For counting larger numbers (particularly of sheep or cattle) pebbles were moved from one pile to another, a practice still followed in some areas. This led to the development of the **abacus,** using beads moving along strings. The origins of the abacus are obscure, and various forms seem to have been put to use independently in different places. The abacus makes use of the idea of place value, and counting in groups. A bead stands for one, or ten, or one hundred, etc., depending on the row it is in.

Counting in other bases followed. The first known user of binary numbers was Francis Bacon in 1623.

John Napier (1550 to 1617)

This Scottish mathematician invented logarithms in 1614 to assist multiplication and division, and a set of rods (Napier's bones) also as an aid to multiplication. Each rod contains a multiplication table. Figure 21.1 shows how they are used.

Blaise Pascal (1623 to 1662)

One of the earliest known calculating machines was designed and constructed by the French mathematician Blaise Pascal in 1642. Using toothed wheels, and a special mechanism for carrying, it was used for tax calculations. Its disadvantage was that it would only add or subtract.

Gottfried von Leibnitz (1646 to 1716)

A further advance in mechanical calculating devices was made when, in 1671, this famous

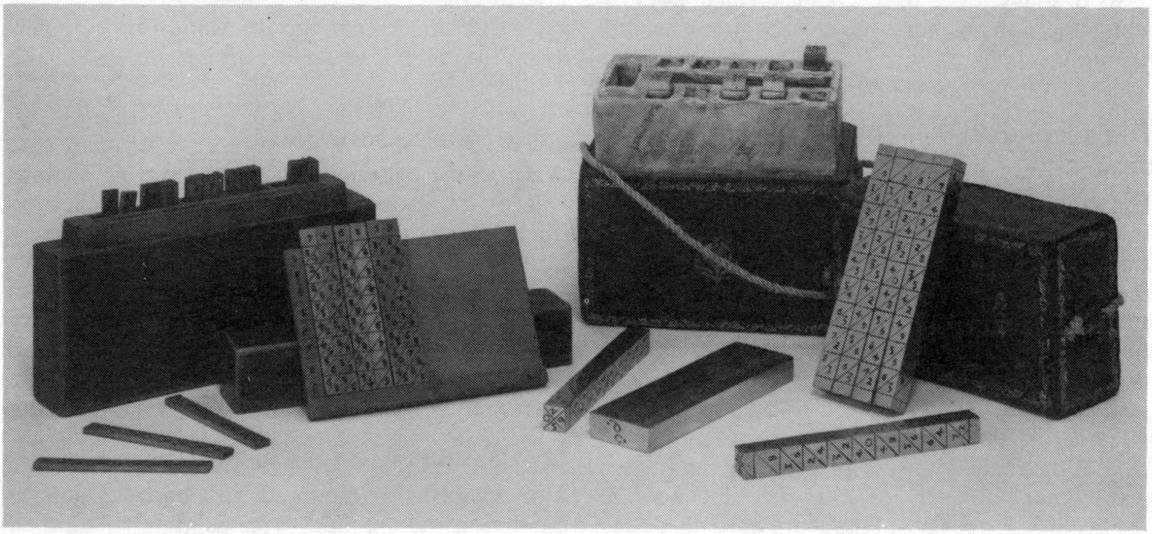

A set of Napier's bones

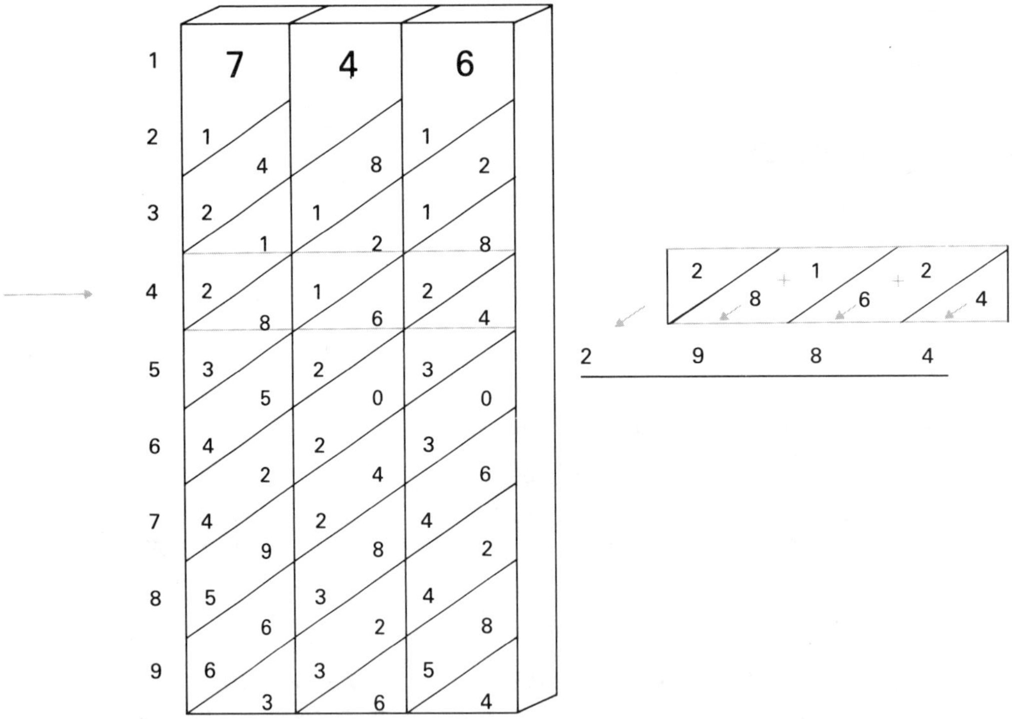

The numbers in the 4th row are added diagonally to give the answer: 2 9 8 4.

Fig. 21.1: The calculation 726 × 4 done using Napier's bones

German philospher and mathematician invented a machine capable of multiplication and division, as well as addition and subtraction. It also used toothed wheels.

The machines of Pascal and Leibnitz formed the basis of many types of mechanical calculators, of which the cash register is the most common current example.

The second phase: Towards information processing

The next phase of computer development moved away from pure calculation, and established the idea of information processing. During this period, manual methods of storing large quantities of information, such as ledger cards, were being developed. Many of these manual processes were later to be replaced by computers.

Joseph Jacquard (1752 to 1834)

One of the first advances was made by the French textile manufacturer Joseph Marie Jacquard in about 1802. Large sets of numbers were needed to enable his looms to weave complex patterns. He devised a system of punching holes in cards to store the numbers, and mechanically reading these numbers by a device connected to the loom. A binary code was used – a hole meant that a warp thread had to be raised, no hole meant that it was not raised.

Jacquard's system soon became very popular. Many looms based on his design are still in use today.

Fairground steam organs

Another use of punched paper to store instructions was on fairground steam organs, from the mid nineteenth century onwards. These organs had a large number of pipes and other instruments, all of which were controlled by holes in a wide roll of paper, as it was wound through the control box of the organ. Different patterns of holes produced different pieces of music, some of which were extremely complex.

Charles Babbage (1792 to 1871)

The English mathematician Charles Babbage combined the method of calculating by toothed gear mechanisms with that of storing information

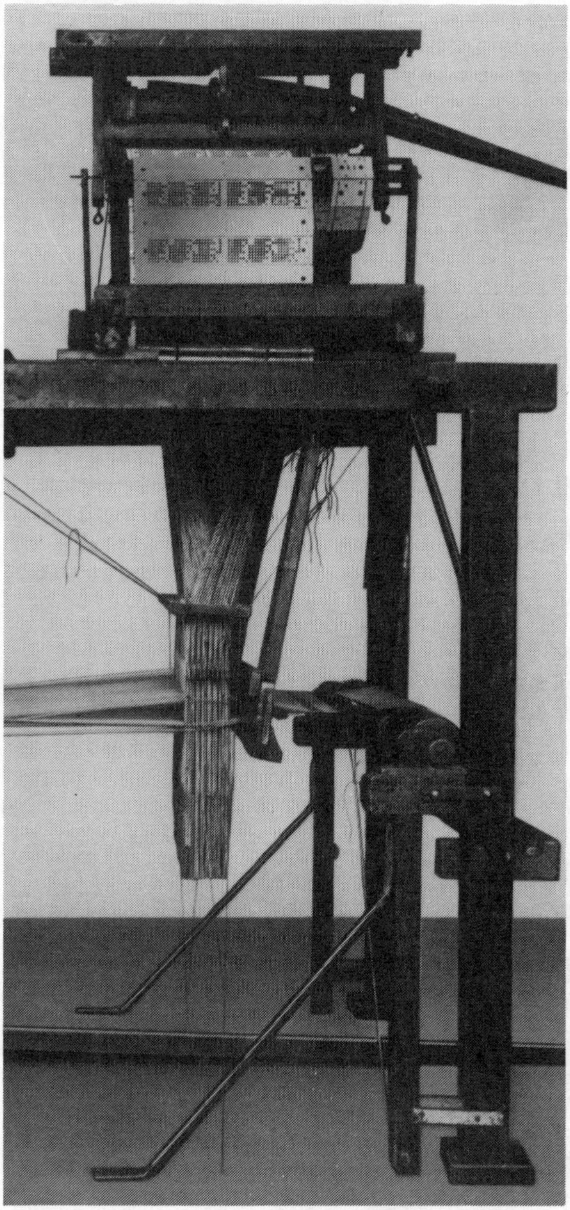

The punched card control device on a Jacquard loom

on punched cards. He also introduced the idea of a program, and of input and output.

His first device, the **Difference Engine,** was based on the idea of differences of a polynomial. Starting with one value of a polynomial, it could calculate others by the various differences. A small working model was built in 1822.

Babbage's second machine, the **Analytical Engine,** designed in 1834, was the first device to use many ideas found in modern computers. A general purpose calculating machine, it had input

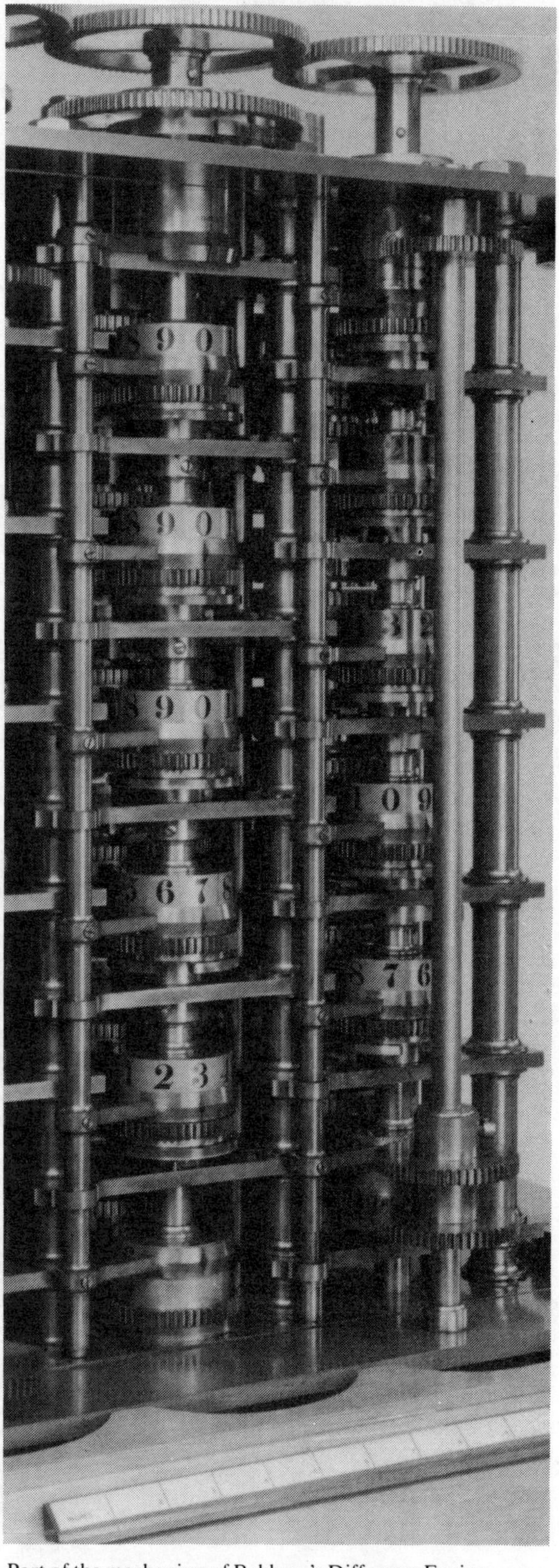

Part of the mechanism of Babbage's Difference Engine

and output devices, and a processing unit (called a **mill**), using toothed wheels. Furthermore, it could be programmed.

Unfortunately Babbage's design proved too difficult to construct during his lifetime. Almost a hundred years passed before many of his ideas were put into practice, on electronic machines.

Countess of Lovelace

One of the few women to feature in the development of computers was Augusta Ada Byron, daughter of the poet Lord Byron, and later the Countess of Lovelace. She wrote detailed notes describing the workings of the Analytical Engine, including programs to be run on it.

George Boole (1810 to 1864)

An important step towards the logical design of computers was made by George Boole in 1847 when he devised a system of algebra which could be used to describe and manipulate logical expressions.

Hermann Hollerith (1860 to 1929)

The application of automatic data processing techniques made a significant advance when Dr. Hermann Hollerith used a punched card system and mechanical calculators (called tabulators) to store and process information for the U.S.A. Census of 1890. It was realized that a manual processing system would not have the results ready before the 1900 Census, but Hollerith's system took only three years, in spite of the increased population, as the table below shows:

	1880	1890
U.S.A. population	50 million	63 million
Time to complete census	7 years	3 years

To market his machines (including card punches, sorters and tabulators) he formed the Hollerith Tabulating Machine Company in 1897. Through a series of mergers, this became part of International Business Machines in 1911.

In the meantime, Hollerith's assistant, Powers, formed his own company which eventually became part of International Computers Limited.

Semi-automatic business machines

Following the work of Hollerith and others at the turn of the century, a large number of machines for

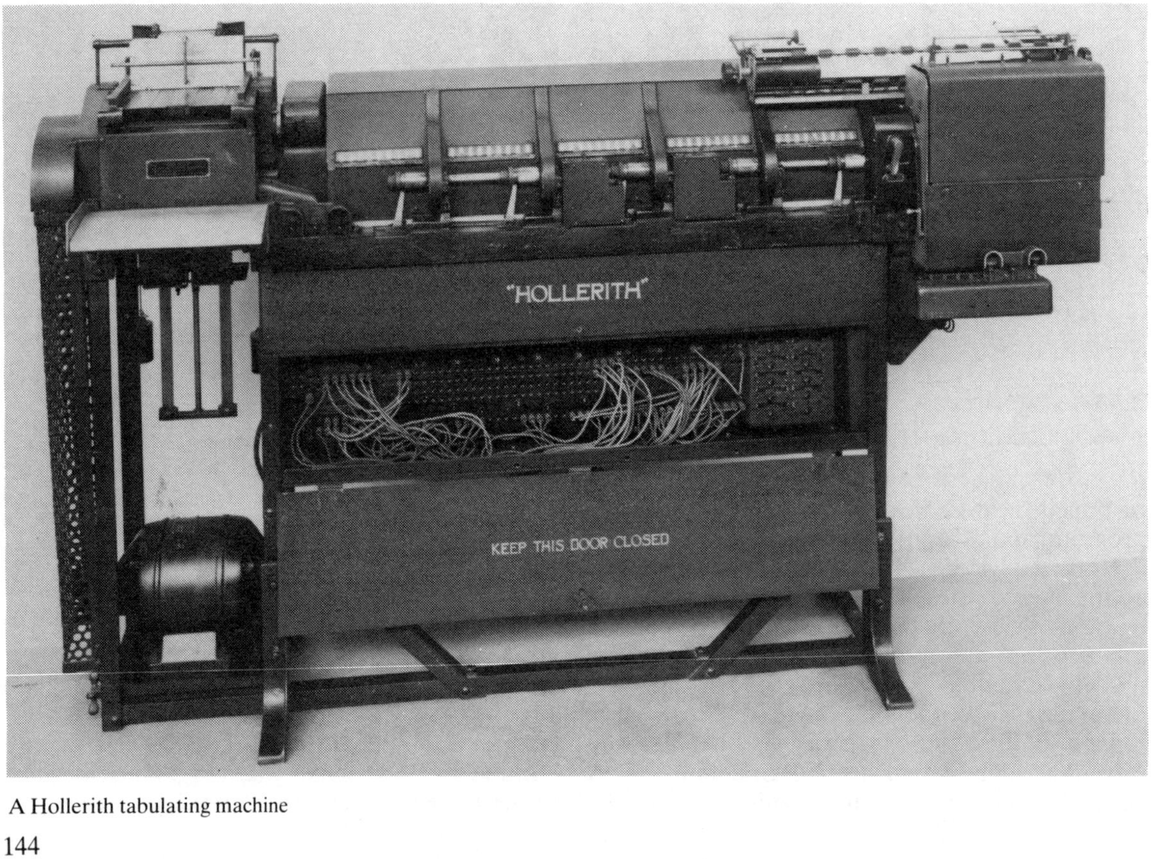

A Hollerith tabulating machine

doing routine commercial work were devised. These machines could perform calculations, and store limited amounts of information. They were driven by electric motors, and used gears and levers to calculate. Input and output was on printed ledger cards, sometimes with magnetic stripes to store data.

Experience of using these machines made it easier for firms to change to electronic machines in the 1950s and 1960s.

Hardware developments

At about this time, there were a number of developments in the field of electronics, which were later to have great significance for computers. In about 1900, recording devices using magnetic tape or magnetic drums were developed by Valdemar Poulsen, and in 1906, the valve was invented by Lee de Forest.

Alan Turing (1912 to 1954)

In 1937, the British mathematician Alan Turing proved that a fairly small set of simple instructions is all that is needed to solve any problem, no matter how complex, as long as it has a logical solution. Thus a simple computing machine, working very fast, can solve problems of great complexity.

Claude Shannon

Following Boole's work, Claude Shannon, an electrical engineer, showed, in 1938, that electrical switching circuits can perform logical operations, and their working can be described by the same algebra as Boole used to describe logical expressions.

The third phase: World war two and beyond

Much progress had now been made along several lines:

- ☐ Information could be stored in a binary code.
- ☐ The logic of combining binary coded information was known.
- ☐ The idea of a program was established, and it was known that simple instructions could be combined to solve complex problems.
- ☐ Electrical devices had been invented which could carry out these processes.

The combination of these separate lines led to the very rapid development of computers after 1940. With the Second World War forcing the pace, a number of pioneering computers were produced in a short space of time.

Konrad Zuse

It appears that several electronic computers, capable of storing programs, were developed during the war by Konrad Zuse, in Germany. The first operational machine, the Z3, was working in 1941, the second, the Z4, was used for design calculations for flying bombs. However these machines were all destroyed by Allied bombing.

Codebreaking at Bletchley Park

At the same time, the British Intelligence Establishment at Bletchley Park, with a staff including Alan Turing and other computer pioneers, developed the COLOSSUS machine. Coming into operation in 1943, it had 1500 valves, and was used to crack Germany's top secret ENIGMA code.

ASCC

Working on an IBM scholarship at Harvard University, U.S.A., Howard Aiken completed the Automatic Sequence-Controlled Calculator (ASCC) in 1944. An electro-mechanical device, using standard tabulating machine parts driven by electric motors, it could store sixty numbers (in base ten) and took four seconds for one multiplication. It had paper tape or keyboard input (for instructions and data) and punched cards or keyboard output. Programs could not be stored.

ENIAC

An early electronic calculating machine was the Electronic Numerical Integrator and Calculator (ENIAC), produced by a team led by J. Presper Eckert and John Mauchly at the University of Pennsylvania in 1946. It had eighteen thousand valves, stored twenty numbers (using base ten) and could add two numbers in two hundred microseconds. Programmed by connecting up a large number of wires, it was used to calculate ballistic trajectories (paths or bombs or rockets), and later for calculations concerned with the development of the hydrogen bomb.

Von Neumann: The general principles of computers

The biggest step forward in computer design since the work of Charles Babbage came when the general requirements of a computer were summarized in 1946 by John Von Neumann. His two main points were:

- ☐ Data and instructions are coded as binary digits and stored together in the computer. No distinction is made between them.

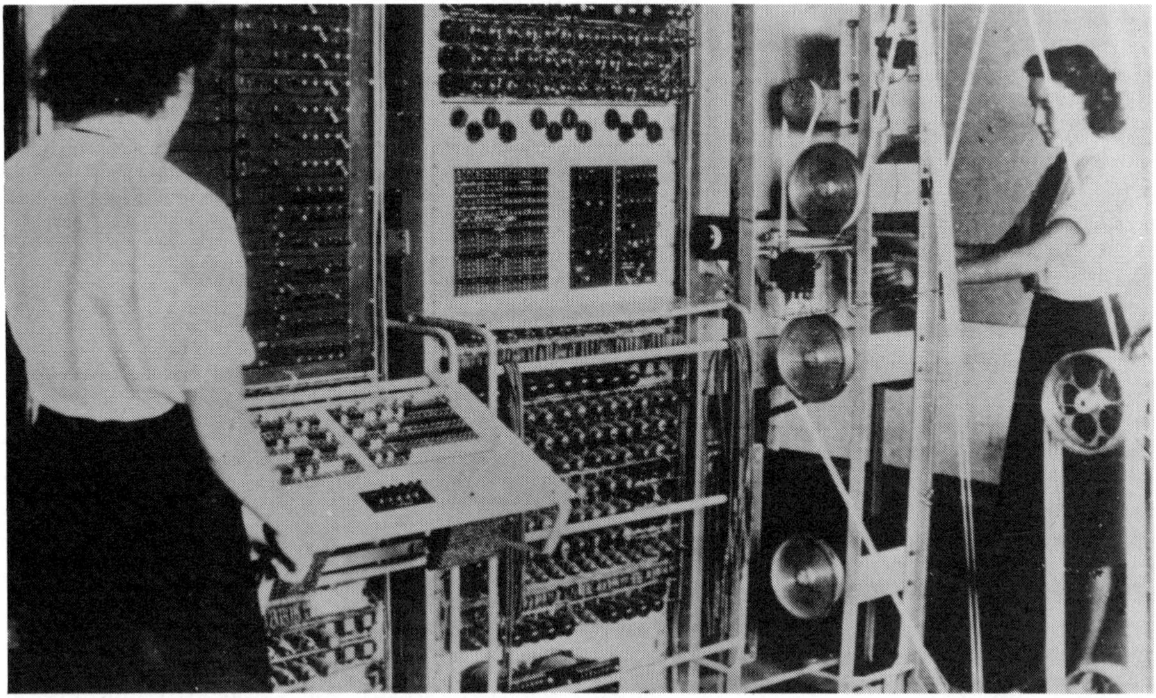

The COLOSSUS computer at work during the Second World War

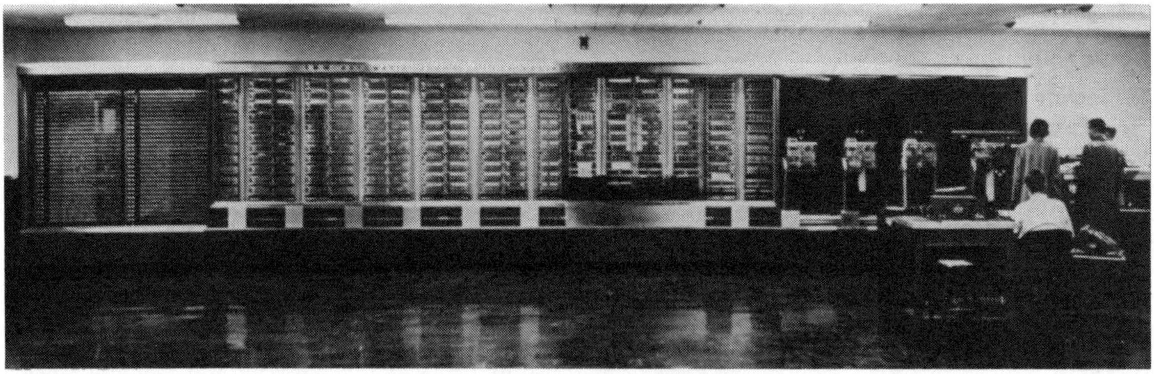

The IBM Automatic Sequence Controlled Calculator at Harvard University in 1944

☐ The computer processes both data and instructions.

Von Neumann's principles have formed the basis of all subsequent electronic computers.

Manchester University mark 1

One of the first computers based on Von Neumann's principles was completed in 1948 by F. C. Williams, T. Kilburn and G. C. Toothill at Manchester University. It was a small general purpose machine, with keyboard input, visual display output, 32 word binary memory, and could store a program. It worked at 1.2 milliseconds per instruction.

EDSAC, EDVAC and ACE

These were general purpose computers with stored program capability, and working in binary. EDSAC (Electronic Delay Storage Automatic Computer) was designed by M. V. Wilkes at Cambridge University. Using 3800 valves, and mercury tubes (called tanks) to store numbers, it ran its first program on 6th May, 1949.

EDVAC (Electronic Discreet Variable Automatic Computer) was developed at the University of Pennsylvania, after the completion of ENIAC. Von Neumann played a major part in its design. It came into operation in 1950.

ACE (Automatic Computing Engine) was built

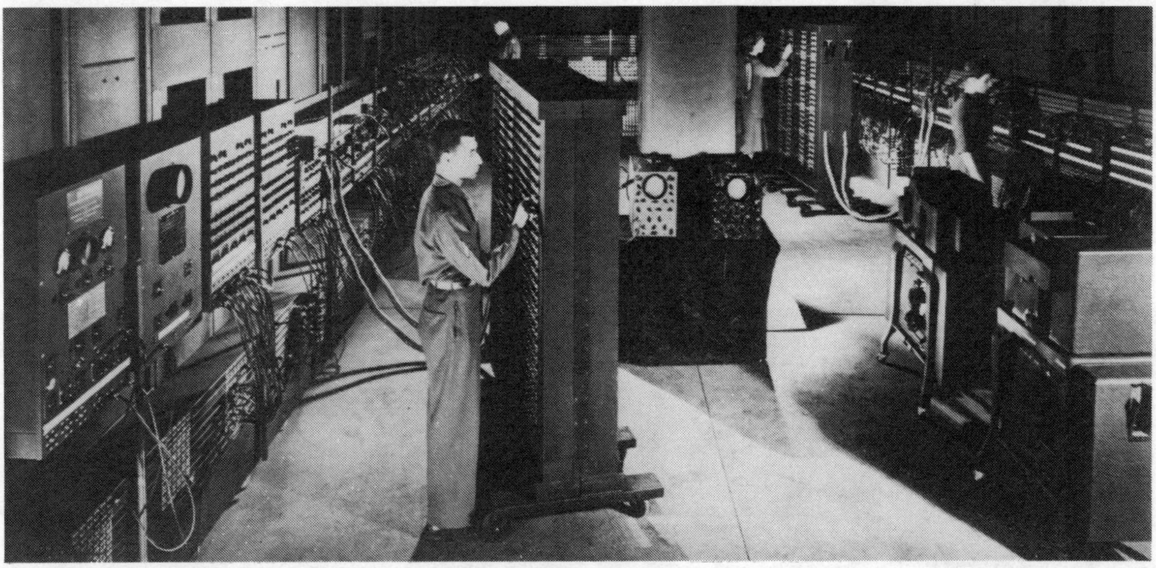

The ENIAC computer in operation

by Wormsley, Turing and Colebrook at the National Physical Laboratory (U.K.) in 1951. It was one of the fastest early computers.

Developments in Europe, Asia and the Far East

By 1950, computers had been completed in Sweden, the Netherlands, Switzerland and West Germany. In the next decade, Denmark, Norway, France, Austria, Belgium, the U.S.S.R., Czechoslovakia, Poland, Japan, Israel, Rumania and India followed suit.

These were mainly small research computers, but all could store programs.

Commercial applications: LEO and UNIVAC

Although the first electronic computers were designed and built at universities and research establishments, their commercial potential was soon realized. Several university workers moved into this field.

In 1951, Lyons Electric Office (LEO), constructed by M. V. Wilkes, began commerical work for J. M. Lyons, the teashop firm. It had puched card or paper tape input, 2048 (2 K) of main store, and output on a line printer or punched cards. It was programmed in machine language, and operated at one thousand instructions per second. An improved version, LEO Mark 2, followed fairly soon afterwards. Several of these computers were built.

In the U.S.A., Eckert and Mauchly formed a company, and produced the first of the UNIVAC (Universal Accounting Machine) series in 1951. UNIVAC 1 was for the U.S.A. Census Bureau. The company later became part of the Remington Rand group.

IBM

The company with the largest share of the world computer market, International Business Machines, was formed in 1911 from three business machine companies (including Hollerith's). Directed by Thomas J. Watson from 1914 to 1956, it initially produced commercial scales, tabulating and time recording equipment.

Its first commercial computer was the IBM 701 in 1952. Because its worldwide network for selling, servicing and leasing business machines was firmly established when computers were first introduced, it was in an ideal position to dominate the world computer market, which it has done consistently. It is one of the largest companies in the world, with profits of 3.1 billion dollars in 1978.

Transistors and the second generation of computers

Once the general principles of computer design had been established, intensive research was aimed at smaller, faster machines. A limitation on all the computers previously mentioned – now known as first generation machines – was their use of valves, which are large, create a large amount of heat, and need frequent replacement.

The invention of the transistor in 1948 by William Shockley signalled the beginning of the second

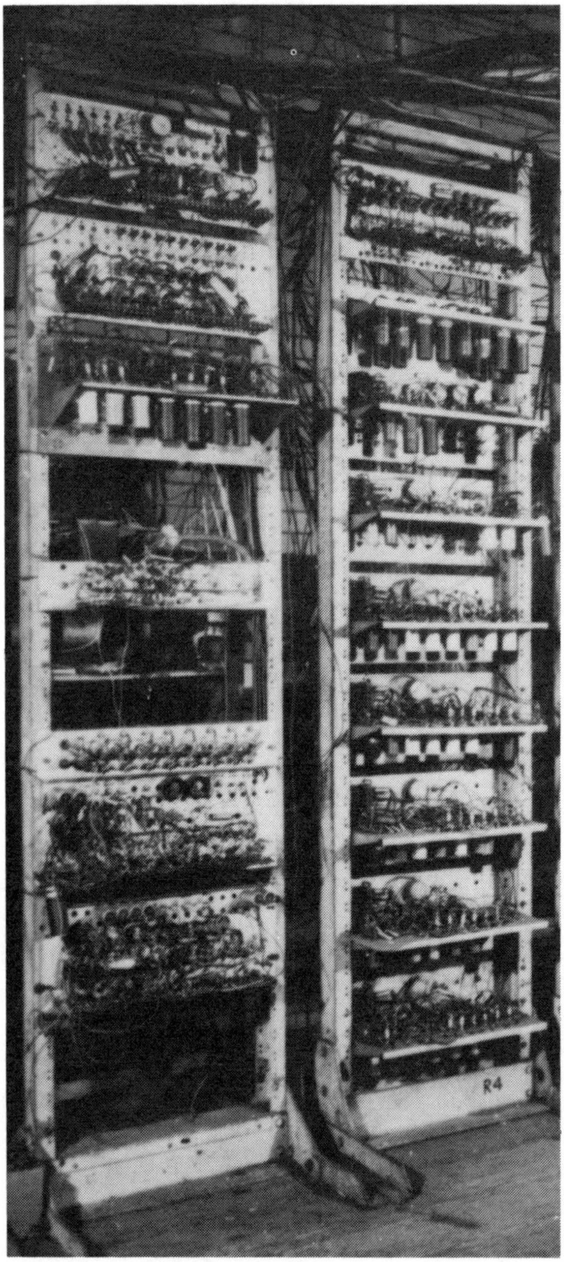

Part of the logic circuits of the Manchester University Mark 1 computer

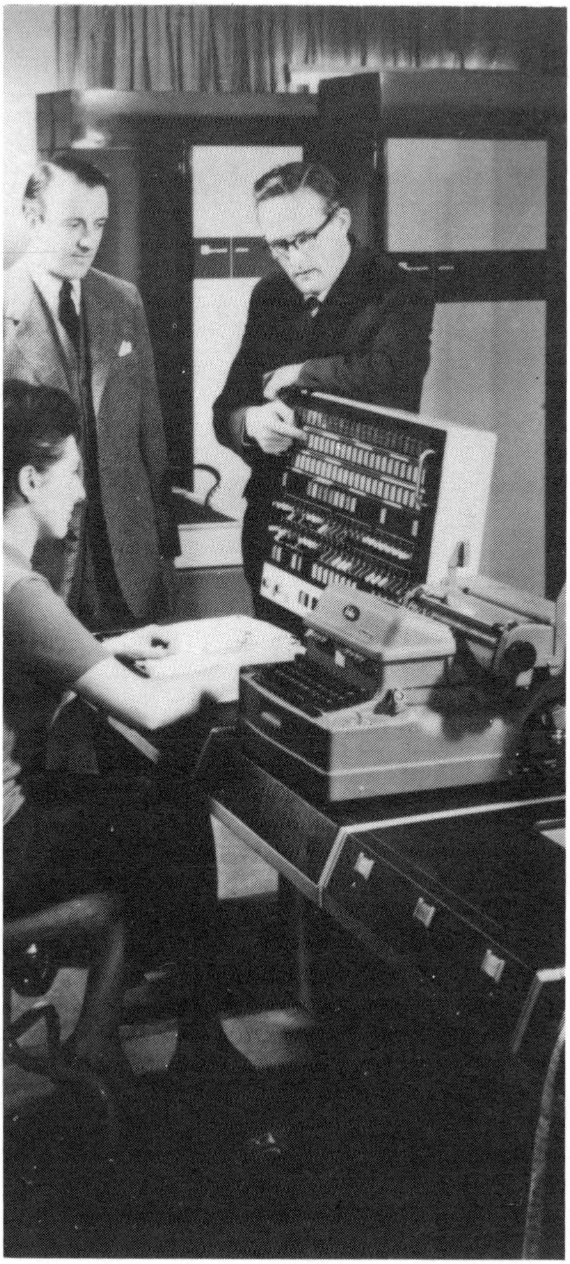

The operator's console of the Atlas computer

generation of computers. First marketed in 1956, early examples of computers using transistors were the TXO from Massachusetts Institute of Technology, the IBM 7000 series, and LEO Mark 3.

A significant development at this time was the ALTAS computer from Manchester University in 1962. A powerful, general purpose machine, it was the first computer to use magnetic disc backing store in such as way that it appeared to have a much larger memory than it actually had. It also had read-only memory for storing constant information.

During the second generation, the idea emerged of a series of computers, with different units which could be interchanged to suit the particular needs of the computer user, and allow for expansion if necessary. Most computer manufacturers now follow this principle.

Computer languages

All the first generation computers had to be programmed in machine code – a slow, laborious process. The first improvement was to replace each binary machine instruction with a code word using letters, and a memory address using letters or decimal numbers. The assembly languages thus formed were translated into machine code by a program called an assembler before processing. (See Chapter 13.)

Very soon afterwards came a much bigger advance with the development of high level languages, the first being FORTRAN in 1957. ALGOL and COBOL were introduced in 1960, with PL1 following in about 1965.

The most recent tendency has been towards increased capability (more done by a single statement) and languages which are easier to use. The educational language BASIC (introduced in 1964) the commercial language RPG and the scientific language APL (1968) are examples of this.

The third generation

A further reduction in size and increase in speed was achieved by the combination of several transistors and other components into integrated circuits. Third generation computers, using these circuits, first became available in 1964, the IBM 360 series being one of the most successful.

Since then, the direction of development has been towards large scale integrated circuits, sometimes equivalent to thousands of components. This has led to even smaller computers, known as microcomputers, with the same capabilities as the large systems of a few years ago. A computer with the same capability as ENIAC could now be contained in a shoebox.

The microprocessor revolution

The most recent phase in the development of computers has been called the **microprocessor revolution.** Starting in about 1972, there has been an increasing output of tiny, cheap microintegrated circuits from a number of manufacturers, mainly situated in California ('Silicon Valley') U.S.A.

These circuits use **large scale integration** (LSI), and contain thousands of components. They are usually about a quarter of an inch square, and very thin. Many of them contain all the components of a CPU: timing circuits, control circuits, an arithmetic and logic unit, and memory cells. Memory sizes are generally 8 K or 16 K of 8 bit bytes.

These tiny circuits can be used in calculators, microcomputers, clocks, cameras, ovens, washing machines and hundreds of other appliances. Because they are so cheap and so plentiful, they are revolutionizing a number of industries, and may affect the living and working habits of millions of people. (See also Project 5, page 162.)

The future

At the time of writing this book, computing is a vigorous and rapidly expanding activity, involving, directly or indirectly, most people in industrial countries. It is quite certain that, in the forseeable future, this growth will continue.

However, the directions of development are not so certain. The pursuit of smaller, faster and cheaper computers will no doubt continue, but whether existing designs and concepts will be extended, or whether new ones will replace them, remains to be seen.

At the present time, the extent of the use of computers is determined by economic factors, and technological developments. In the near future it seems likely that the further spread of computers will become a political issue.

Exercise 21

1 Write down the meanings of the following words of phrases:
Napier's bones; mill; tabulator; COLOSSUS; ENIGMA; ASCC; ENIAC; EDSAC; EDVAC; ACE; LEO; UNIVAC; IBM.

2 (a) Who wrote the first computer program?
(b) Who worked on a scientific and a commercial computer in Britain?
(c) Who made the major contribution to computer logic?
(d) Who invented the transistor?
(e)Who first summarized the general requirements of computers?

3 (a) List three contributions to computers made by Alan Turing.
(b) Which ideas in computing were first thought of by Charles Babbage?
(c) What did UNIVAC 1 and Hermann Hollerith have in common?

4 Which early computer(s):
(a) used base ten numbers?
(b) was designed but not built at the time?
(c) did not have a stored program capability?
(d) had transistors?
(e) was called a tabulator?

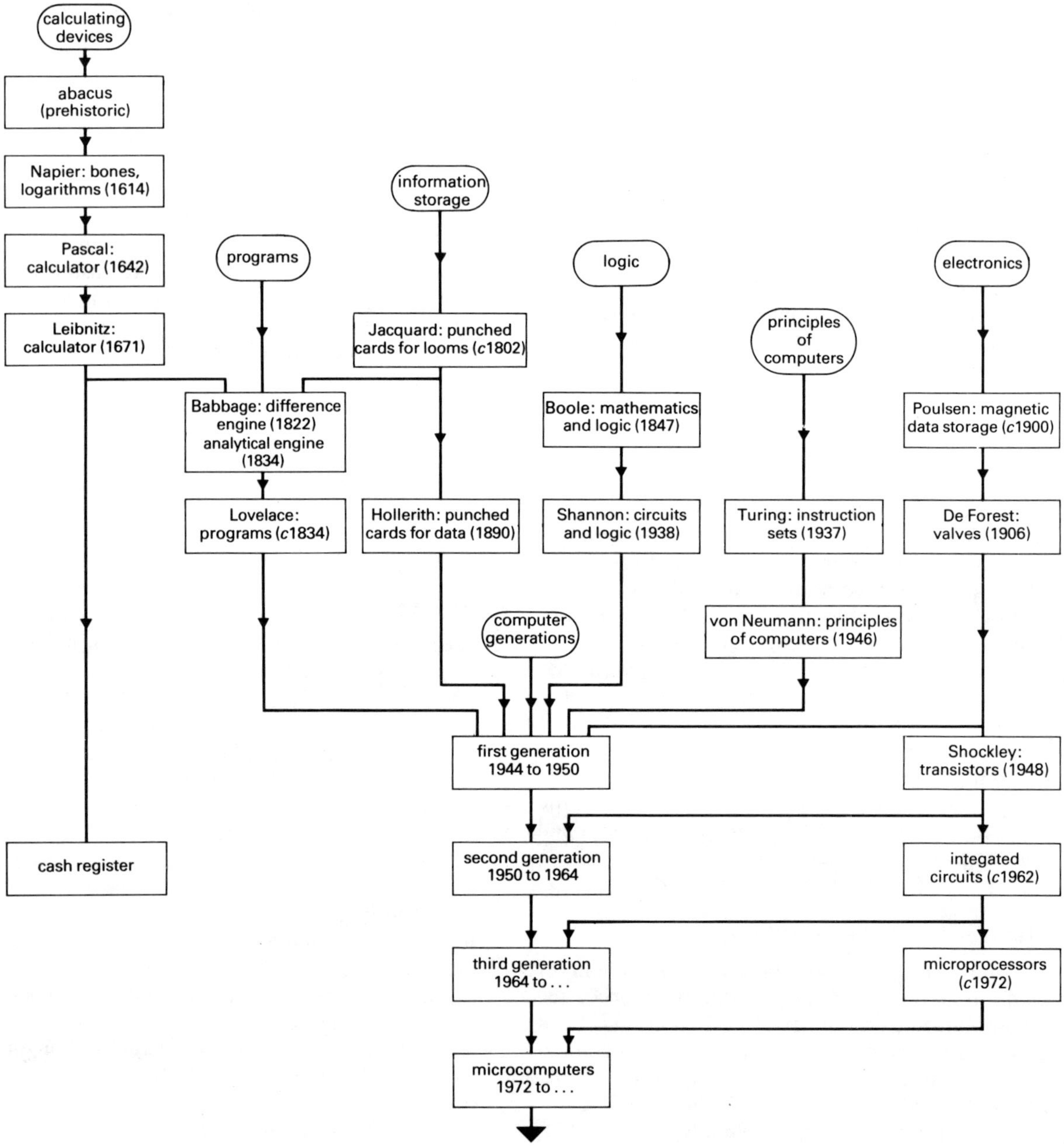

Fig. 21.2: The computer family tree

5 Summarize the development of information storage on punched cards.

6 Summarize the development of computer logic.

7 In what ways was ENIAC different from EDVAC?

8 Make a list of machines which could qualify for the title 'the world's first computer'. Giving your reasons, award the title to one of them.

9 Copy and complete the following passage fitting the names Babbage, Hollerith, Leibnitz, Lovelace, Napier, Odhner, Oughtred, Pascal, and Powers into the correct places:

'One of the first aids to calculation was the invention of logarithms by . . .. This was developed to the slide rule by . . .. The first mechanical aid was . . .'s calculator. This was improved by . . . who used the stepped wheel principle which was further refined by . . .. The first attempt at a programmable machine was the Analytical Engine of . . . which was programmed by . . .. In the United States census of 1890 . . . stored information on cards and he and his assistant . . . went on to form the computer firms which later became IBM and ICL respectively.' (MREB 76)

10 Copy the sentences below and fit ASCC, EDSAC, ENIAC, and LEO into the most appropriate spaces:

One of the first commercial computers was . . ..
One of the first electronic computers was . . ..
One of the first automatic computers was . . ..
One of the first stored program computers was . . .. (MREB 77)

11 Explain, with reasons, how the advent of the transistor revolutionized computer design in the 1950s. (UCLES 76 I)

12 (a) What major data processing problem caused the introduction of punched cards as a means of data storage?
(b) When did this take place? (AEB 78 specimen)

13 Write an account of the main changes in the hardware of computer systems from 1950 to the present day. (OLE 76 II)

22

The social effects of computers

Computers have already had very far-reaching effects on society. If the present rate of growth of computing continues, these effects will become even more significant. Indications are that by 1990, computing will have become the world's largest single industry.

The widespread introduction of computers has been described as the second industrial revolution. The social changes that it is bringing about are as large, and potentially as damaging, as those brought about by the first industrial revolution.

There are several issues that are already giving cause for concern:

- ☐ The effect of computers on employment and unemployment.
- ☐ The loss of privacy caused by storing vast quantities of easily accessible personal information in data banks.
- ☐ The use of computers by some governments and police forces to store information on citizens for political reasons.
- ☐ These and other issues relate to the central theme: The kind of society that computers are helping to create.

Employment and unemployment

Much hostility towards computers has been based on the fear of widespread unemployment resulting from their introduction. One of the earliest examples of this was the burning of Jacquard's punched-card operated looms by the weavers of Lyons. Computers are often installed as part of automated production systems requiring a minimum of operators, resulting in the loss of many jobs. This has happened, for example, in many steelworks.

On the other hand, computers do create jobs. They are more skilled and better paid, though fewer in number than those they replace. Many activities could not continue in their present form without computers, no matter how many people were employed. Examples are the cheque clearing system of major banks, and the weather forecasting system.

When a firm introduces computers, a few new people are usually employed in key posts (such as operations manager) while other staff are re-trained as operators, programmers and data preparation staff. After the new system has settled down, people

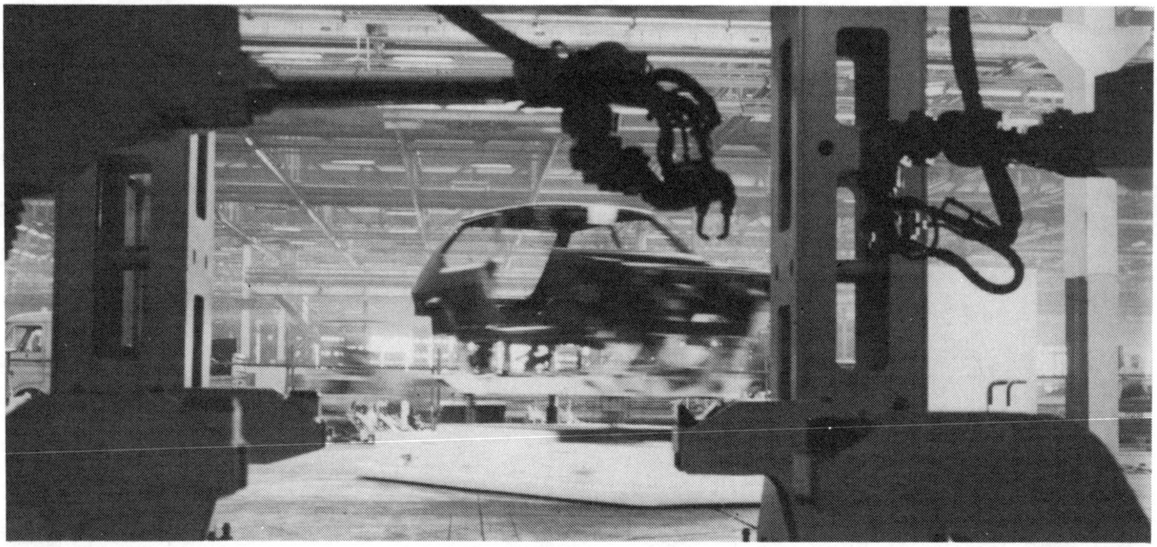

Computer-controlled equipment in a Fiat car assembly plant

in non-computer jobs are not always replaced when they leave, resulting in a decrease in the number of employees. This decrease is sometimes offset by a substantial increase in the activity of the firm, resulting from the introduction of computers.

Trade unions

The attitudes of trade unions towards computers vary. There is fear of widespread unemployment, and of the takeover of many jobs by computer trained workers, making promotion for older workers, not skilled in the use of computers, more difficult. In early 1977, the British Transport and General Workers Union announced its intention to close its own data processing department because 'computers put people out of work'.

On the other hand, many trade unionists see the drift towards computers as inevitable. They feel that their contribution to greater efficiency and productivity will improve the condition of the whole economy, and lead to the creation of more jobs. This view was endorsed by the British Prime Minister, James Callaghan, in January, 1979, when he made the point that new technologies hold the key to increased productivity, which will benefit the economy in the long run.

There has been a recent drive by several trade unions to recruit members from data processing personnel. A significant proportion of computer operators, programmers, systems analysts and data processing managers are trade union members.

Women working with computers

At present, virtually all data preparation staff are women, but most other data processing jobs are held by men. Most of the people working in the design, selling and maintenance of computers are men, while computer manufacture employs a considerable number of women.

Data preparation is undoubtedly one of the least pleasant aspects of working with computers. It is impossible to compare women's wages with men's wages in this area, as men are rarely employed. This amounts to a degree of discrimination against women.

On the other hand, a small but significant number of women do have jobs in other areas of computing, often in senior positions. It remains to be seen whether their numbers in this field of work will increase.

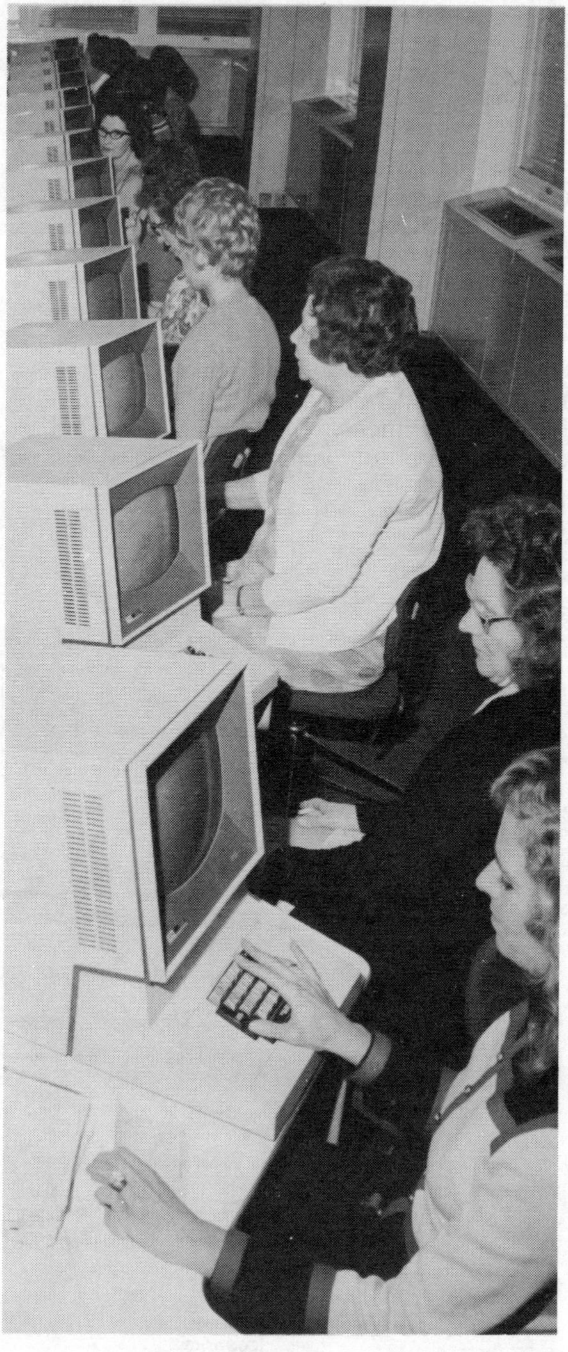

Women data preparation staff at work at the National Westminster Bank in London

Privacy

At present, a large amount of personal information is held on computers. This amount is rapidly increasing. Information held on computers about an average person might include: salary records, social security records, bank account details, insurance policies, gas, electricity, telephone and other business accounts, health records, motor vehicle and television licences, police and criminal records. See Figure 22.1.

Some difficult questions are raised by the use of computers to store this personal information:

- ☐ How much information is to be stored?
- ☐ Who is to have access to the information?
- ☐ How can unauthorized access be prevented?
- ☐ What is to prevent information which is supplied for one purpose, from being used for another?

At present, the information is stored on a number of different computers, some controlled by the government, others by local authorities, others by private companies. The most serious abuse of privacy could arise if these computers were connected. Detailed information on many aspects of a person's life would then be instantly available.

Concern has been expressed in many countries about abuses of personal information stored on computers. In most of these countries, steps are being taken to control the storage of, and access to this information.

The Younger commission

In Britain, a Parliamentary Commission of Enquiry (the Younger Commission) into the whole matter of privacy reported in 1972. Its main finding was that there were no major abuses of privacy at the time, but that the potential existed for them.

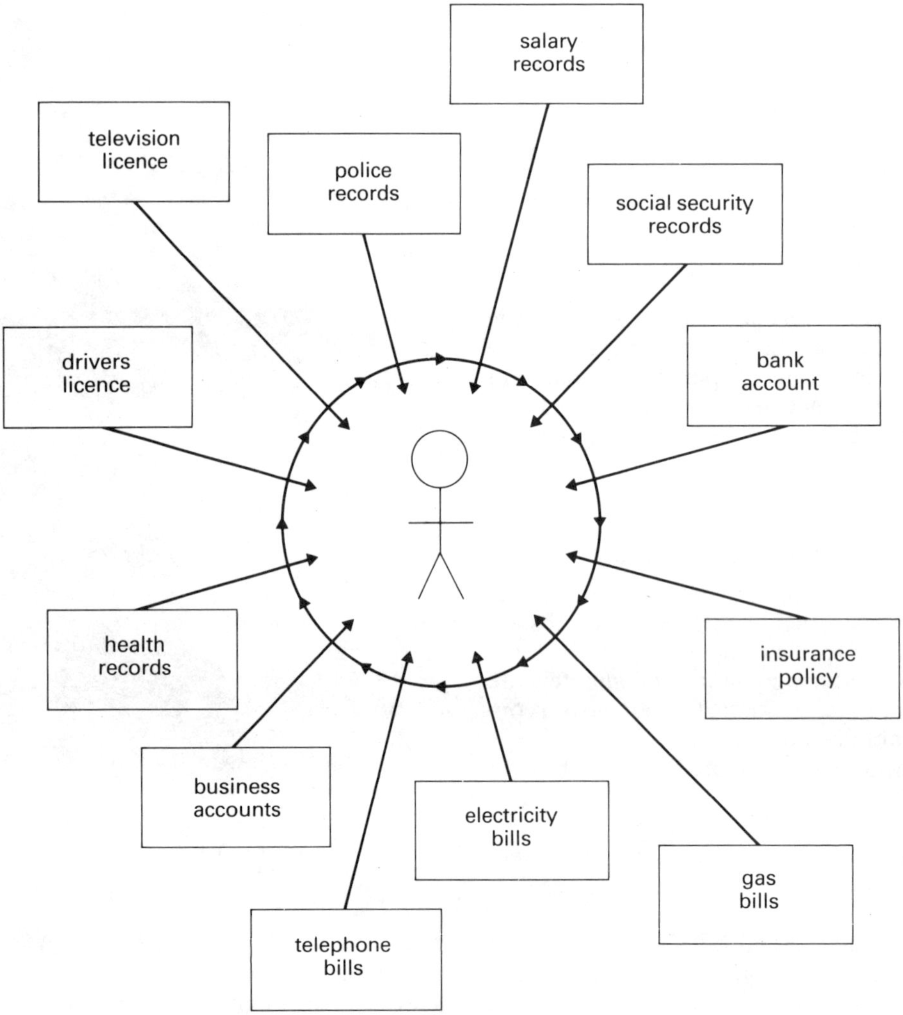

Fig. 22.1: The nightmare: a network of linked computers providing details of all aspects of a person's life

The data protection committee

In December 1975 the British government published a White Paper on computers and privacy. It announced its intention to make laws to regulate the storage of information on computers. A Data Protection Committee was set up in July 1976 to consider evidence and make recommendations about legislation. Its eleven members included a journalist, a trade union secretary, a local authority official and two university professors.

The Committee made its report in July 1978. It recommended that an independent authority, the Data Protection Authority, should be set up to regulate the collection and processing of personal data on computers. All users of such information would register with the authority.

Permission would have to be obtained before information gathered for one purpose could be used for another prupose, or be exchanged between computers. Unauthorized possession of information would be an offence.

People giving information about themselves should have a right to know what it will be used for, and who will see it. Most important, people should have a right to see and correct information concerning themselves.

Privacy laws in other countries

Sweden has had a Data Act since 1973. Rights to information date back to 1806, and are part of the Swedish constitution. In the U.S.A, the Freedom of Information Act was passed in 1966, and strengthened by amendments in 1974. The act gives U.S. citizens the right to inspect their own personal files held by police and other government departments.

Security of data

Related to the issue of privacy of information is the issue of unauthorized access to information. Most computer installations have various security measures. Computers and data storage media are in secure areas, to which only certain people have access. Codes and passwords are often needed to gain access to information.

However, there is considerable doubt about the effectiveness of these measures against the determined (and often well-informed) intruder. There have been several major thefts of information on magnetic media, and much unauthorized access no doubt goes on undetected. (See also the project on computer crime on page 165.)

Conclusion

Privacy of information stored on computers is a problem, not of the future, but of the present. Although it affects everyone, there has been no major public outcry yet. Most of the concern about the issue, and proposals for action on it, have come from within the computer industry itself.

Computers and political control

Computers are the ideal way for secret police to store information on terrorists, spies and other opponents of the government of the particular country. There is evidence that computers are being used in this way in several South American and African states, and with some success in West Germany against East German spies.

Pressure is being exerted by humanitarian groups on computer manufacturers, urging them to stop supplying computers for these purposes. The difficulty is to determine the use to which a computer will be put, and preventing a computer, which has been sold for one purpose, from being used for another.

The British Special Branch Computer

At a secret location somewhere in London, the British Special Branch computer went on-line in August 1978. The system provides immediate access to over two million personal records in a complex cross-indexed database. According to the Home Office, the data concerns crime, criminals and their associates, and matters relating to national security.

Users of the information are the Special Branch, the Fraud Squad, the Drug Squad, immigration authorities and the Criminal Intelligence Unit. Only a small proportion of the records are on people with criminal records. The majority are simply 'persons of interest'. At present there appear to be no restrictions on the information stored in this system.

The computer image

The first computers were developed at university research establishments, during and after the Second World War, against a background of high level science, weapons development and secrecy. As most people did not understand how they worked, or what they could (and could not) do, they acquired a mysterious, almost sinister image. The way computers have been portrayed in some science fiction books and films has not helped.

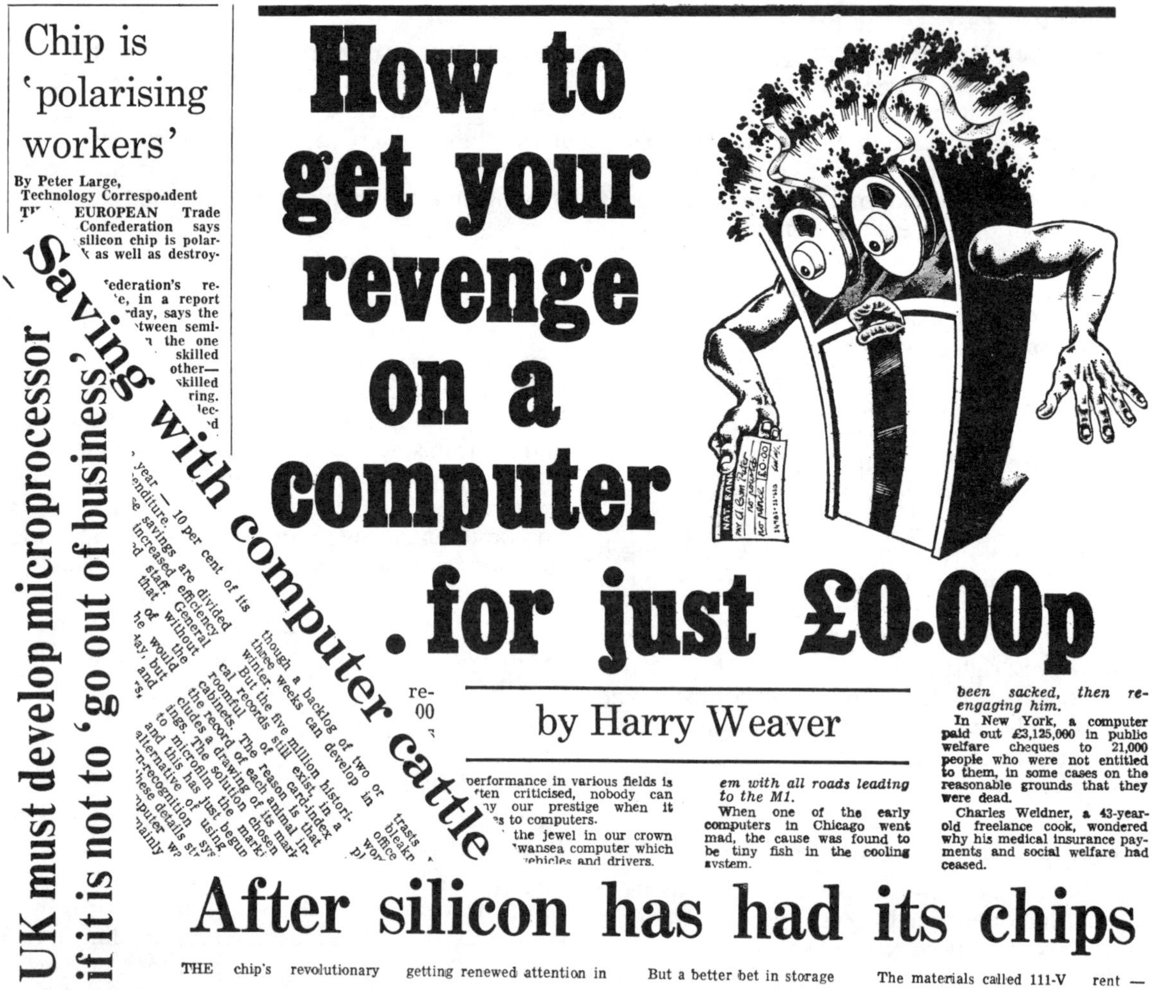
Chip is 'polarising workers'
By Peter Large, Technology Correspondent
How to get your revenge on a computer for just £0.00p
by Harry Weaver
Saving with computer cattle
UK must develop microprocessor if it is not to 'go out of business'
After silicon has had its chips

Computers in the news

As computers have become more widespread, their capabilities and limitations have been better understood. An increasing number of people work directly or indirectly with them. In addition, digital watches and pocket calculators have brought a small part of computer technology within reach of most people. All this has helped dispel the mystery surrounding computers, and give them a more down-to-earth image.

However some uncertainty persists, and it remains to be seen whether people's apprehensions are justified.

The computerized society

The overall impact of computers must be judged by the kind of society they are helping to create. Computers imply efficiency, convenience and high standards of work. They are an essential part of an affluent society.

On the other hand computers lead to conformity and increase the monotony of many everyday tasks. They help quicken the pace of twentieth-century living, increasing the strain felt by many people.

The growth of computing cannot continue unchecked. From time to time, decisions will have to be made placing limits on the intrusion of computers into some areas of life. The more people there are who are well informed about computers, the easier these decisions will be to make.

Exercise 22

1 Make a list of the information which would probably be stored on computers about a person who has a bank account, insurance policy, driver's licence and works for a company using a computerized wages system.

*2 Give your opinion on the question of privacy and computers, and your recommendations for action to be taken.

3 Find out whether any local firms or factories have recently installed computers, and what effect this has had on the number (and type) of jobs available.

4 Give your opinion on the question of unemployment caused by the introduction of computers.

5 List any applications of computers where you think that the adverse effects outweight the advantages. Mention any future applications where you think this will happen. Give reasons for your answers.

6 List some books or films which you think have contributed to the sinister image of computers.

7 Try to find out which countries use computers to store political iformation, and of any incidents which have resulted from this use of computers. Give your opinion on the matter.

*8 'Now what I want is, Facts. Teach these boys and girls nothing but Facts. Facts alone are wanted in life. Plant nothing else, and root out everything else.'

Charles Dickens *Hard Times*

These words were first published by Charles Dickens in 1854. State, with reasons, the extent to which you think computers are making them come true.

*9 Karl Marx wrote of socialists gaining control of countries by gaining control of the means of production. A century later, control of a country can be achieved by gaining control of the means of data processing.

Write an essay giving your opinion on these statements.

10 The following paragraph appeared in a newspaper:
'During the last few years computers have been gradually taking over the world. The power which they have over people is very great. Information about everyone in the country is stored on computers. We have no idea whether this information is correct or not, and it cannot be checked. Once the information is put on to a computer it is there for ever, and there is no way of changing it. It is common knowledge that computers are always making mistakes, and no one knows what the computer will do next with this information.'

Write a letter to the paper which published the article, saying why you agree or disagree with the points raised. (YREB 77 I)

11 Write about the use of computers for storing and processing information about people. Refer to the advantages of computer methods over manual methods and the benefits that arise. Refer also, from the point of view of the individual, to some of the dangers that arise. (EAEB 78 II)

23

Projects

Projects on topics related to computers are required by most examination boards. Several areas of this book, notably the chapters on applications, history and social implications of computers, provide information useful as a starting point for a project. This chapter provides some further suggestions for projects, as well as information which may be of general interest.

A wide variety of topics is covered. Each project contains a brief summary of the topic, together with some questions and ideas for further investigation.

Projects

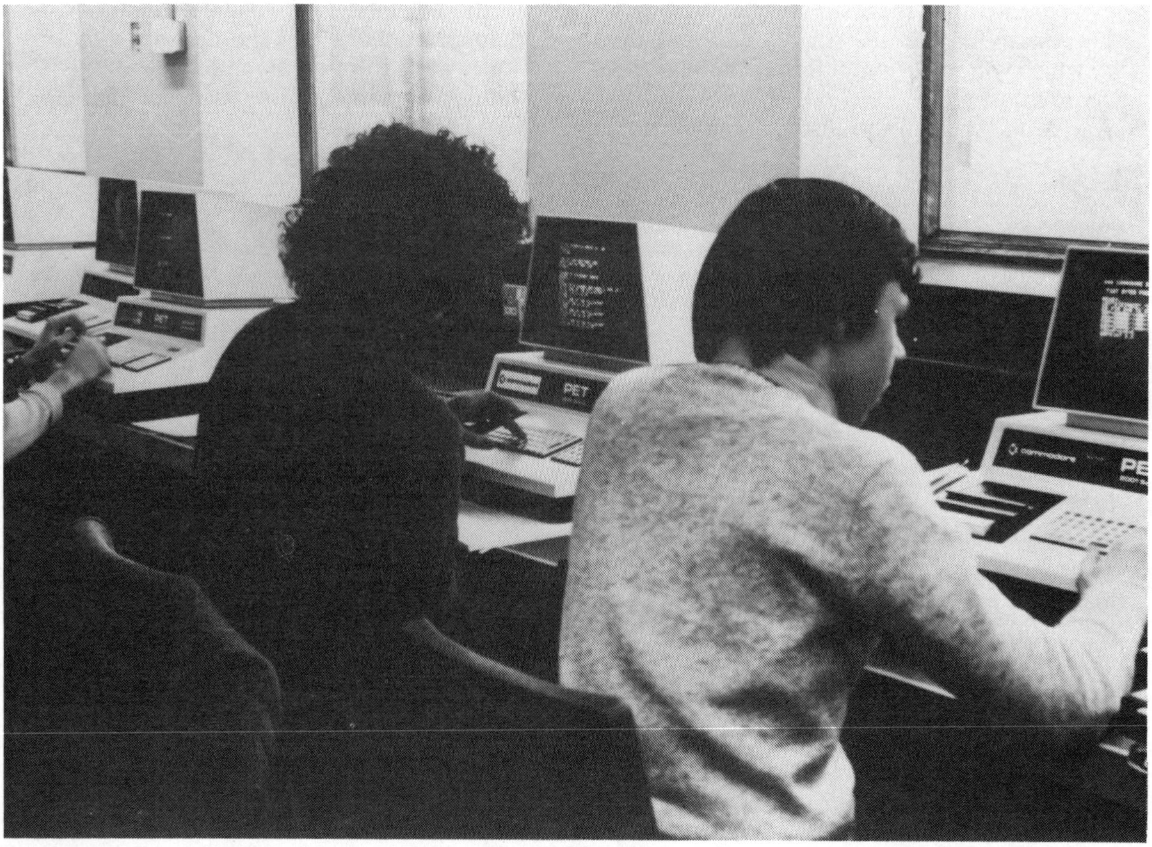

Strathclyde University students at work on Commodore Pet microcomputers

Project 1: New hardware developments

In the effort to produce faster, cheaper and more powerful computers, new hardware developments are announced almost daily. Some recent examples are:

- ☐ Visual display screens using minature laser beams and liquid crystals.
- ☐ Solid state devices having more than two stable states (a return to base ten computers?).
- ☐ Computer output on moving holograms (three dimensional laser pictures).
- ☐ Magnetic bubble memories, using very small magnetized areas to store data.
- ☐ Using materials at very low temperatures in computers. This reduces electrical resistance to almost zero.
- ☐ Complete central processors on a single chip. See project 5: The Microprocessor Revolution.

Questions

1 Find out about other new hardware developments, and more detail about those mentioned above.
2 Predict which ones you think will be widely used, and which will not.
3 Suggest some further hardware developments.

Project 2: Computing in the U.S.S.R.

Although much of the original development of computers took place in Britain and the U.S.A., Communist countries, particularly the U.S.S.R. and more recently China, have made considerable progress. They now have well established computer industries.

This project concerns the development of computers in the U.S.S.R. and Eastern Europe. The next project is about computers in China.

The East/West balance of computers: (December, 1974)

Development of computers in Russia and Eastern Europe has been much slower than in the West. There are far fewer computers (see Table 23.1), and they are generally older and less powerful. Many first and second generation computers are still in operation. The state of development is at least five years behind that of the West.

This slower progress has been partly due to the lack of communication between East and West about computers, particularly during the Cold War. Even now, government permission must be obtained for each Western computer sold to a Communist country. The other major reason for slow development is that Communist countries have preferred to develop their own computers, rather than rely on imported technology.

Work on computers began in the U.S.S.R. in the early 1950s, apparently against some opposition. The emphasis was on scientific and military applications, and has been ever since. Ten first generation URAL 1 computers did the calculations for the first Sputniks in 1957.

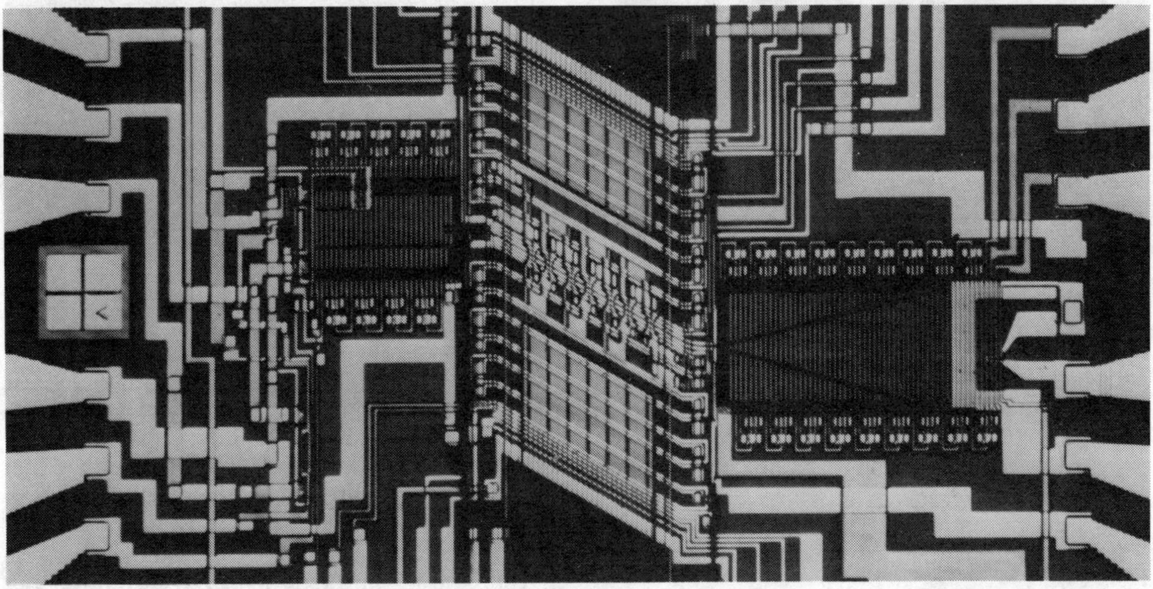

An experimental magnetic bubble chip

Table 23.1

Country	Population (million)	Installed computers	Computers per million people
West			
U.S.A	211.9	168800	797
Japan	109.7	30095	274
West Germany	62.0	20860	337
U.K.	56.2	15520	276
France	52.5	13064	249
Total	492.3	248339	504
East			
U.S.S.R.	252.1	12500	50
East Germany, Poland, Hungary, Czechoslovakia, Romania, Bulgaria	104.8	2935	28
Total	356.9	15435	43

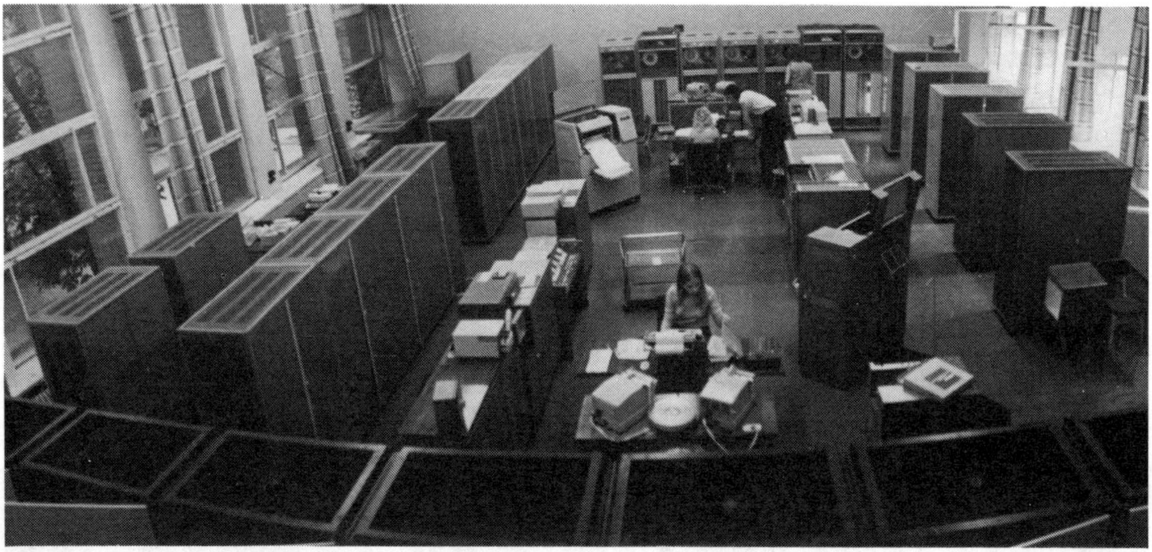

The computing centre in the Tartu State University, USSR

In 1969 an agreement was made between Russia and the Eastern European countries to produce a unified range of computers. The larger series appears to be very similar to the IBM 360 range, even using much the same machine language, and costing about the same. There have been delays in producing an equivalent to the IBM 370 series. The smaller range of computers resembles the PDP series.

Manufacture of the various units of these computers is shared between Russia and her European allies.

In contrast to the poor hardware performance, there is a very high standard of programming. Many advances in programming techniques that have been used throughout the world have originated in Russia or Eastern Europe.

At the present time, sales of Western computers in communist countries remain few, currently about one hundred medium or large computers a year.

Communist countries lack foreign currency to buy the computers, and the fear of computers being used for military purposes has prevented many sales (such as a large weather forecasting computer to Russia in 1977). However, the Russian tourist agency Intourist has an IBM 370 for hotel room reservations, and the airline Aeroflot has a Univac seat reservation system. The airlines of the other Eastern European countries work on a combined booking system based on Univac computers.

Undoubtedly the major computer application is to military uses. For example, the defection, in 1977, of a Russian Foxbat fighter pilot with his plane disclosed a sophisticated on-board electronic guidance system. Most non-military computers are used in scientific research or industrial management.

It appears that the trends described here will continue for the foreseeable future. Communist bloc computing activity will be characterized by a small, uniform range of computers, very little co-operation with the West, and a strong emphasis on military applications.

Questions

1 Try to find out more about computing in Russia and Eastern Europe.
2 List the main similarities and differences between computing in the East and in the West.
3 List some advantages and disadvantages of a unified range of computers.
4 A recent report claims that 'there is a vast market for Western computers in Communist countries'. Give your opinion.

Project 3: Computing in China

China was engulfed in the revolution which brought the Communists to power (1949) while the first steps in the development of electronic computers were being made in the West. Until the breakdown of relations between Russia and China in 1960, computers and computer staff were mainly supplied by Russia. There were also a few computers from the West.

After 1960, work started on developing original Chinese computers. 1967 saw the first all-Chinese computer in operation. It was a large second generation machine. The third generation arrived in 1973, with the first Chinese computer to work at more than one million operations per second. Smaller computers went into production in 1974, with the Great Wall 203, followed shortly afterwards by the medium range DJS 18 and DJS 130.

The largest computers are used for scientific purposes, particularly earthquake research. The smaller models are used in industry. Principal applications are computer aided design, and computer control of machine tools. Computerization is not aimed at increasing profit, as in the West, but

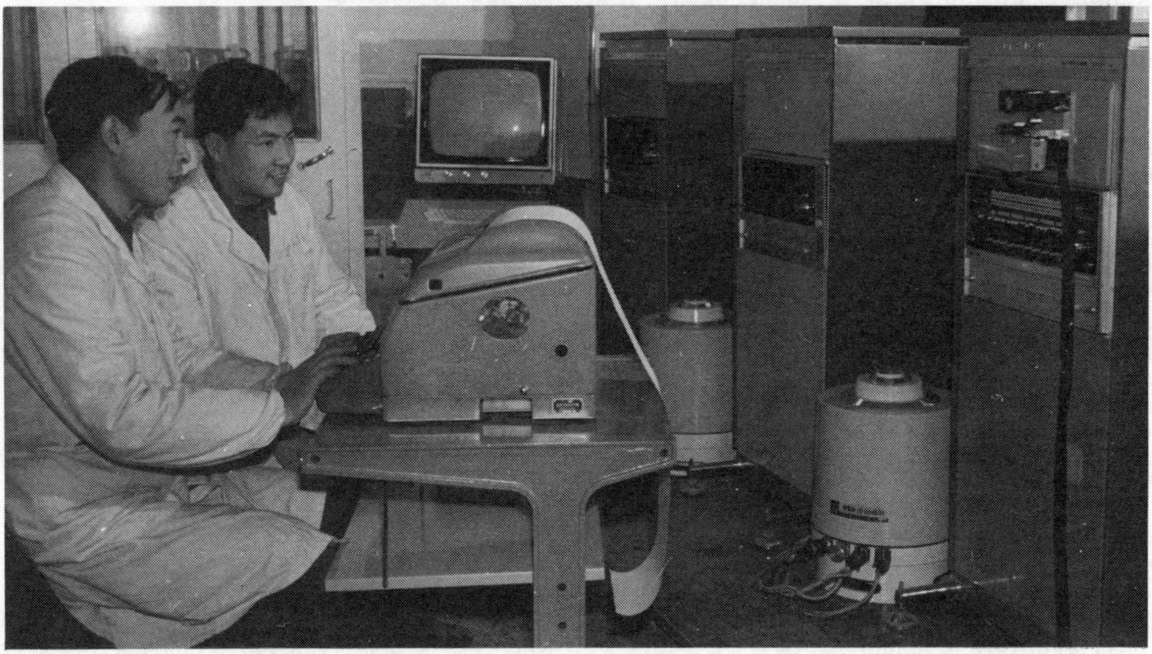

A DJS 130 computer produced by the Soochow Radio Factory, China

at increasing productivity.

In spite of these advances, development of computing in China has been much slower, and on a much smaller scale, than corresponding development in the West.

Questions

1 Try to find out more about computing in China, particularly the effect which computers are having on the Chinese way of life.
2 Towards the end of 1978, China embarked on a 'Great Leap Outwards'. This involved establishing diplomatic and trade relationships with Japan, the U.S.A. and other countries. Find out what effect this is having on computing in China.
3 Give your opinion of the way in which computer design and applications will develop in China, and the impact it will have on Chinese Society.

Project 4: Computers in the Third World

There are hardly any computers in developing countries. Major problems of these areas such as malnutrition, lack of basic amenities, underemployment and lack of employment opportunities would not be solved by their widespread introduction. In addition, there is little local knowledge of high technology, and no servicing facilities. Above all, there are very few tasks suited to computerization.

One exception is population census work, a task often undertaken with the assistance of the United Nations Development Programme, which frequently supplies computers and trained staff for the purpose. The U.N. had spent £16 million on this project by the end of 1974.

The computers used are generally small, simple, reliable machines. They are often given to the country after the census. About thirty countries have so far made use of this facility.

Other applications in Third World countries include public administration (Mongolia), studying epidemics (Argentina), population growth surveys (Santiago, Chile), computer technology research (Bombay, India). All of these have been sponsored by the United Nations.

Computers in the oil producing countries

The big increase in oil prices in 1974 has brought enormous sums of money into oil producing countries such as Saudi Arabia, Kuwait and Venezuela. Several of these countries have embarked on ambitious programmes to raise the standard of living of their people. Many of these projects involve computers.

Large, expensive computer systems are being bought from the U.S.A. and European countries. Computer staff are being attracted to the oil states by high salaries, often tax free.

Questions

1 Find out other ways in which computers are being used in developing countries.
2 Suggest any activities in Third World countries which you think would benefit from the assistance of computers.
3 List some disadvantages of using computers in developing countries.
4 In your opinion, what will be the extent of computing in developing countries in twenty years time?
5 'Computers bring progress, and progress brings prosperity.'
Discuss this statement in relation to computers in developing countries.

Project 5: The microprocessor revolution

For a brief introduction to the topic, see page 149. Find out more about microprocessors and their impact from newspapers and magazines, radio and television programmes and literature supplied by manufacturers.

Questions

1 Select one or two common makes of microprocessor and find out
(a) how many components they have,
(b) what their function is, (c) their price.
2 Find out as many applications of microprocessors as you can.
3 Suggest further applications, and also some areas where you think they would not be useful.
4 Much attention is being given to the social effects of microprocessors.
(a) Find out what effects have already become evident (for example the effect they are having on Swiss watch manufacturers).
(b) Find out what effects are being predicted, both in the short term and the long term.
(c) Give your own opinion of the social effects of microprocessors.

Project 6: Personal computing

Personal computers first saw the light of day in 1977, and may take a mere ten years to become as common in homes as T.V. sets.

Personal computers are microcomputers designed for home use. With microprocessors based on a

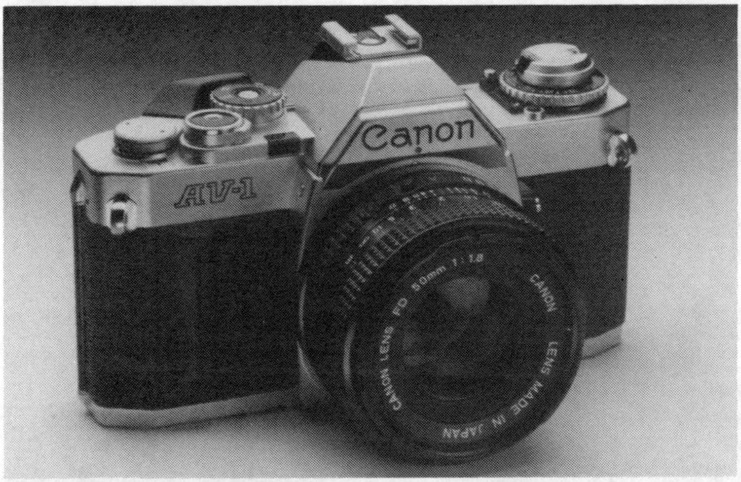

A camera which incorporates a microprocessor

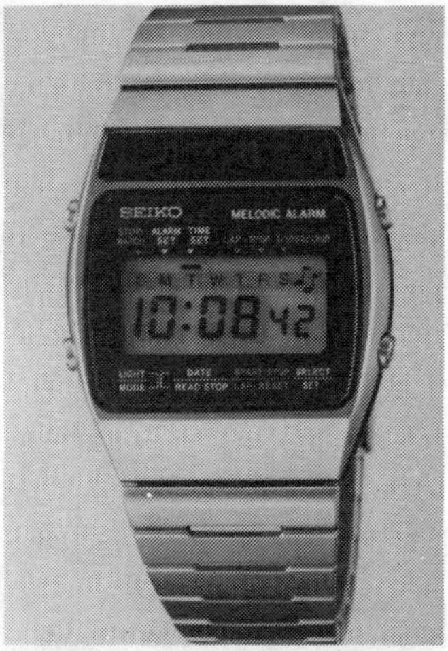

A microprocessor-controlled digital watch

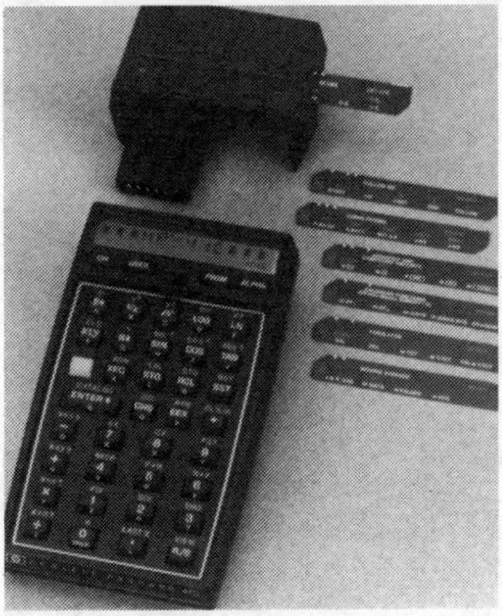

A Hewlett-Packard programmable calculator, with magnetic cards for storing programs

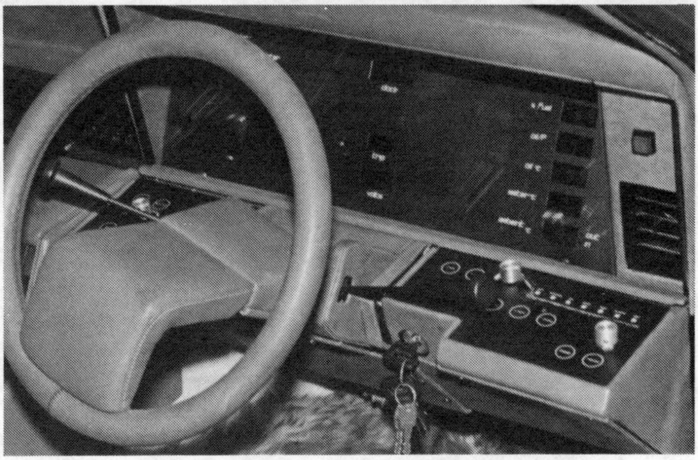

Electronic dashboard display in an Aston Martin Lagonda

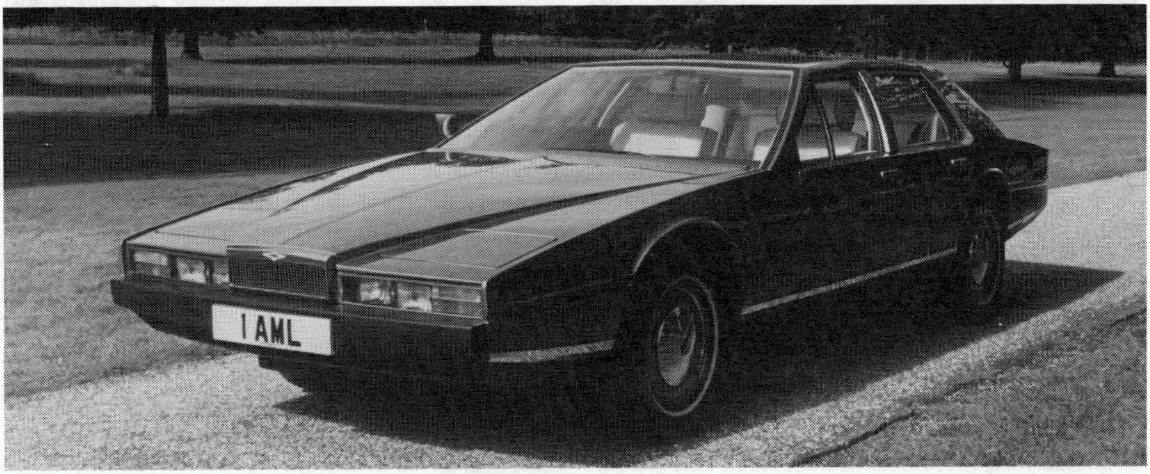

An Aston Martin Lagonda, with electronic controls

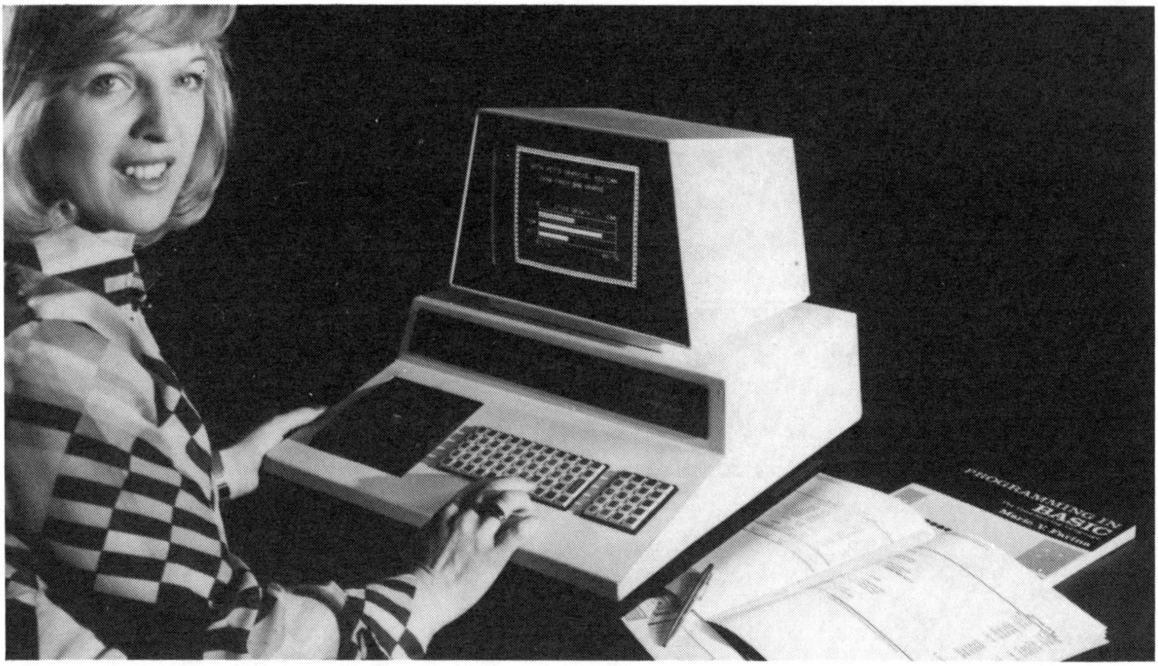

A Commodore Pet microcomputer in use

single integrated circuit, they are versatile, fast, easy to use, and cheap.

They have a keyboard input and visual display output. The simplest models use an assembly language, slightly larger ones can accept a high level language, usually BASIC. Most come supplied with a variety of ready-to-use programs. Some are capable of extending to include cassette tape and magnetic disc backing store, printers and links via a telephone line to a large computer.

Fierce competition amongst a number of manufacturing firms has led to steadily increasing capabilities and decreasing prices. It appears that the large computer manufacturers will soon enter this potentially huge market.

Computers have invaded laboratories, offices, hospitals, factories, ships, aircraft and spacecraft. It remains to be seen whether they will succeed in their final invasion – of the home.

Questions

1 Find out details about some personal computers which are currently available, in particular:
memory size; wordlength;
type of input and output;
program language(s) used;
what standard programs are supplied with them;
to what extent they can be extended; price.

2 Decide which type you would prefer, if you were to buy one. Give reasons for your choice. Alternatively, give your reasons for rejecting all of them.

3 Give your opinion of the way in which personal computing will develop, and the effects it will have.

Project 7: The cost of computers

A major reason for the rapid spread of computers is their decreasing cost. At a time when virtually all other costs (especially wages) are rising rapidly, hardware costs are falling. There is a steady flow of new products with greater capacity at hardly any extra cost.

There are several reasons for the decreasing costs. As computers are made in larger numbers, the research and development costs are spread more widely. Accumulated experience in intergrated circuit technology has led to much cheaper components. Perhaps most important of all, IBM, whose prices determine much of those of the rest of the industry, has a policy of keeping prices low, even to the extent of selling new computers initially at a loss.

The initial expense of buying a large computer can be avoided by leasing the system, usually for a fixed amount per month which includes maintenance costs. This practice is becoming slightly less common as users prefer to mix units from different manufacturers to make up their system.

For these reasons the major cost of a data processing department is the staff salaries. Low hardware costs mean that staff can be paid well, but increases the temptation to have more hardware and fewer staff.

Questions

1 Find out the cost of buying various small, medium and large computers.
2 Find out the leasing costs of these systems.
3 A data processing department contains:
☐ a medium sized computer (say an ICL 2903), with three disc drives, a card reader, a line printer and two VDU screens for direct data entry.
☐ a data processing manager
☐ a computer operator
☐ two data preparation staff

(a) Find out the cost of buying the computer (or a suitable equivalent).
(b) Find out (or estimate) the annual maintenance cost.
(c) Find out reasonable salaries for the staff.
(d) Estimate the additional costs (stationery, electricity, etc.) for a year.
(e) From these figures, estimate the total cost of running the data processing department for a year.

4 Repeat question **3** for a different sized data processing department.

Project 8: Computers and disabled people

Many physically handicapped people are in all other ways suited to working with computers, particularly as programmers or data preparation staff. The main obstacles have been the reluctance of employers to taken them on, despite their competence at a task, and, in some cases, their need for slightly modified equipment.

A recent initiative has been made by the computer industry to provide more jobs for handicapped people. Funds have been raised to finance administration and publicity for the effort, and to modify equipment.

One promising scheme is for handicapped people to work at home, writing programs or preparing data on a contract basis. This will enable them to work at their own pace.

Questions

1 Find out what progress has been made in the effort to provide computer jobs for handicapped people.

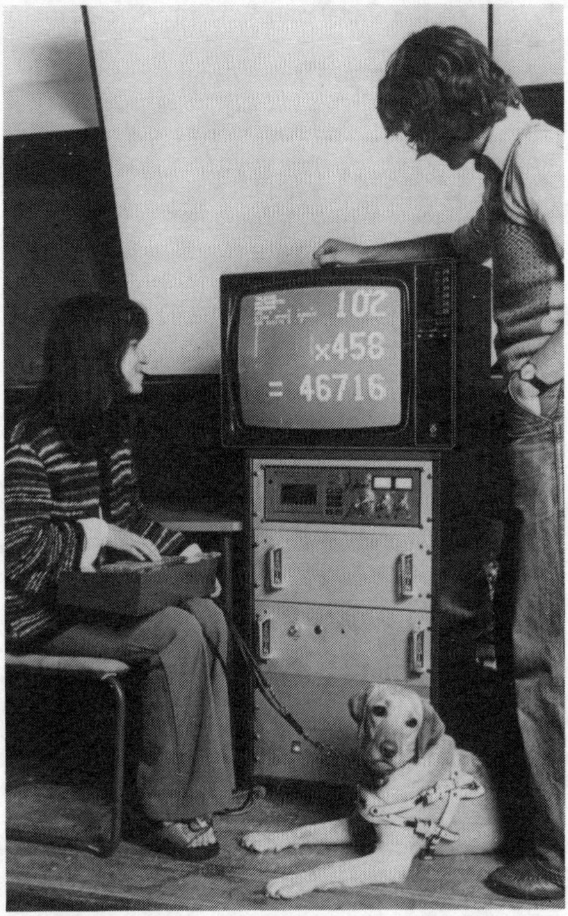

Julia Howlett, director of St Margarets Software Limited, demonstrating her arithmetic project for backward and disabled children, which includes spoken output. Julia Howlett is completely blind.

2 Suggest what further steps might be taken in this direction.

Project 9: Computer crime

Computers provide intriguing new opportunities for criminal activities, both by computer staff and outsiders. Dishonest practices are generally concealed in a mass of routine data, and although a number of cases have been reported, it is not known how many have been (or still are) undetected.

Criminal activities include falsifying input data, inventing fictitious accounts, altering programs, rewiring hardware, changing MICR figures on cheques, and even creating phantom companies to buy or sell goods.

The amounts involved vary from tens to millions of pounds. The British average is thought to be in the £10000 to £50000 range. The U.S.A. figure is higher.

For those who have been caught, the penalties have been fairly light, usually just dismissal. For those prosecuted, there have been suspended sentences, fines or a few months in jail. In many cases, charges have not been laid to avoid bad publicity.

A typical case is that of a multinational company, with two foreign subsidiary companies. Programmers at the head office created a phantom company to buy goods from the one subsidiary and sell them to the other. They made £150000 profit in two and a half years.

Measures to combat computer crime include more thorough restriction of access of unauthorized people to computer installations, stricter job segregation (programmers may not handle input data, etc.), careful documentation of programs, and increased vigilance by data processing managers.

Questions

1 Find out about other cases of computer crime which have been reported. Write descriptions of some cases.
2 Do you think that computers make some crimes easier?
3 Suggest additional ways in which computer crime might be prevented.

Project 10: When things go wrong

'It won't happen here', or even 'it won't happen again' seems to be the prevailing attitude of computer staff, intent on keeping programs running and customers satisfied.

However it has happened, and will continue to happen – fires, floods, bombing, building collapses, and power fluctuations have damaged or destoyed a number of computer installations, occasionally with loss of life. In addition to the cost of replacing equipment, large losses are caused by disruptions to the processing of programs.

Fires have been caused by electrical faults, arson, or bombs, or have spread from outside areas. The fumes from burning plastic insulation materials are particularly hazardous. Many computers have fireproof safes for data, and carbon dioxide extinguishers (water causes as much damage as fire).

Flooding has been caused by rivers overflowing their banks, or massive leaks from roofs. Corrosion has ruined much equipment, though data has generally remained intact. Ceiling collapses have damaged equipment, and dust in the air delayed restarting.

Power surges have caused computers to malfunction. A particularly bad period in Britain was January, 1974, during the three-day week, especially at 10.30 p.m. as millions of people switched off their T.V. sets.

Some plans have been made to cope with these emergencies: vital data is duplicated and copies stored at another site, computer centres have standby agreements to use other computers if their own is put out of action, and fire protection measures are becoming stricter. The idea of a disaster centre is being pursued, and of training staff by simulated emergencies.

Questions

1 Find out about some accidents that have happened to computers, particularly how long it took to resume normal working, the amount of processing that was lost, and the cost.
2 Find out what fire precautions are in force at local computers, and what plans they have to continue operations if their computers were put out of action.
3 Suggest additional ways of preventing fires and other damage to computers.

* Project 11: Simulating the IMC-1 in BASIC

The frequent mention of the IMC-1 model computer gives rise to a tempting possibility. Is it possible to make one? In most cases, the answer is definitely no. The diagrams of the IMC-1 are deceptively simple, with no details of the control and timing logic circuits shown.

However, a more practical possibility is to write a computer program in BASIC (or any other suitable language) to simulate the behaviour of the IMC-1. An IMC-1 simulation program must do the following:

- ☐ Input a program in IMC-1 machine code (i.e. in binary) and load it into position in the IMC-1 memory. The address of the start of the program will also have to be input.
- ☐ Reserve an area in the IMC-1 memory for data. The start and end address of the data will have to be input.
- ☐ Accept input data for the program when it is required, or store the data ready for input.
- ☐ Dry run the program, showing the contents of the accumulator and memory data cells at each step.

☐ Store and print the results output by the program.
☐ Carry out suitable checks and print error messages if necessary.

Writing a program of this nature is a considerable challenge, but not beyond the capability of anyone with a thorough grounding in BASIC. A terminal is the most suitable method of input, though off-line processing is quite possible. Here are a few ideas which may be useful:

1 All binary numbers are best stored in character form. For example the list M$(31) could be used to store the contents of the memory cells, with the index as the address (from 0 to 31). In this way, zeros at the beginning of a number are not lost, and all words stay 8 bits long.
2 As some operations are best carried out in binary, and others in decimal, a defined function for converting from binary to decimal, and one for converting from decimal to binary, are essential.
3 The part of the program to carry out each of the eight operations in the IMC-1 instruction set is best written as a set of subprograms. During the dry run, once the operation code has been decoded, control is passed to the appropriate operation subprogram by an ON . . . GOSUB statement.
4 It is an idea to print the contents of the memory (**a core dump**) at the start and end of the program, or if an error has occurred.
5 A considerable enhancement to the IMC-1 machine language is achieved by changing the 0 0 0 operation code to mean GO TO. For example the instruction 0 0 0 1 0 1 1 0 means 'go to the instruction in memory cell 22'.

   This instruction can still be used as an END instruction by repeatedly transferring control to itself. This would be achieved by the above instruction if it already was in memory cell 22.

Project 12: The future of computers

Electronic computers have changed extremely rapidly in the thirty years of their existence. It is certain that this rapid change will continue. Actual predictions are a mixture of speculation and long-term planning. There are several areas of progress: hardware developments, new program techniques, new applications and consequently the social effects of all of these.

Hardware will continue to get smaller, faster and cheaper. Integrated circuits will combine more and more components in a single chip. The present limit of a quarter of a million components to one chip will no doubt be exceeded. Processing speeds are expected to exceed 500 million instructions per second in the near future. Technologies such as lasers and very low temperature electric circuits will be further explored, and incorporated into computer design.

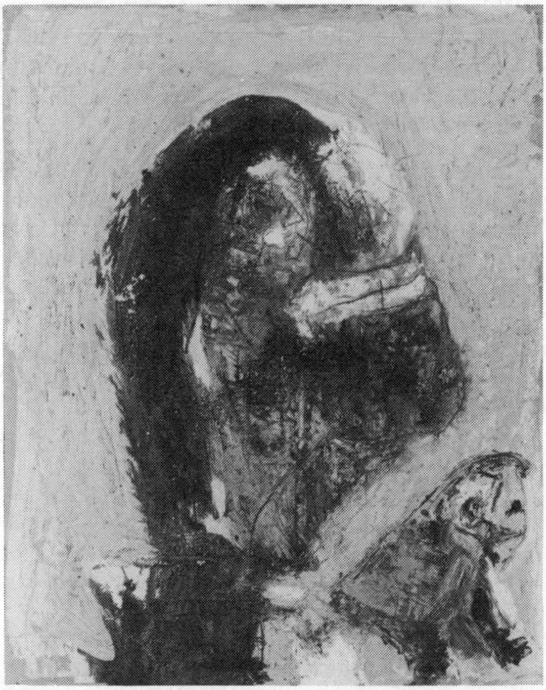
'Timid Proud Person' by Asger Jorn

Large computers will be linked, to form networks of computers. Britain may eventually have a national computer grid, rather like the national electricity grid. Microcomputers may be included in the control systems of motor cars, washing machines, stoves and heating systems. A more distant development might combine computers with digital watches, using the watch display for input and output, and linked if necessary to a nearby CPU by radio.

An alternative view

A dissenting view is that computers are steadily eroding the quality of life, and the basic needs of the majority of the world's people are more important than the luxuries of the few. Computers are widening the gap between rich and poor nations. The following points emphasize this view:
☐ How relevent are computers in the home, when two billion people live in slums with four to six people per room?

☐ Will electronic funds transfer benefit the three billion people who do not have a bank account?
☐ Communicating with electronic equipment hampers communication between people, and stifles direct experience of events.

Program developments will undoubtedly include ever wider applications, and an increased demand for reliability, as processes become more and more dependent on computers, with less manual backup should the computer fail. Tasks performed will become increasingly tailored to needs of the user, and less restricted by the computer hardware. Computers that can process high level languages directly are a possibility.

The use of computers will become even more widespread. Cash will be virtually eliminated by an electronic financial transaction system. Almost all information storage, processing and communication will be done by computers. There will be widespread use of computer-controlled automation in industry. There may well be no more postal service, and hardly any unskilled jobs in industry.

The limits? Computers use very little energy, and cause very little pollution. Costs are steadily falling. None of these factors should restrict the growth of computers in the near futue. The only present possibility is that of a strong shift of public opinion against computers, causing a reduction in their use. Unless this happens, it is fairly certain that by the turn of the century, computing will have become the world's largest single industry.

Questions

1 Find out about future development of
(a) computer hardware, particularly new technologies,
(b) computer programming,
(c) applications of computers.

2 Make some predictions of your own about the future of computers.

3 Comment on the social effects of the various future developments.

4 The development of motor cars started about fifty years before the development of electronic computers.
(a) Find out some details about the development of motor cars, particularly speed, cost and fuel consumption.
(b) Find out about the speed, cost and power consumption of computers, as they have evolved.
(c) Compare your findings for motor cars and computers. Does the information on cars give any insight into the future of computers?

*5 The British General Election of 2001 is to be fought between the Conservation Party and the Progressive Party. The Conservation Party advocates protection of the environment, and a return to a way of life with a lower level of technology. The Progressive Party favours continued development of high technology.

The British population is stable at 63 million, North Sea oil has run out, unemployment is 26%, inflation 12%. Britain exports food, owing to a computer assisted food production system.
(a) Write an election manifesto for each party.
(b) Which party would you support? Give your reasons.
(c) Which party do you think will win? Give your reasons.

A survey of the future

A survey was carried out by Computer Weekly magazine to find out when its readers thought that certain developments would occur. The results were published in May 1977.

Readers were asked to put a date, or the word 'never' next to several possible computer developments. The dates were averaged, and the percentage deciding on never was calculated, for each development. Here are some results:

Development	Average expected date	% never
1 Complete computer on one integrated circuit	1980	0.5%
2 Widespread use of computers in cars for minor functions (fuel economy, headlight intensity)	1981	1%
3 Widespread use of teaching programs for children and adults on home terminals	1985	1%
4 50% of homes in U.K. with teletypes or VDU's	1985	4%
5 Widespread use of computers in public interviewing (hospitals, social security etc.)	1987	5%
6 Widespread use of computers in cars for major functions (steering, speed control).	1988	6%

7 Widespread use of pocket terminals with radio links to computers.	1989	8%
8 Most software developments undertaken by computers (automatic programming).	1990	5%
9 Postal service largely replaced by communication between word processors.	1990	9%
10 Computer program beats world chess champion for the first time.	1990	10%
11 Average working week reduced to 20 hours because of widespread automation	1994	21%
12 Major breakthrough in the field of artificial intelligence, leading to computer self-awareness	1999	18%

Questions

1 Fill in your own estimates of when these applications will take place. Write 'never' if you do not think the application will happen.

2 Obtain estimates from other people, and find the average date, and the percentage who think that the application will not happen. Compare your results with those quoted, and comment.

24

Revision exercise

This exercise contains questions which combine information from different parts of the book. All the questions are from past examinations in Computer Studies.

1 (a) Figure 24.1 shows a logic circuit that will give an output of 1 if $A = 0$, $B = 1$, $C = 0$, $D = 1$ and 0 for all other inputs.

Copy the diagram and make the circuit work by filling in the circles with any of the following words; AND, OR, NOT.

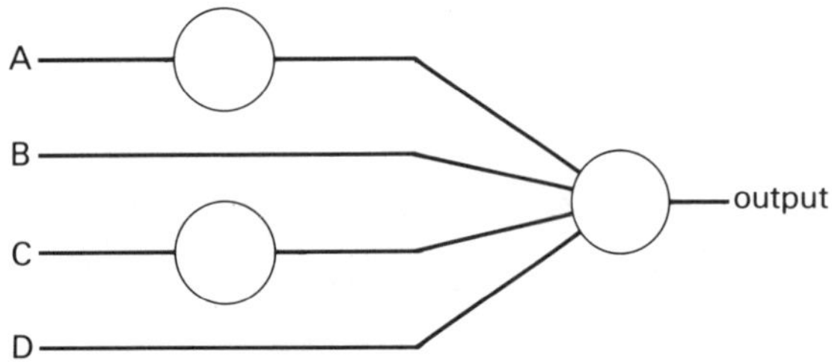

Fig. 24.1

A computer stores instructions in a 10 bit word with the four most significant bits holding the instruction code and the remaining six holding the address.

How many different instructions are possible?

How many different addresses are possible?

Explain the following terms: fetch phase, execute phase, processor cycle.

Explain what part the logic diagram (Figure 24.1) plays in the execute phase.

(b) What is compilation?

Explain what **compilation errors** and **execution errors** are and what effect they have on the running of a program. For each one, give an example that you have discovered during your own programming and say what needs to be done to correct the error. (MREB 76)

2 If a mistake occurs in a computer system, it is usually for one of the reasons that are listed below:

(a) mechanical or electrical failure
(b) operating errors (c) programming errors
(d) basic design fault of the system that is being run on the computer
(e) errors when the data is copied onto the input medium.

For each of these *five* things (i) explain how the errors occur, (ii) say what precautions should be taken to lessen the chances that such errors can occur. (MREB 76)

3 Copy and complete the table in Figure 24.2 by working through the flowchart.

Flowchart 2

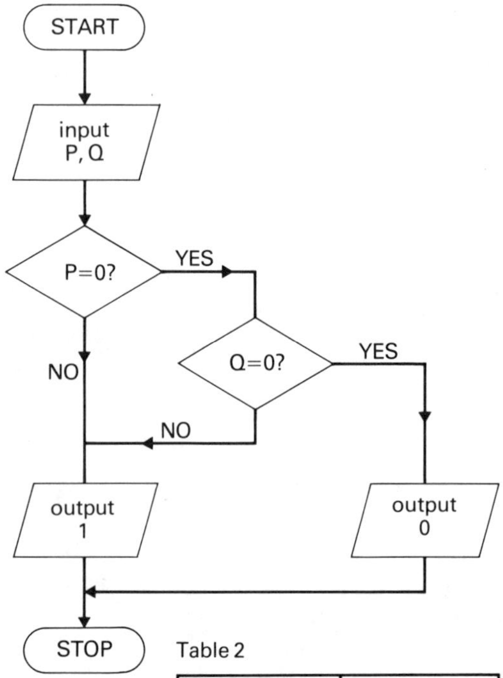

Table 2

input		output
P	Q	
0	0	
0	1	
1	0	
1	1	

Fig. 24.2

Copy and complete the following sentence:
This is the truth table for . . .? (MREB 77)

4 Describe a typical scientific computer installation of the early 1950s, and contrast it with one of the 1970s. Include in your description the hardware you would see, the kinds of jobs the computer would be doing, and the personnel who would be working with it. (OLE 77 II)

5 Explain what is meant by 'data banks'.

Give TWO examples to show how they can be used for the benefit of people in general.

Give TWO reasons why data banks could cause harm or disadvantage. (EAEB 76 I)

6 'The first electronic digital computers were used for calculating. Today's computers cope with the information explosion.'

Comment on this statement. Say what developments in computing have assisted this trend. Illustrate your answer by describing briefly an application in which the computer is used as an information processor rather than as a calculator. (EAEB 76 I)

7 Computers are used to prepare gas and electricity bills. Write a brief note about two checking procedures which can be made during data processing to avoid incorrect bills being sent out. (EAEB 76 II)

8 Write brief notes on (a) the difference between a calculator and a computer, (b) the impact of the early Hollerith card on data processing. (UCLES 75 II)

9 Explain how a computer system, linked to the cash tills, might help in the management of a supermarket. (UCLES 76 I)

10 Place each of the following items under the appropriate heading to indicate whether it is classed as **hardware** or **software** in a computer installation. The first one is done for you. (YREB 75 I)

magnetic disc	program
line printer	core store
subroutine	card reader
compiler	magnetic tape unit
library programs	

Hardware	**Software**
magnetic disc	. . . .

11 Nowadays a great deal of computer time is devoted to information storage and retrieval rather than to the performance of calculations.
(a) Outline *three* advantages of this use of computers.
(b) Give *three* examples of the use of computers for information storage and retrieval. (YREB 77 I)

12 Explain the meaning of the following terms:
(a) data preparation, (b) object program, (c) diagnostics, (d) address,
(e) 16-bit word. (YREB 77 II)

13 The types of program listed below are often included in the computer software provided for use on a large computer.
compiler, assembler, operating system, utility program, application package.
(a) Why are they necessary?
(b) Describe the main features of each.
(c) Name the type of software from the list above which you would expect to be used for the following jobs (i) copying a program automatically onto a magnetic tape, (ii) sending a message to the operator that the line-printer requires more paper, (iii) working out the payroll of a company, (iv) translating a FORTRAN program into machine code. (YREB 77 II)

14 A factory is to computerize its payroll. Every week the name, code number, and number of hours worked by each employee is input to the computer which automatically produces the printed wage slips.
(a) What information about each employee must be permanently held on backing storage in order for the above to be done?
(b) In what ways will this information need to be amended from week to week in order to make sure that it is up to date? (WMEB 74 I)

15 (a) In computing, what is a file?
(b) Give an example of a file.
(c) What structure must the file have so that it may be searched by the binary search technique?
(d) Name one other operation apart from searching which is also often carried out with files. (WMEB 74 II)

16 (a) Three people *A*, *B* and *C* vote whether they think a pop record will be a HIT or a MISS. Rearrange the boxes in Figure 24.3 and draw in connecting lines with arrows so that if two or three people vote HIT the word HIT is output but if only one or none vote HIT then the word MISS is output.
(b) The logic diagram in Figure 24.4 shows a circuit made up from four logic gates, two of which are AND gates and two of which are OR gates.

If the circuit is to operate in the same way as the flowchart in (a) with HIT represented by 1 and MISS by 0, say which of the logic gates must be

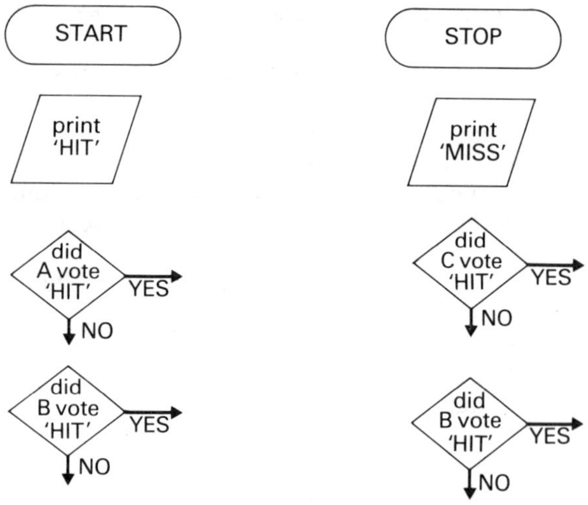

Fig. 24.3

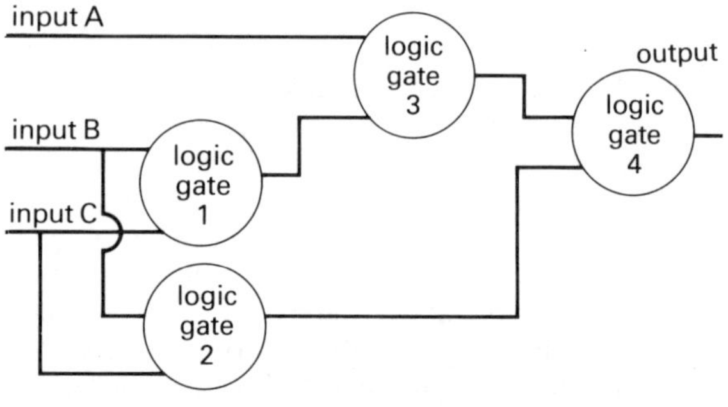

Fig. 24.4

the AND gates and which must be the OR gates. (WMEB 74 II)

17 What items of equipment would need to be provided for a computer controlled system of traffic flow in a large town (a) in the street, (b) at the control centre?

Describe briefly how the system would work and what steps might be taken to keep traffic flowing in the event of a serious road accident. (WMEB 75 I)

18 (a) How many different arrangements of holes are possible on seven-channel paper tape?
(b) What is meant by 'odd parity'?
(c) If only the arrangements which have odd parity can be used to represent characters, how many characters can be represented on seven-channel tape?
(d) What is the purpose of parity? (WMEB 75 II)

19 A company buys motor car spares in bulk from the manufacturers, stores them in a large central warehouse, and then distributes them to garages upon receipt of an order form. The company employs several hundred people and plans to install a computer

List *three* activities for which the company may wish to use the computer and describe briefly for *each* activity how the computer system might operate. (WMEB 75 II)

20 (a) What is information retrieval?
(b) Why is it important nowadays?
(c) Give an example of an information retrieval system.
(d) In using an information retrieval system explain what is meant by a keyword. (WMEB 76 I)

21 Describe briefly the twos complement method of representing integers (positive and negative) in storage locations.

Illustrate your answer by listing all the possible bit patterns which can occur in a 3-bit cell and the numbers they would represent in the twos complement system.

Show how the calculation $3 + (-1) = 2$ is performed in the twos complement system with 3-bit cells. (WMEB 76 II)

22 A list of English words in alphabetical order is stored in a computer.
(a) Describe the binary search method of searching this list in order to find a given word.
(b) What advantage does the binary search method have over the method where the search starts at the beginning and looks through the list in order, one word at a time, until the given word is found?
(c) If each English word in the list has its French translation stored with it, why would it be easier to use the list to translate from English into French rather than the other way round? (WMEB 76 II)

23 The information in the table represents a machine code program in a certain computer.

Location	Function	Address
50	01	100
51	02	101
52	04	102
53	03	103
54	04	104
55	05	55

The computer has the following instruction code:

01n: load contents of address n to Accumulator
02n: add contents of address n to Accumulator

03n: subtract contents of address n from Accumulator

04n: copy contents of Accumulator to store n

05n: jump to address n for next instruction

If locations 100, 101 and 103 contain the numbers +7, +29 and +149 respectivity, describe what the program does. (AEB 78 specimen)

24 Figure 24.5 shows a simple piece of decoding logic.

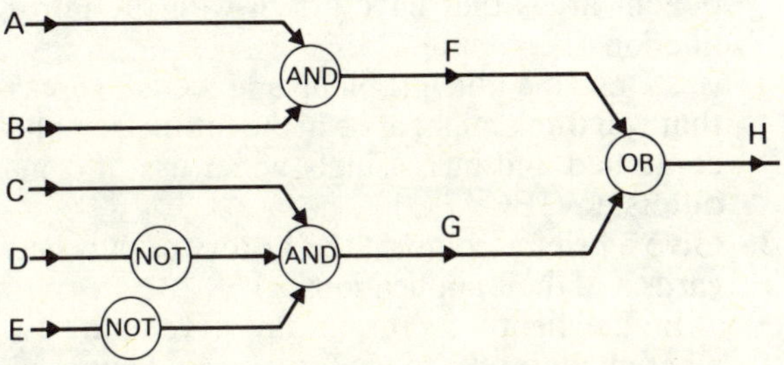

Fig. 24.5

Complete the table below, in order to find the value of H for each of the inputs listed. (AEB 78 specimen)

A	B	C	D	E	F	G	H
1	1	0	1	1			
0	1	1	0	0			
0	0	1	0	1			
1	1	1	1	1			
1	0	0	1	1			
1	1	1	0	0			

25 Design a document which could be used as a source for punching a card which would enable a library to capture all the information which is needed about a borrower. Indicate which parts would have to be punched and which are merely for the guidance of the librarian.

What checks for accuracy do you think that the library should carry out (a) manually and (b) during computer processing? (AEB 78 specimen)

26 An information file on criminals has been constructed to show whether or not each criminal has the following characteristics:

1 Taller than 5 feet
2 older than 21 years
3 younger than 40 years
4 female
5 male
6 bald

Part of the file is given by:

Characteristic	1	2	3	4	5	6
Criminal 1	1	0	0	0	1	1
Criminal 2	0	1	0	1	0	1
Criminal 3	0	0	1	1	0	0

(a) (i) Give a description of each of the three criminals, explaining carefully how you decided to interpret the code. (ii) How many criminals could have distinct codes? (iii) Suggest a more efficient coding system and explain how it should be interpreted.

(b) Draw a flowcart to show how you would search this file to extract the names of criminals who are under 21, have no hair, are male and less than 5 feet tall. (AEB 78 specimen)

27 Information is often presented in a compact form by coding. For example, on a school time-table the coding 29 ERW CS1 might be used where 29 is the room number, ERW gives the teacher's initials and CS1 gives the subject and set.

Choose one of the following codes and explain briefly what information is given by each character group in the code.

(a) A car registration number **CAA 274P**
(b) A national grid reference **SN 203 080**
(c) A post code **SK8 7BS.** (EAEB 77 I)

28 Read the following passage and answer the questions below using the information given.

'The personnel file of a company with 10000 employees is first punched on standard 80 column cards. Each employee record is 250 characters. The card file is then transferred to magnetic tape. The working storage of the computer can hold 1700 characters at any one time. The computer has a 400 cards per minute reader. Punched cards are sold in boxes of 2000 costing £2.60 per box. The average keypunch operator works at a speed of 5000 characters per hour.'

(a) How many cards are needed for each employee record?
(b) What will be the total cost of the boxes of cards?
(c) How many records can be written to the tape in one transfer?
(d) How long will it take to read the card file?
(e) How many hours will it take to punch the cards? (EAEB 77 I)

29 'John and Mary Brown rent a Midshire council house and have two young children, Peter and Jane. John has a bank account. He owns and drives a car. They rent a television set from a large rental company and are buying a cooker and deep freeze on hire purchase. The children have just had the first of two immunization injections. Mary unfortunately suffers from a serious kidney disease.'

In the above passage it can be seen that there may be at least nine instances in which data about the Brown family is stored in computer files.

(a) Write down *seven* of these and in each case say briefly what information may be stored and by whom and for what purpose it is used.

(b) In what way, if any, could computer files be used, (i) if Mr. Brown's car was stolen, (ii) if a potential kidney donor died in an accident, (iii) if Mr. and Mrs. Brown wanted to borrow money for a washing machine? (EAEB 77 I)

30 Draw a flowchart to play the game of conkers using the following rules:

Two people *A* and *B* play.

A has first strike.

A and *B* alternate turns until one conker breaks completely from its string.

If on striking, the strings intertwine, the player whose strike it was is allowed one further turn.

If on striking, one of the conkers and string falls to the ground, the striker has an extra turn.

The game continues until one conker breaks completely and the winner is the player with the conker intact. (WJEC 77 CSE)

Before answering questions 31, 32 and **33, read the following brief description carefully.**

One computer installed in a commercial organization was described as having a central processor, 512 K words of main store, with six disc units, four magnetic tape units, six VDU's for data entry, card reader, two line printers and a communications processor controlling twenty terminals.

The company is involved in supplying metal and plastic spare parts etc., to shops, and maintains a database of all these parts which is constantly updated. In addition, a variety of other applications are run on the machine, including a weekly and monthly payroll.

31 What backing store does this computer installation have?

32 What backing store would you expect to use for (a) the database, (b) the payroll?

Give a reason for each.

33 What device connected with the installation would be used for (a) interrogating the database, (b) performing calculations? (WJEC 77 O)

34 Write *short* notes on *three* of the following (indicate the main differences and give an example to illustrate the meanings):

(a) software and hardware,
(b) on-line and off-line working,
(c) software packages and library sub-routines,
(d) system analysis and programming,
(e) computer operations and data preparation operations. (WJEC 77 O)

35 (a) State *briefly, three* problem areas and *three* benefit areas that have arisen with the introduction of computers.

(b) Describe the problem and benefit areas that you think might arise in the future from the continued and increasingly wider use of computers. (WJEC 77 O)

36 Give a brief account of the history of punched cards and their applications.

In the light of present-day developments, what might be the likely future use of punched cards? Give your reasons. (OLE 77 II)

37 Write down in order the stages in the production of a program, from the first idea to its general use. (OLE 78 I)

38 Software can be classified into six categories:

(a) assemblers	(d) applications packages
(b) compilers	(e) operating systems
(c) utility programs	(f) supervisory (executive) programs

(i) Give *two* examples of an applications package.

(ii) What are the essential differences between an assembler and a compiler?

(iii) Say which of the categories (a–f) of software each is the following is:
a sort program;
a program which tells the operator if a peripheral is broken; a program used to test circuits in the computer; a program that records how long each user has used the computer.

(iv) Give examples, with a brief explanation, of *two* situations where an operating system is necessary. Explain how an operating system can help to reduce errors.

(v) Explain the difference between the work of a systems programmer and an applications programmer. (MREB 78)

39 You have been asked to take a small party on a guided tour of a computer installation, visiting the data preparation area and the computer room.

Write notes to help you to talk about the various people, their jobs, and the equipment you may expect to see. (EAEB 78 I)

40 The flowchart (Figure 24.6) is designed to provide information from data which are input as indicated.

(a) Suggest an appropriate entry for the decision box which has been left blank.

(b) Explain the purpose of your suggested entry.

(c) What information is provided by the output from this flowchart? (JMB 78)

41 (a) Choose *one* application of a data bank which you have studied and explain (i) how the data are efficiently captured, (ii) how the data are kept up to date, (iii) how the information can be used as a result of the rapid access which the computer affords.

(b) Explain the concern which the ordinary citizen may feel as a result of the increasing use of data banks containing personal information.

Outline some of the steps which could be taken to dispel this concern. (JMB 78)

42 A firm that has not used a computer before has ordered one for delivery in a year's time. State any *three* things that the firm ought to be doing to prepare for the arrival of the computer. (MREB 77)

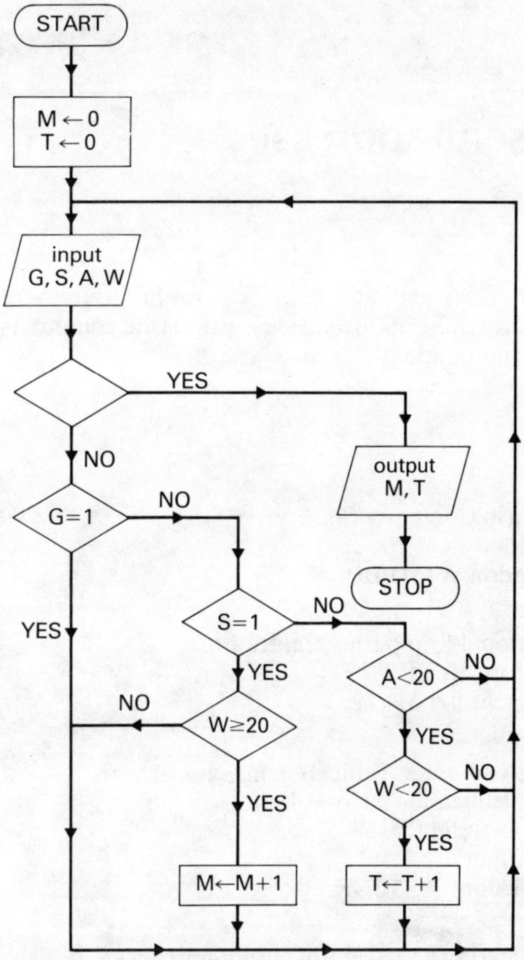

G values represent the sex: male (1) female (0).
S values represent martial status: married (1) single (0).
A values are the ages in years.
W values are the number of working hours per week.

Useful addresses

The following addresses are useful sources of information about various aspects of computers and computing:

British Computer Society
13 Mansfield Street
London W1M 0BP

National Computing Centre Ltd
Oxford Road
Manchester M1 7ED

ICL Computer Education in Schools
The Educational Consultant
60 Portman Road
Reading
Berkshire RG3 1NR

Education and Scientific Programmes
IBM United Kingdom Ltd
101 Wigmore Street
London W1H 0AB

Bank Education Service
10 Lombard Street
London EC3V 9AT

Police National Computer Unit
Room 352
Horseferry House
Dean Ryle Street
London SW1P 2AW

Nascom Minicomputers
121 High Street
Berkhamsted
Herts. HP4 2DJ

Computer Weekly Magazine
Dorset House
Stamford Street
London SE1 9LU

Computing Magazine
Computing Europe
53/55 Frith Street
London W1A 2HG

Educational Computing Magazine
30/31 Islington Green
London N1

Personal Computer World Magazine
Sportscene Publishers (PCW) Ltd
14 Rathbone Place
London W1P 1DE

Glossary

abacus an early calculating device using beads moving on strings.
absolute address the address of a storage location as determined by the computer hardware.
access to locate data, usually on a file.
accoustic coupler see *modem.*
accumulator a register in the arithmetic and logic unit of a CPU, which stores data while it is being processed. Amongst other things, it stores the results of steps of calculations.
address a number which specifies the location of a cell in a computer memory.
address decoder a logic circuit which recognizes an address and sends a pulse of electricity to the control switch at the memory cell addressed.
address modification (or indexing) the process of changing the address part of a machine instruction.
alphabetic (character) a letter which can be input or output by a computer.
alphanumeric (character) a letter or a number.
analogue computer a computer which represents data by a physical quantity, such as voltage.
analogue-to-digital converter (ADC) the interface between an analogue and a digital unit in a hybrid computer.
applications package a complete, documented program for a computer application.
applications programmer a person who writes programs for applications of computers, usually in commerce or industry.
arithmetic and logic unit (ALU) part of the CPU of a computer, where calculations and logical operations are done.
assembler a program which converts programs in assembly language to machine language.
assembly language (or low level language) a programming language were each instruction corresponds to one machine code instruction.

backing store storage for large quantities of data outside the CPU of a computer.
balance (of an account) the amount of money owing on, or contained in, the account.
baud a data transmission rate of one bit per second.
batch processing a type of operating system where programs are run in batches, or a type of data processing where data is processed in batches.
batch total a check total used in data validation.
binary base two.
binary coded decimal (BCD) each digit of a decimal number is converted separately to binary.
binary search a common method of accessing a data item from a set of data which is in numeric or alphabetic order.
bistable device a computer component which has only two stable states.
bit binary digit (0 or 1).
block a set of data items stored together on backing store, and normally transferred as a unit.
Boolean expression see *logic expression.*
branching transferring control from one part of a computer program to another part. Branching may be conditional or unconditional.
bubble sort a common sorting process where small numbers 'float' to the top of the list.
buffer a register which stores data while it is being transferred from one device to another.
byte a set of bits which together represent one character.

cell a storage space in a computer memory.
central processing unit (CPU) the unit of a computer in which processing of data takes place.
channel see *track.*
character a letter, number or symbol which can be input, stored and output by a computer.
character code a binary code for characters.
character set the set of characters which can be input, stored and output by a computer.
check digit an extra number or letter placed on the end of a data item for checking purposes.
chip see *integrated circuit.*
clock pulse a pulse of current at regular time intervals, controlling the timing of a process.
clock pulse generator a hardware device in the control unit of a CPU, which generates clock pulses.
commissioning starting up and testing a new computer.
compilation changing a source program in a high level language into an equivalent object program in machine language.
compilation error an error in a high level language program which is detected by the compiler.
compiler a program which changes a source program in a high level language into an equivalent object program in machine language.
computer a machine, controlled by a stored program, which automatically accepts and processes data, and supplies the results of the processing.

computer architect a person who designs computers.

computer bureau a company which does data processing for other companies.

computer operator a person who operates a computer.

computer output on microfilm (COM) a method of photographing computer output onto microfilm.

computer log a record, produced by the operating system of a computer, of all the work done on the computer.

constant a quantity which stays the same throughout a computer program.

continuous (representation of data) a representation which can represent all values of the data. (Compare with *discrete* representation of data.)

control switch a solid state switch controlling the flow of data in a data channel.

control unit part of the CPU of a computer which controls the step-by-step running of the computer.

core plane a layer of ferrite cores in a core store.

core store a computer memory consisting of ferrite cores.

counter a variable which controls the number of times a program loop is repeated.

current instruction register (CIR) a register in the control unit of a CPU, which stores the machine instruction currently being procesed.

cycle time the time for one instruction cycle.

cylinder the tracks in a magnetic disc pack which can be accessed by a read/write head in one position.

data information in a form which can be stored on, and processed by a computer.

database a structured set of data, used by more than one computer application.

data capture obtaining information for use in data processing

data channel (or data highway) a set of wires, inside a computer, along which data flows.

data control staff people who supervise the collection and preparation of data for input into a computer.

data highway see *data channel.*

data preparation preparaing data for input into a computer, by punching it onto cards or paper tape.

data preparation staff people who punch and verify cards or paper tape, or operate direct data entry terminals.

data processing (DP) a general phrase which describes the work done by a computer.

data processing department in an organization which uses a computer, the people who work directly with the computer.

data processing manager (DPM) the person in charge of a data processing department.

data processing system people, programs and a computer working together to do data processing.

debugging eliminating all the errors in a program.

deck a set of punched cards.

decoder a logic circuit which recognizes one or more combinations of inputs.

delay register a register which stores one or more bits for a short space of time.

destructive readout a method of reading data from a computer memory which clears the memory cell in the process.

device (or unit) a piece of equipment which forms part of a computer. A device does one specific task, such as input or output.

diagnostic error message a message output by a computer when an error has occurred. The message identifies the type of error.

digital computer a computer which stores and processes data in the form of digits. Most computers are digital computers.

digital plotter an output device which produces graphs or drawings. It does not move continuously, but in small steps.

direct access (data storage) see *random access.*

direct data entry (DDE) input data is typed directly onto a magnetic tape or magnetic disc.

discrete (representation of data) a representation which can only represent certain values of the data. (Compare with *continuous* representation of data.)

distributed array processor (DAP) a CPU which is capable of processing a large number of data items simultaneously.

distributed processing processing shared in a computer amongst several CPU's or intelligent terminals.

documentation a written description of how a program works. Also see *user documentation.*

dot matrix printer a type of output device which prints characters by patterns of dots.

double length word two words in a computer memory joined together and manipulated as a single word.

dry run carrying out each step of a program or flow diagram by hand, and writing down the results at each step.

electronic data processing (EDP) data processing involving the use of a computer.

electronic funds transfer (EFT) a method of transferring money between banks, using computer terminals.

end-of-data marker (or rogue value) a number or set of characers which indicates the end of a set of data.

end-of-field marker
end-of-record marker
end-of-file marker one character on a data storage medium which marks the end of the field, record or file.

error message a message output by a computer when an error has occurred. Also see *diagnostic error message.*

even parity the total; number of 1's in a word or byte is an even number.

exchangeable disc pack a magnetic disc pack which can be removed from a magnetic disc drive, and exchanged for another pack.

execute (phase) the second part of an instruction cycle. The current machine instruction is carries out.

execution error (or run time error) an error in a program which is detected while the program is running.

executive program see *operating system.*
exponent the power of two of a floating point number.

ferrite core a small ring of soft iron used to store one bit in some computer memories.
fetch (phase) the first part of an instruction cycle. The machine instruction to be processed is fetched from the memory.
field an area on a data storage medium which contains one item of data.
file a structured collection of related data.
file directory a set of data describing the structure of a file, and enabling records to be located in the file.
file librarian a person in charge of all the magnetic tapes and discs at a computer centre.
fixed point number a number with the decimal or binary point in a fixed position.
flip-flop a logic circuit which is always in one of two states. It is most commonly used to store one bit.
floating point number a method of representing very large or very small numbers on a computer. The number is represented as a binary fraction (the *mantissa*) multiplied by a power of 2 (the *exponent*).
floppy disc a single, lightweight magnetic disc.
flow diagram (or flowchart) a diagram consisting of a set of boxes, joined by arrows, describing the steps of a process.
frame the storage area for one character on paper or magnetic tape. It is a single row of bit positions across the width of the tape.
front-end processor a CPU which controls the flow of data to and from another CPU, or other CPU's.
full adder a logic circuit which adds two input bits, and a previous carry bit, producing a sum and a carry output.

gate a logic element which acts as a solid state switch. A gate opens to pass on a pulse of electricity, or closes to stop it.
generation (of computers) a group of computers using the same kind of hardware technology.
generation (of a file) when a file is updated, a new generation of the file is created.
GIGO Garbage In, Garbage Out. If wrong input data is processed by a computer, the output will be wrong.
grandfather/father/son principle keeping the current version, as well as the two previous versions of a magnetic tape, to guard against accidental loss of data.
graphical display unit a terminal, resembling a VDU, on which graphs and pictures can be displayed.
graph plotter see *digital plotter.*

half adder a logic circuit which adds two input bits, producing a sum and a carry output.
hard copy printed input or output data.
hardware the components and devices which make up a computer.
hash total a check total used in data validation.
hexadecimal (numbers) base sixteen numbers.
high level language an application oriented programming language, which does not correspond to the machine code of any computer.
hybrid computer a computer containing digital and analogue units.

immediate access (storage) data storage in the memory of a CPU.
indexing see *adress modification.*
index register a register which stores a word used in address modification.
indirect addressing the memory address part of a machine instruction locating a memory cell which contains the address of the data item required by the machine instruction.
information retrieval the process of recovering specific information from a database.
input (verb) to supply data or programs to a computer
input (noun) the data or programs supplied to a computer.
input device a device which accepts input data and converts the data into the pattern of electrical pulses used by a CPU.
installation engineer the person who supervises the installation of a new computer.
instruction cycle a sequence of steps which processes one machine instruction. The sequence is repeated for the next instruction, forming a cycle.
instruction register (IR) see *current instruction register.*
instruction set the set of operation codes in a machine language.
integrated circuit (or chip) a solid state electronic circuit equivalent to a number of transistors and other components.
intelligent terminal a terminal which is capable of a certain amount of processing.
interactive processing data processing where some work is done by the user, and some by the computer.
interface the point of contact between one device and another, or a device which links two other devices.
interrupt a temporary halt in the processing of a program, while some other operation takes place.
invoice a written record of a purchase of goods.

K a unit of memory size. 1 K = 1024 ($=2^{10}$).
key a data item in a record, used to identify or locate the record.
key-to-disc (input) see *direct data entry.*

large scale integration (LSI) describes an integrated circuit containing more than 1000 logic elements.
library subprogram see *utility routine.*
light pen a device which draws lines on the screen of a graphical display unit.
line printer an output device which prints one complete line at a time.
log see *computer log*

logic circuit an electric circuit containing logic elements and performing a logic operation.
logic element a computer component which performs a logic operation.
logic expression (or Boolean expression) a set of symbols describing a logic circuit.
loop a part of a computer program which is repeated a number of times.
low level language see *assembly language.*

machine code see *machine language.*
machine language a programming language consisting of instructions in a binary code. The instructions control the hardware of a computer directly.
macro-instruction an instruction which is carried out by a set of other instructions.
magazine the housing for a set of magnetic cards.
magnetic ink character recognition (MICR) reading characters, printed in magnetic ink, by a specially designed device.
main program the part of a program which accesses the subprograms.
main store see *memory.*
maintenance engineer a person who inspects and repairs computers.
mantissa the fraction part of a floating point number.
master data data which is used for reference by a data processing system.
medium a material on which data is stored.
megabyte a unit of information storage capacity. 1 megabyte = 1 million bytes.
memory (or main store) part of the CPU of a computer, where the data and programs are stored, which are in use at the time.
memory address part of a machine code instruction, locating the data item to be used by the instruction.
merge to combine data from two sources.
microcomputer a computer built up around a microprocessor.
microfilm reader a device which enlarges a page of microfilm onto a screen.
microfiche a postcard-sized piece of film which contains about 200 pages of microfilm.
micro-instruction an instruction forming part of a microprogram.
microprogram a set of instructions which open and close the appropriate control switches to carry out a machine instruction.
microprocessor a single integrated circuit containing the control unit, ALU and sometimes the memory of a central processor.
microsecond one millionth of a second.
mill an early name for a central processing unit.
millisecond one thousandth of a second.
minicomputer a small computer, most commonly contained in one unit.
modem (or accoustic computer) a *mod*ulator/*dem*odulator, the device which links a terminal to a telephone line.
modifier bit one bit in a machine code instruction which determines whether or not the memory address is to be modified.
module a part of a computer program, written and tested separately before being combined with other modules.
modulo check a method of calculating or testing a check digit.
most significant (digit or bit) the digit or bit with the highest place value in a number.
multi-access a mode of operation of a computer which allows CPU time to be shared amongst a number of terminals, so that each terminal appears to be using the whole computer all the time.
multiplexer a hardware device which shares CPU time amongst a number of terminals.
multiprogramming (or multitasking) a mode of operation of a computer where CPU time and memory space are shared amongst several programs.
multitasking see *multiprogramming.*

nanosecond one thousand millionth of a second.
normalization shifting the mantissa and adjusting the exponent of a floating point number so that the most significant bit of the mantissa contains a 1.
numeric (character) a number which can be input, stored or output by a computer.
***n*-type (semiconductor)** a semiconductor with a surplus of electrons.

object program a program in a machine language, produced by a compiler or assembler from a source program in a high level or assembly language.
octal (numbers) base eight numbers.
odd parity the total number of 1's in a word or byte is an odd number.
off-line (device) a device, such as a card punch, not connected to the CPU of a computer.
ones complement a binary representation of numbers. A negative number is represented by negating each bit of the corresponding positive number.
on-line (data processing) data processing where there is a direct link between the user and the computer.
on-line (device) any device connected to the CPU of a computer.
operating system a program, or set of programs, which co-ordinates the running of all the units of a computer, and provides communication between the computer and the person operating it.
operation code part of a machine code instruction, specifying the type of operation to be carried out.
operation decoder a logic circuit which recognises each different operation code and sends pulses of electricity to all the control switches which carry out the particular operation.
operations manager the person in charge of the day-to-day running of a computer.
operation table see *truth table.*
operator's console a device used by a computer operator to send instructions to a computer, and the computer to send messages to the operator.

optical character recognition (OCR) reading printed characters by optical means, on a specially designed device.

output (noun) the data which is printed or displayed by a computer after processing.

output (verb) to print or display the results of data processing.

output device a device which converts data in the form of electrical pulses from a CPU into printed or displayed characters.

overflow the error which occurs when a computer produces a number which is too large for it to store. (Also see *underflow*.)

overflow bit the bit in the output register of a serial or parallel adder which stores the carry from the most significant bit.

packing density the number of characters per inch (or centimetre) on magnetic tape or magnetic discs.

parallel adder a logic circuit which adds all the bits of two input numbers.

parallel central processors two or more central pro cessors working together in the same computer.

parallel computer a computer which does all its processing one byte or word at a time. (Also see *serial computer*.)

parity bit an extra bit placed on the end of a byte or word for checking purposes. (Also see *even parity*, and *odd parity*.)

parity check a test to see if the parity bit of a byte or word is correct.

peripheral a device connected to the CPU of a computer, for input, output or backing store.

place value the value of a bit or digit, depending on its position in the number.

***p-n* junction** the boundary between *p*-type semiconductor and *n*-type semiconductor in a transistor or integrated circuit.

printout printed output from a computer.

program a set of instructions to a computer.

program counter see *sequence control register*.

program library a set of utility routines permanently stored on a computer for access by other programs.

program maintenance making changes in a computer program from time to time in the light of experience or changing circumstances.

programmer a person who writes, corrects, maintains and documents computer programs. (Also see *systems programmer* and *applications programmer*.)

process an operation, or set of operations, carried out by a computer.

***p*-type (semiconductor)** a semiconductor with a shortage of electrons.

random access (data storage medium) a storage medium where the data can be accessed equally quickly regardless of its position on the medium.

random access memory (RAM) solid state memory circuits, in which the data at any location can be accessed equally quickly.

range check a validation check to see if data lies within a certain range.

read-only memory (ROM) memory circuits storing data which can be accessed but not altered.

read/write head a device which transfers data to or from a magnetic storage medium.

real time processing data processing where the computer must keep up with some other process, which it monitors or controls.

receipt a written record of a sum of money paid to a firm.

record a set of related data items on some storage medium. A set of records forms a file.

register a set of flip-flops storing a byte or a word, for a specific purpose.

remote access access to a computer from a distant site, using a terminal.

remote job entry a type of operating system which allows programs to be input and output from remote sites.

research engineer a person who invents and tests new devices for use in computers.

reset (phase) the step of an instruction cycle during which the SCR is increased by 1, ready for the next instruction.

rogue value see *end-of-data marker*.

rounding (a binary number) reducing the number of bits representing a number, and adding 1 to the last retained bit if the first discarded bit is 1.

rounding error the error caused by rounding.

run time error see *execution error*.

sector a portion of a track on a magnetic drum or disc.

semiconductor materials materials such as silicon or germanium which can be made to conduct a carefully controlled amount of electricity.

sequence control register (SCR) a register in the control unit of a CPU which stores the address of the next machine instruction to be processed.

sequential file a file in which all the records are in alphabetic or numeric order.

serial access (data storage medium) a storage medium where the time required to access a data item depends on the position of the data item on the medium.

serial adder a logic circuit which adds the bits of two input numbers one pair at a time.

serial computer a computer which does all its processing one bit at a time. (Also see *parallel computer*.)

shift to move all the bits of a byte or word to the left or to the right.

shift leader a person in charge of a shift of computer operators and data preparation staff.

sign bit a bit used to indicate the sign of a number. In most cases, 0 means positive, 1 means negative.

sign-and-magnitude code a binary code for numbers where one bit represents the sign and the remaining bits represent the magnitude of the number.

single program operation an operating system which allows a computer to run one program at a time.

software another word for *programs*.

software writer (or systems programmer) a person who writes systems software for computers.

source documents documents, usually written by hand, from which input data is prepared

source program a program in a high level language, or assembly language, which is input into a compiler or assembler.

special (character) a punctuation mark or other symbol (not a letter or number) which can be input or output by a computer.

standard form (numbers) a method of storing very large or very small numbers in base ten.

statement (of an account) a document which shows all the transactions over a period of time, and the balance of an account.

statement (of a program) a program in a high level language consists of a set of statements. Each statement usually corresponds to several machine instructions.

subprogram (or subroutine) a part of a program, performing a specific task, which is accessed (usually several times) from the rest of the program.

subroutine see *subprogram.*

switching circuit a way of representing a logic circuit, by means of a network of switches.

system an assembly of parts functioning as a whole.

systems analyst a person who plans how work is to be done on a computer.

systems flow diagram a flow diagram, usually drawn by a systems analyst, which describes all the stages of a data processing operation.

systems programmer see *software writer.*

systems software the set of programs which enable the hardware and machine code of a computer to do useful work.

tabulator a mechanical device used for commercial calculations.

tag sort a method of sorting the records of a file, by sorting the keys of the records first.

teletypewriter (teletype) a terminal where input and output are typed, as on an ordinary typewriter.

terminal a device providing a direct link between a computer and a person using it.

test data data which is used to test a program for errors.

threshold size (of pulse) the smallest pulse of electricity which affects the magnetisation of a ferrite core.

trace to monitor the progress of a program, usually by outputting the contents of certain storage locations at various stages of the execution of the program.

track a circular zone for storing data on a magnetic disc or drum, or a row of punching positions along the length of paper tape.

transaction file a file used to update a master file.

transaction record a record of a business transaction, usually an invoice or a receipt.

transistor a solid state electronic component used in many computers, usually as a logic element.

truncation reducing the numbers of bits in a number, to make it fit into a shorter storage location.

truncation error the error caused by truncation.

truth table (or operation table) a table showing all the combinations of inputs and outputs of a logic element or logic circuit.

twos complement a binary representation of numbers. The most significant bit represents a negative quantity.

underflow the error which occurs when a computer produces a number too small for it to store. (Also see *overflow.*)

unit see *device.*

update to alter information so as to bring it up to date.

user a person or a group of people who use a computer.

user documentation a description, written by a programmer for the benefit of a user, of how a program works.

user program a program, usually in a high level language, written by or for a user of a computer.

utility routine (or library subprogram) a program or subprogram for some common process, permanently stored on a computer for access by other programs.

validate to check input data before using it in processing.

variable a quantity which changes its value during the running of a computer program.

verify to check that punched cards or paper tape have been punched correctly.

vet see *validate.*

visual display unit (VDU) a terminal where input and output are displayed on a screen rather like a television screen.

word a set of bits treated by a CPU as a single unit.

wordlength the number of bits in a word.

word processing writing, correcting, storing and sending letters, legal documents, newspaper articles etc. by computer.

write permit ring a ring attached to a spool of magnetic tape. If the ring is removed, no data may be written onto the tape.

wrap-around carry a bit carried from the most significant place of a number to the least significant place.

Answers

Exercise 1

1 See Glossary of Terms

2

	Input	Process	Output
(a)	Recipe, ingredients	Mix and put in oven.	Cake.
(b)	Plans, materials.	Cut parts, assemble, paint.	Plane.
(c)	Name, address, number of calls, charges per call.	Calculate amount to pay.	Bill.
(d)	Seeds, soil water, fertiliser, sunlight.	Plant, care for, harvest.	Vegetables.
(e)	Faulty car.	Decide what is wrong, obtain spares, fit parts.	Car in working order.

3 Stages as described in correct shapes of box.

4 **(a)** Yes, very precisely **(b)** Yes, but the answer might be wrong **(c)** No **(d)** No **(e)** Yes, with about 75% accuracy.

*5 Several relevant points can be made, including: **(a)** Information which is not worth remembering is not worth storing in any other way. **(b)** Computers relieve people from having to remember fairly trivial information, and free them to concentrate on more worthwhile matters. **(c)** There is some truth in the assertion that vast quantities of information are created simply because the facilities exist for storing it.

Exercise 2

1 See Glossary of Terms.
2 ALU, memory, control unit.
3 CPU.
4 Input devices, output devices, backing store, terminals.
5 Control unit of the CPU (*NOT* operator's console).
6 Computer manufacturers will often supply literature with photographs.

Exercise 3a

1 See Glossary of Terms.
2 bank branch codes
school subject codes, form codes etc.
National Insurance code numbers
code names of wartime operations
book subject codes
telephone exchange STD codes

3 **(a)** BYTE
(b) 1 0 0 0 0 1 1 0 0 0 1 0 1 0 1 1 0 1 1 0 0 1 0 1

4 **(a)** 1 0 0 1 0 0 0 1 **(b)** 0 1 0 1 0 1 1 0
(c) 0 1 0 0 1 0 0 1 0 0 1 1 **(d)** 94 **(c)** 87 **(f)** 647

5 **(a)** 0 0 1 0 0 1 1 1 **(b)** 1 0 1 1 1 1 0 1
(c) 0 1 1 1 0 1 0 1 **(d)** 54 **(e)** − 38 **(f)** − 93
(g) 127 and − 127

6 **(a)** 0 1 1 0 1 1 **(b)** 1 1 0 0 1 1 **(c)** 0 1 1 1 1 1
(d) 18 **(e)** − 5 **(f)** − 2

(g)

store 7:	0 0 0 1 1 1
reverse bits:	1 1 1 0 0 0
add 1, gives − 7:	1 1 1 0 0 1
store 15:	0 0 1 1 1 1
add − 7 and 15:	(1) 0 0 1 0 0 0 = 8

(h)

store 18:	0 1 0 0 1 0
reverse bits:	1 0 1 1 0 1
add 1, gives − 18:	1 0 1 1 1 0
store 28:	0 1 1 1 0 0
add − 18 and 28:	(1) 0 0 1 0 1 0 = 10

(i)

store 22:	0 1 0 1 1 0
reverse bits:	1 0 1 0 0 1
add 1, gives − 22:	1 0 1 0 1 0
store 19:	0 1 0 0 1 1
add − 22 and 19:	1 1 1 1 0 1 = −3

(j) 31 and − 32

7 **(a)** 0 1 1 0 1 1 **(b)** 1 1 0 0 1 0 **(c)** 0 1 1 1 1 1 **(d)** 18
(e) − 4 **(f)** − 1

(g)

store 7:	0 0 0 1 1 1
reverse bits, gives − 7:	1 1 1 0 0 0
store 15:	0 0 1 1 1 1
add − 7 and 15:	1 0 0 0 1 1 1
and overflow bit:	1
	0 0 1 0 0 0 = 8

(h) store 18: 0 1 0 0 1 0

reverse bits, gives – 18: 1 0 1 1 0 1

store 28: 0 1 1 1 0 0

add – 18 and 28: 1 0 0 1 0 0 1

and overflow bit: 1

0 0 1 0 1 0 = 10

(i) store 22: 0 1 0 1 1 0

reverse bits, gives – 22: 1 0 1 0 0 1

store 19: 0 1 0 0 1 1

add – 22 and 19: 1 1 1 1 0 0 = – 3

(no overflow bit to add)

8 **(a)** 2 **(b)** 4 **(c)** 8 **(d)** 64 **(e)** 256 **(f)** 2^n

9 **(a)** 0 1 0 0 1 0 1 1 **(b)** 0 1 0 1 0 0

(c) The first number is wrong (odd parity is being used).

10 **(a)** 0 0 1 1 0 0 0 1 1 1 1 1 0 0 0 0 0 0 0 1 1 1 1 1 0 1 0 1 0 1 0 0

(b) 0 0 1 0 1 0 0 1 1 1 1 1 0 0 0 0 0 0 1 0 1 1 1 1 0 1 1 0 0 1 0 0

(c) 01/05/61

11 **(a)** 0 0 0 1 1 1 0 1 **(b)** 1 1 0 1 0 0 0 0

(c) 1 0 0 1 1 0 0 1

(d) 47 **(e)** – 90 **(f)** – 47

(g) store 13: 0 0 0 0 1 1 0 1

reverse bits: 1 1 1 1 0 0 1 0

add 1, gives 13: 1 1 1 1 0 0 1 1

store 68: 0 1 0 0 0 1 0 0

and – 13 and 68: (1) 0 0 1 1 0 1 1 1 = 55

(h) store 27: 0 0 0 1 1 0 1 1

reverse bits: 1 1 1 0 0 1 0 0

add 1, gives 27: 1 1 1 0 0 1 0 1

store 53: 0 0 1 1 0 1 0 1

add – 27 and 53: (1) 0 0 0 1 1 0 1 0 = 26

11 **(i)** store 58: 0 0 1 1 1 0 1 0

reverse bits: 1 1 0 0 0 1 0 1

add 1, gives – 58: 1 1 0 0 0 1 1 0

store 79: 0 1 0 0 1 1 1 1

add – 58 and 79: (1) 0 0 0 1 0 1 0 1 = 21

(j) from – 128 to 127

*__12__ *Note:* There are several alternative codes for the sign. The codes + = 1 0 1 0 and – = 1 0 1 1 have been used in these answers.

(a) 0 1 0 1 1 0 1 0 **(b)** 1 0 0 1 1 0 1 1

(c) 0 1 0 0 0 0 1 0 0 0 0 1 1 0 1 0

(d) 0 0 1 0 0 0 0 1 1 0 0 1 1 0 1 1

(e) 0 0 0 0 0 1 0 1 0 1 1 1 1 0 1 1

(f) 301 **(g)** – 2 **(h)** 892

Exercise 3b

1 See Glossary of Terms.

2 **(a)** 52 **(b)** 670 **(c)** 777 **(d)** 21 **(e)** 2347

3 **(a)** 1 1 1 1 0 0 **(b)** 1 1 0 0 0 1

(c) 0 0 1 0 1 1 0 1 0 **(d)** 0 0 1 1 0 1 0 1 1

(e) 1 0 0 1 1 1 0 1 0

4 **(a)** 65 **(b)** C5 **(c)** 25FA

5 **(a)** 0 1 1 1 0 0 0 1 **(b)** 0 1 1 1 1 1 1 0

(c) 1 0 1 0 1 1 1 1 **(d)** 0 0 0 1 0 0 0 0 0 0 1 1

(e) 0 0 1 1 0 1 0 1 1 0 1 1

6 8

7 6

8 **(a)** $\frac{7}{8}$ **(b)** $\frac{17}{32}$ **(c)** $\frac{3}{8}$ **(d)** $-\frac{1}{8}$ **(e)** $-\frac{7}{16}$

9

	-1	$\frac{1}{2}$	$\frac{1}{4}$	$\frac{1}{8}$	$\frac{1}{16}$	$\frac{1}{32}$
(a)	0	0	0	1	1	0
(b)	0	0	1	0	1	0
(c)	0	1	0	0	0	1
(d)	1	1	1	0	0	0
(e)	1	1	1	0	0	1

10 $\frac{31}{32}$

11 **(a)** 5 **(b)** 24 **(c)** 28 **(d)** – 48 **(e)** $\frac{3}{16}$ **(f)** $\frac{7}{32}$ **(g)** $-\frac{3}{64}$ **(h)** $\frac{5}{8}$

12

	mantissa				**characteristic**			
	$\pm$	$\frac{1}{2}$	$\frac{1}{4}$	$\frac{1}{8}$	$\pm$	4	2	1
(a)	0	1	1	0	0	0	1	0
(b)	0	1	1	0	0	0	1	1
(c)	0	1	0	1	0	1	0	0
(d)	1	1	1	1	0	1	0	0
(e)	0	1	0	0	1	0	0	1
(f)	0	1	0	1	1	0	0	1
(g)	0	1	1	0	1	0	1	1
(h)	1	1	0	1	1	0	1	1

13 **(a)** $\frac{7}{8} \times 128 = 112$ **(b)** $\frac{1}{2} \times \frac{1}{128} = \frac{1}{256}$

14 **(a)** 95 **(b)** – 107 **(c)** – 106 **(d)** $-\frac{21}{128}$ **(e)** $-\frac{107}{128}$

(f) – 4 (note that it is not normalised)

Comment: A binary number stored in a computer cannot be converted to base ten unless it is known which code is being used.

Exercise 3c

Negative numbers:

1	5	**2**	– 1	**3**	1	**4**	– 5	**5**	– 3	**6**	2
7	– 6	**8**	– 5	**9**	– 3	**10**	– 6	**11**	– 6	**12**	0

Exercise 3d

Binary numbers:

1 12, 15, 18

2 1 1 0 1, 1 0 0 1 1, 1 1 0 1 1

3 1 0 0 0 1, 1 0 1 1 0 0, 1 0 1 0 1 0, 1 1 1 1 0, 1 1 0 0 1 1

Exercise 4

1 See Glossary of Terms.
2 $4 \times 1024 \times 24 = 98304$
3 64
4 The half pulses travel through other cores without affecting their magnetisation. Only the core in which they combine to exceed the threshold pulse size is affected. This arrangement considerably reduces the number of wires needed to thread the cores.
5 Any cell in the memory can be accessed immediately.
6 Post codes, Cinema seat numbers, Aeroplane flight numbers, Building room numbers, etc.

Exercise 5

1 See Glossary of Terms.
2 *Advantages:* saves paper, easy to correct, magnetic discs can be re-used
Disadvantages: the data can only be accessed by the computer (whereas punched cards can be read along the top), magnetic discs can be accidentally erased.
3 Any suitable combinations of fieldwidths of total width not exceeding 80 characters.

Exercise 6

1 See Glossary of Terms.

2

			C	
	D		C	
	D E		C E	
	D E	I	C E	
O	D E	I	C E	etc.

No.

3 Chain type. The paper moves as soon as the number has been printed. The next number occurs fairly soon on the chain.
4 Wage slips, salary cheques, gas and electricity bills, O Level and CSE certificates, etc.
5 A whole line is printed at a time. Several letters may be printed simultaneously.
6 Microfilm is much less bulky, and may soon become cheaper than output paper.

Exercise 7

1 See Glossary of Terms.
2

Serial Access	Random Access
magnetic tape	magnetic discs
cassettes	magnetic drums
	magnetic cards
	floppy discs

3 **(a)** 60 bytes (approximately, other answers depend on this figure)
(b) 150 megabytes
(c) 5 discs
(d) 37500000 seconds = 10417 hours
= 1302 working days
4 Because of the very high packing density of the data, expansion or contraction from changes of temperature would make it impossible to read.
5 500000 punched cards
6 **(a)** serial **(b)** direct **(c)** direct **(d)** serial

Exercise 8

1 See Glossary of Terms
2 As fast as the operator can type.
3 **(a)** VDU **(b)** graphical display unit **(c)** teletype **(d)** VDU **(e)** graphical display unit **(f)** VDU **(g)** teletype

Exercise 9a

1 See Glossary of Terms.

2

A	B	C
0	0	1
0	1	0
1	0	0
1	1	0

3

A	B	C	D
0	0	0	0
0	0	1	0
0	1	0	0
0	1	1	0
1	0	0	0
1	0	1	0
1	1	0	0
1	1	1	1

4

A	B	C
0	0	0
0	1	1
1	0	1
1	1	1

5

A	B	C	D
0	0	0	1
0	0	1	0
0	1	0	1
0	1	1	1
1	0	0	1
1	0	1	0
1	1	0	1
1	1	1	0

6

A	B	C	D
0	0	0	0
0	1	1	1
1	0	0	1
1	1	0	1

7

A	B	C	D
0	0	0	1
0	1	1	1
1	0	0	0
1	1	0	1

8 An OR gate.
9 and 10 Figure 9.41.

Exercise 9b

1 **(a)** $C = \sim(A \vee B)$ $\qquad c = \overline{(a + b)}$
(b) $D = (A \wedge B) \vee C$ $\qquad d = (a.\ b).\ c$

(c) $C = \sim(\sim A \wedge \sim B)$ $\qquad c = \overline{(\bar{a}.\ \bar{b})}$

(d) $D = (\sim A \wedge B) \vee \sim C$ $\qquad d = (\bar{a}.\ b) + \bar{c}$

(e) $C = (A \vee B) \wedge \sim A$ $\qquad c = (a + b).\ \bar{a}$
$D = A \vee B$ $\qquad d = a + b$

9

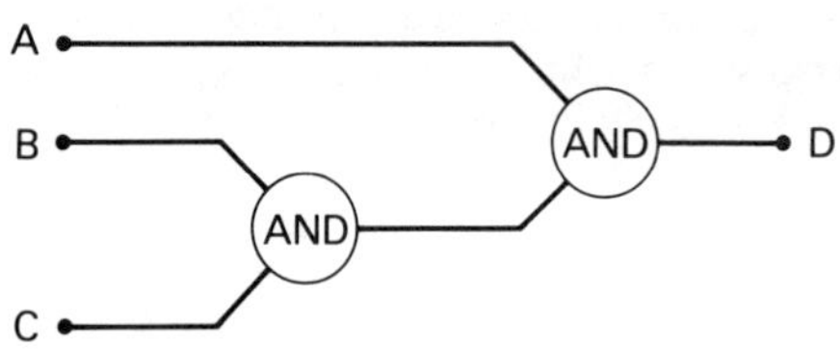

10

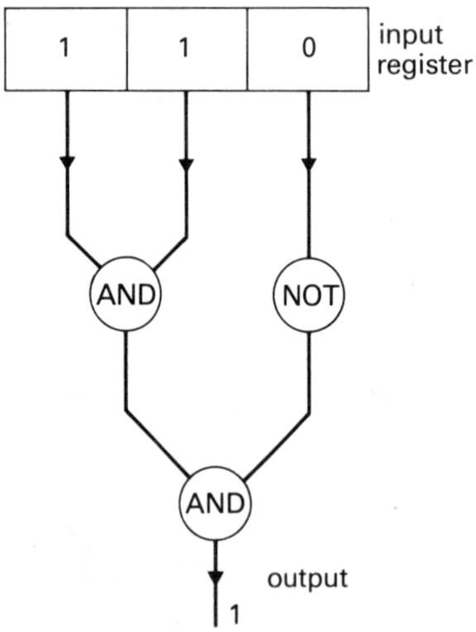

Fig. 9.41

(f) $C = \sim A \wedge B$ $c = \bar{a}. b$

$D = \sim A \vee B$ $d = \bar{a} + b$

2 Figure 9.42

3 Operation tables:

(a) Inputs / Output

A	B	C	D
0	0	0	0
0	0	1	1
0	1	0	0
0	1	1	0
1	0	0	0
1	0	1	1
1	1	0	0
1	1	1	1

(b) Inputs / Output

A	B	C	D
0	0	0	1
0	0	1	0
0	1	0	0
0	1	1	0
1	0	0	0
1	0	1	0
1	1	0	0
1	1	1	1

(c) Inputs / Output

A	B	C	D
0	0	0	1
0	0	1	1
0	1	0	1
0	1	1	0
1	0	0	1
1	0	1	1
1	1	0	1
1	1	1	1

(d) Inputs / Output

A	B	D
0	0	0
0	1	1
1	0	1
1	1	0

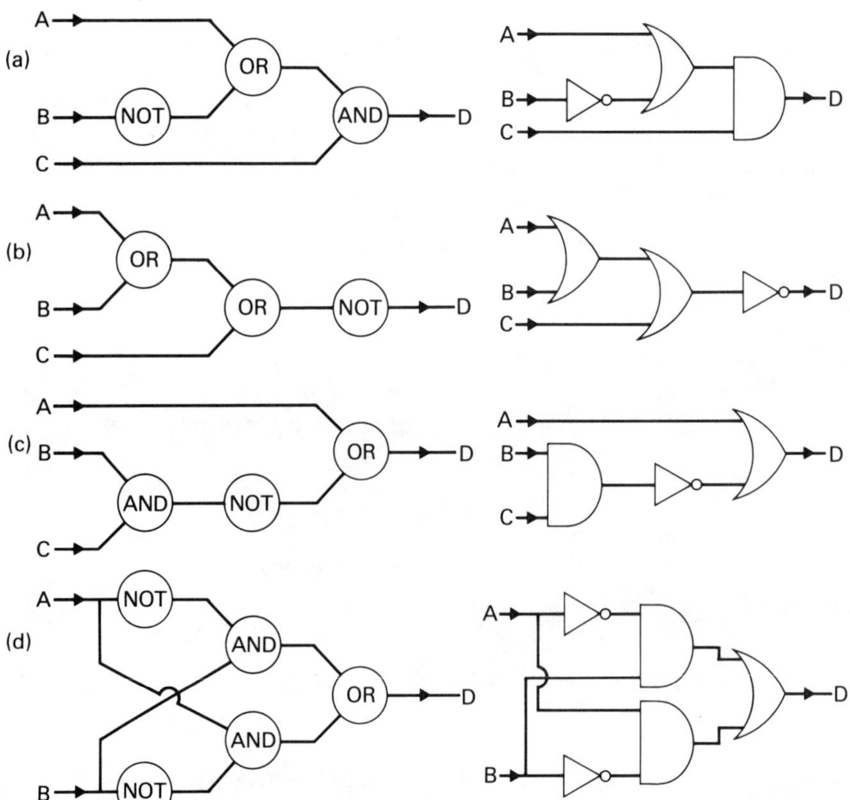

Fig. 9.42

4 Figure 9.43

5 **(a)** (A OR B) AND (C OR D)
(b) A OR (B AND C) OR D

6 **(a)**

Input			**Output**
A	B	C	D
0	0	0	1
0	0	1	1
0	1	0	0
0	1	1	1
1	0	0	1
1	0	1	1
1	1	0	1
1	1	1	1

(b)

Input			**Output**		
A	B	C	D	E	F
0	0	0	0	0	0
0	0	1	0	1	1
0	1	0	0	1	1
0	1	1	0	1	1
1	0	0	1	1	1
1	0	1	1	1	1
1	1	0	1	1	1
1	1	1	1	1	1

(c)

Input			**Output**		
A	B	C	D	E	F
0	0	0	0	0	0
0	0	1	0	0	0
0	1	0	1	0	1
0	1	1	0	0	0
1	0	0	0	0	0
1	0	1	0	1	1
1	1	0	0	0	0
1	1	1	0	0	0

Possible use: a decoder to recognise input signals 0 1 0, or 1 0 1

Exercise 10a

1 See Glossary of Terms.

2

Input			**Output**	
A	B	Previous carry	Sum	Carry
0	0	0	0	0
0	0	1	1	0
0	1	0	1	0
0	1	1	0	1
1	0	0	1	0
1	0	1	0	1
1	1	0	0	1
1	1	1	1	1

3 and 4 Figure 10.9

5 Figure 10.10.

*7 Twelve bits.
Example:

```
           111111
          x111111
          -------
           111111
          111111
         111111
        111111
       111111
      111111
     ------------
     111110000001
```

Exercise 10b

1 See Glossary of Terms.

2 **(a)** − 512 to 511 **(b)** − 2048 to 2047
(c) − 32768 to 32767 **(d)** -2^{n-1} to $2^{n-1}-1$

3 **(a)** 0.634, 23.815, 0.000, 3.61
(b) 0.0101, 10.0110, 0.0010, 10.001
(c) 0.62, 0.80, 67.42, 41.70
(d) 0.101, 1.011, 10.100, 1.001

4 Answer = 0.011110 Truncated = 0.0111
Error = 0.00001 = $\frac{1}{32}$

5 **(a)** $\frac{1}{12}$
(b) $\frac{2}{3} = 0.1010$
$\frac{7}{12} = 0.1001$ −
0.0001 = $\frac{1}{16}$, error = $\frac{1}{12} - \frac{1}{16} = \frac{1}{48}$
(c) $\frac{2}{3} = 0.1011$
$\frac{7}{12} = 0.1001$ −
0.0010 = $\frac{1}{8}$, error = $\frac{1}{8} - \frac{1}{12} = \frac{1}{24}$
(d) In this case, rounding increases the error.

6 **(a)**

```
    .111          100
  × .110        + 010
  ------        -----
     000          110
    1110        -----
   11100
  ------
  101010
  ------
```

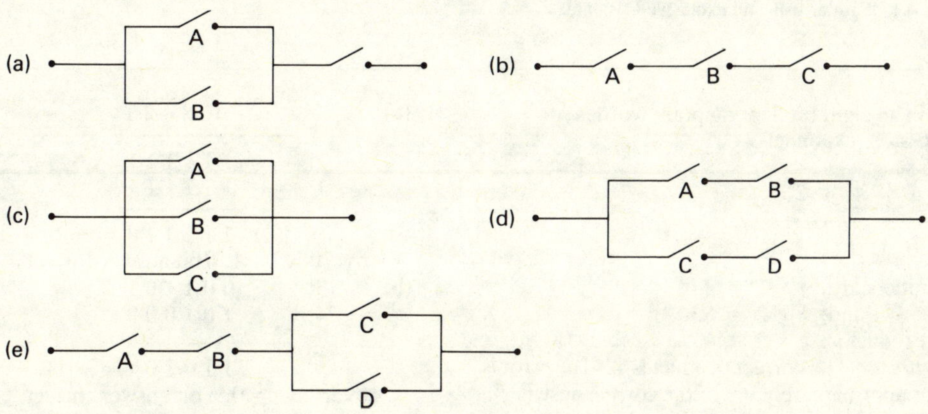

Fig. 9.43

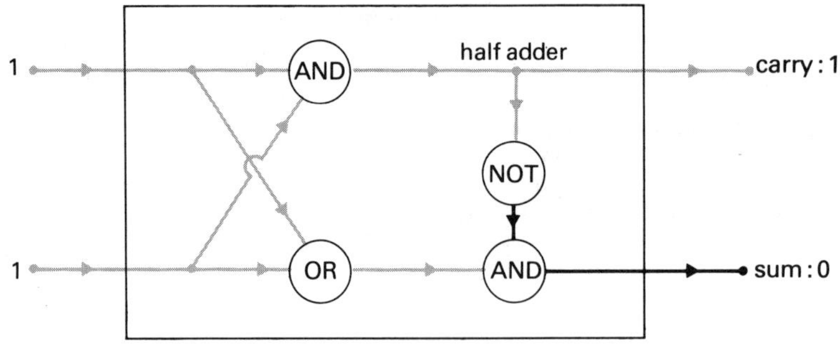

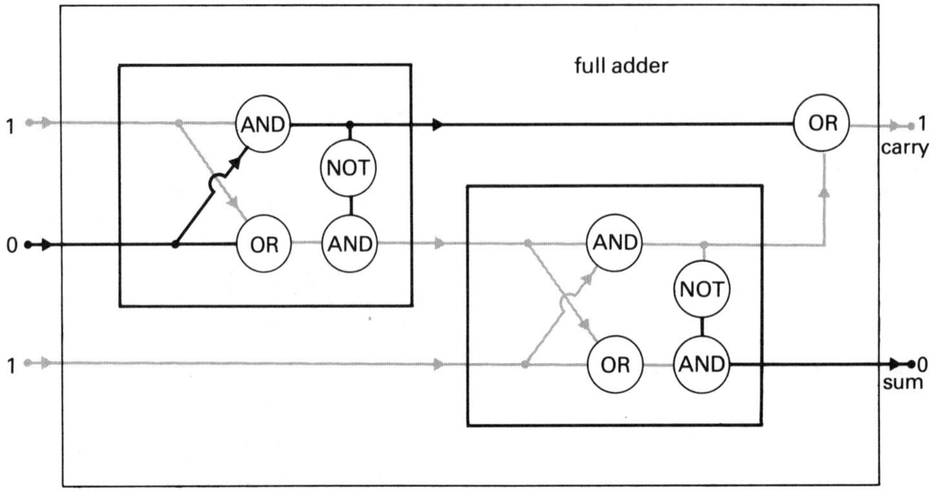

Fig. 10.9

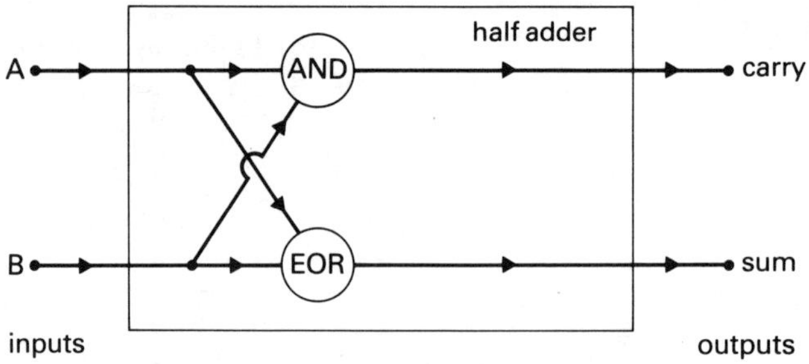

Fig. 10.10: A half adder using an exclusive OR gate

Anwer in an eight bit floating point word is

mantissa				**exponent**			
$\underline{\pm}$	$\frac{1}{2}$	$\frac{1}{4}$	$\frac{1}{8}$	$\underline{\pm}$	4	2	1
0	1	0	1	0	1	1	0

(b) Numbers are: $\frac{7}{8} \times 2^4 = 14$
and: $\frac{3}{4} \times 2^2 = 3$
Product is: $\frac{5}{8} \times 2^6 = 40$
Comment: The correct product is 42. The error is 2, or approximately 5% of the correct answer.

***7 (a)**

	− 32 16 8 4 2 1
− 1:	1 1 1 1 1 1
− 1:	+ 1 1 1 1 1 1
	(1) 1 1 1 1 1 0 = − 2

overflow = 1, 6 bit answer correct.

(b)

13:	0 0 1 1 0 1
− 24:	+ 1 0 1 0 0 0
	1 1 0 1 0 1 = − 11

overflow = 0, 6 bit answer correct.

(c) 18: 0 1 0 0 1 0
15: + 0 0 1 1 1 1

1 0 0 0 0 1 = − 31
overflow = 0, 6 bit answer incorrect.

(d) − 25: 1 0 0 1 1 1
17: + 0 1 0 0 0 1

1 1 1 0 0 0 = − 8
overflow = 0, 6 bit answer correct.

(e) − 11: 1 1 0 1 0 1
− 29: 1 0 0 0 1 1

(1) 0 1 1 0 0 0 = 24

overflow = 1, 6 bit answer incorrect.
Comment: On its own, the overflow bit does not indicate whether or not the answer is correct.

Exercise 11a

1 See Glossary of Terms.

2 (a)

Address binary	decimal	Machine instruction	Decoded instruction
0 1 0 1 0	10	0 0 1 0 0 0 0 0	INP
0 1 0 1 1	11	1 0 0 1 0 0 0 0	STO 16
0 1 1 0 0	12	1 0 1 1 0 0 0 0	ADD 16
0 1 1 0 1	13	1 0 0 1 0 0 0 1	STO 17
0 1 1 1 0	14	0 1 0 0 0 0 0 0	OUP
0 1 1 1 1	15	0 0 0 0 0 0 0 0	END
1 0 0 0 0	16		
1 0 0 0 1	17		

(b) The program inputs a number, doubles it by adding it to itself, and outputs the result.

(c) Dry run, using the number 23 for input data:

Binary machine instruction	Decoded machine instruction	Contents of accumulator and memory cells Acc	Cell 16	Cell 17
0 0 1 0 0 0 0 0	INP	23		
1 0 0 1 0 0 0 0	STO 16	23	23	
1 0 1 1 0 0 0 0	ADD 16	46	23	
1 0 0 1 0 0 0 1	STO 17	46	23	46
0 1 0 0 0 0 0 0	OUP	46	23	46
0 0 0 0 0 0 0 0	END	46	23	46

3 (a) and **(b)**

Address binary	decimal	Machine instruction	Dedcoded machine instruction
1 0 0 0 0	16	0 0 1 0 0 0 0 0	INP
1 0 0 0 1	17	1 0 0 1 1 1 0 0	STO 28
1 0 0 1 0	18	0 0 1 0 0 0 0 0	INP
1 0 0 1 1	19	1 0 0 1 1 1 0 1	STO 29
1 0 1 0 0	20	0 0 1 0 0 0 0 0	INP
1 0 1 0 1	21	1 0 0 1 1 1 1 0	STO 30
1 0 1 1 0	22	0 1 1 1 1 1 0 0	LOA 28
1 0 1 1 1	23	1 0 1 1 1 1 0 1	ADD 29
1 1 0 0 0	24	1 0 1 1 1 1 1 0	ADD 30
1 1 0 0 1	25	1 0 0 1 1 1 1 1	STO 31
1 1 0 1 0	26	0 1 0 0 0 0 0 0	OUP
1 1 0 1 1	27	0 0 0 0 0 0 0 0	END
1 1 1 0 0	28		Storage for first input number
1 1 1 0 1	29		Storage for second input number
1 1 1 1 0	30		Storage for third input number
1 1 1 1 1	31		Storage for total

(c) Dry run using the numbers 3, 19 and 51 for input data:

Binary machine instruction	Decoded machine instruction	Contents of accumulator and memory cells Acc	Cell 28	Cell 29	Cell 30	Cell 31
0 0 1 0 0 0 0 0	INP	3				
1 0 0 1 1 1 0 0	STO 28	3	3			
0 0 1 0 0 0 0 0	INP	19	3			
1 0 0 1 1 1 0 1	STO 29	19	3	19		
0 0 1 0 0 0 0 0	INP	51	3	19		
1 0 0 1 1 1 1 0	STO 30	51	3	19	51	
0 1 1 1 1 1 0 0	LOA 28	3	3	19	51	
1 0 1 1 1 1 0 1	ADD 29	22	3	19	51	
1 0 1 1 1 1 1 0	ADD 30	73	3	19	51	
1 0 0 1 1 1 1 1	STO 31	73	3	19	51	73
0 1 0 0 0 0 0 0	OUP	73	3	19	51	73
0 0 0 0 0 0 0 0	END	73	3	19	51	73

***4**

Address binary	decimal	Machine instruction	Decoded machine instruction
0 0 1 0 0	4	0 0 1 0 0 0 0 0	INP
0 0 1 0 1	5	1 0 0 1 1 0 0 0	STO 24
0 0 1 1 0	6	0 0 1 0 0 0 0 0	INP
0 0 1 1 1	7	1 0 0 1 1 0 0 1	STO 25
0 1 0 0 0	8	0 0 1 0 0 0 0 0	INP
0 1 0 0 1	9	1 0 0 1 1 0 1 0	STO 26
0 1 0 1 0	10	1 1 0 1 1 0 0 1	NEG 25
0 1 0 1 1	11	1 1 1 1 1 0 0 0	ADI 24
0 1 1 0 0	12	0 1 0 0 0 0 0 0	OUP
0 1 1 0 1	13	1 0 1 1 1 0 1 0	ADD 26
0 1 1 1 0	14	1 0 0 1 1 0 1 1	STO 28
0 1 1 1 1	15	0 1 0 0 0 0 0 0	OUP
1 0 0 0 0	16	0 0 0 0 0 0 0 0	END
1 1 0 0 0	24		Storage for first input number
1 1 0 0 1	25		Storage for second input number

1 1 0 1 0	26	Storage for third input number
1 1 0 1 1	27	Storage for result

Note: The addresses used above are only by way of example. Any consistent set of addresses is acceptable.

Exercise 11b

1 See Glossary of Terms.
2 **(a)** $2^4 = 16$ **(b)** 2
(c) $2^6 = 64$ **(d)** $2^{12} = 4096$
(e) $4096 + 64 = 4160$ (provided the address decoder is large enough)
3 **(a)** 126 **(b)** 799

Exercise 12

1 See Glossary of Terms.
2 **(a)** 0 0 1 0 0 1 1 0,unless there has been a transfer of control. **(b)** 0 0 0 0 1 1 1 0
3 **(a)** See table below **(b)** 0 0 1 1 0 1 1 0
4 1 0 0 0 0
5 100 nanoseconds
6 Accumulator
7 It depends where the numbers are just before the addition. If one is already on the accumulator, then one instruction is sufficient. If both are in the memory, then two instructions (plus one to store the answer) are needed. If one or both of the numbers are on backing store, then the whole process will take much longer.

Exercise 13a

1 See Glossary of Terms.
2 **(a)**

Program		Dry run Accumulator	A	B
IN		7		
STORE	A	7	7	
MULTIPLY	A	49	7	
STORE	A	49	49	
IN		3	49	
STORE	B	3	49	3
MULIPLY	B	9	49	3
ADD	A	58	49	3
OUT		58	49	3
HALT		58	59	3

Data: 7 3

Table for question 3(a)

Instruction		SCR	CIR	Accumulator	Contents of memory cells for data Cell 1 1 0 0 0	Cell 1 1 0 0 1	Cell 1 1 0 1 0
INP	FETCH	00001100	00100000				
	EXECUTE	00001100	00100000	01000010			
	RESET	00001101	00100000	01000010			
STO 24	FETCH	00001101	10011000	01000010			
	EXECUTE	00001101	10011000	01000010	01000010		
	RESET	00001110	10011000	01000010	01000010		
INP	FETCH	00001110	00100000	01000010	01000010		
	EXECUTE	00001110	00100000	00001100	01000010		
	RESET	00001111	00100000	00001100	01000010		
STO 25	FETCH	00001111	10011001	00001100	01000010		
	EXECUTE	00001111	10011001	00001100	01000010	00001100	
	RESET	00010000	10011001	00001100	01000010	00001100	
NEG 25	FETCH	00010000	11011001	00001100	01000010	00001100	
	EXECUTE	00010000	11011001	11110011	01000010	00001100	
	RESET	00010001	11011001	11110011	01000010	00001100	
ADI 24	FETCH	00010001	11111000	11110011	01000010	00001100	
	EXECUTE	00010001	11111000	00110110	01000010	00001100	
	RESET	00010010	11111000	00110110	01000010	00001100	
STO 26	FETCH	00010010	10011010	00110110	01000010	00001100	
	EXECUTE	00010010	10011010	00110110	01000010	00001100	00110110
	RESET	00010011	10011010	00110110	01000010	00001100	00110110
OUP	FETCH	00010011	01000000	00110110	01000010	00001100	00110110
	EXECUTE	00010011	01000000	00110110	01000010	00001100	00110110
	RESET	00010100	01000000	00110110	01000010	00001100	00110110
END	FETCH	00010100	00000000	00110110	01000010	00001100	00110110
	EXECUTE	00010100	00000000	00110110	01000010	00001100	00110110

(b) The program inputs values of A and B, and outputs the value of $A^2 + B^2$.

3 Program

Program		Dry run Accumulator	Total
IN		9	
STORE	TOTAL	9	9
IN		14	9
ADD	TOTAL	23	9
STORE	TOTAL	23	23
IN		11	23
ADD	TOTAL	34	23
STORE	TOTAL	34	34
IN		8	34
ADD	TOTAL	42	34
OUT		*42*	34
HALT		42	34

Data: 9 14 11 8

4 Program

Program		Dry run Accumulator	P
IN		5	
STORE	P	5	5
IN		3	5
MULTIPLY	P	15	5
STORE	P	15	15
OUT		*15*	15
ADD	P	30	15
ADD	P	45	15
OUT		*45*	15
HALT		45	15

Data: 5 3

5 Program

Program		Dry run Accumulator	A	TOTAL
IN		2		
STORE	A	2	2	
MULTIPY	A	4	2	
STORE	TOTAL	4	2	4
IN		6	2	4
STORE	A	6	6	4
MULTIPLY	A	36	6	4
ADD	TOTAL	40	6	4
STORE	TOTAL	40	6	40
IN		3	6	40
STORE	A	3	3	40
MULTIPLY	A	9	3	40
ADD	TOTAL	49	3	40
STORE	TOTAL	49	3	49
IN		5	3	49
STORE	A	5	5	49
MULTIPLY	A	25	5	49
ADD	TOTAL	74	5	49
OUT		74	5	49
HALT		74	5	49

Data: 2 6 3 5

6 Program

Program		Dry run Accumulator	LEN	BRD	AREA
IN		17			
STORE	LEN	17	17		
IN		9	17		
STORE	BRD	9	17	9	
MULTIPLY	LEN	153	17	9	
STORE	AREA	153	17	9	153
LOAD	LEN	17	17	9	153
OUT		17	17	9	153
LOAD	BRD	9	17	9	153
OUT		9	17	9	153
LOAD	AREA	153	17	9	153
OUT		153	17	9	153
HALT		153	17	9	153

Data: 17 9

Exercise 13b

1 See Glossary of Terms.

2 (a) The program inputs one number. If the number is 100 or more, it is output, otherwise it is not.

(b) Program

	Program		Dry run with input 150 Accumulator	N	Dry run with input 99 Accumulator	N
	IN		150		99	
	STORE	N	150	150	99	99
	SUBTRACT	+ 100	50	150	− 1	99
	JINEG	END	50	150	− 1	99
	LOAD	IN	150	150		
	OUT		**150**	150		
END	HALT		150	150	− 1	99

Questions 3, 4 and 5 closely resemble examples 5, 6 and 7 respectively.

3 The second number is subtracted from the first one. If the difference is negative, then the first number is smaller. Otherwise the second number is smaller.

	Program		Dry run Accumulator	A	B
	IN		31		
	STORE	A	31	31	
	IN		27	31	
	STORE	B	27	31	27
	LOAD	A	31	31	27
	SUBTRACT	B	4	31	27
	JINEG	X	4	31	27
	LOAD	B	27	31	27
	OUT		**27**	31	27
	JUMP	END	27	31	27
X	LOAD	A			
	OUT				
END	HALT		27	31	27

Data: 31 27

4

	Program		Dry run First Acc	X	Second Acc	X	Third Acc	X
START	IN		3		8	3	−1	512
	JINEG	END	3		8	3	−1	512
	OUT		**3**		**8**	3		
	STORE	X	3	3	8	8		
	MULTIPLY	X	9	3	64	8		
	MULTIPLY	X	27	3	512	8		
	OUT		**27**	3	**512**	8		
	JUMP	START	27	3	512	8		
END	HALT						−1	512

Data: 3 8 −1

5 This program is dry run for the first, second and last input numbers only. (see table below)

Table for question 5

	Program		Dry run First Acc	TOTAL	COUNT	Second Acc	TOTAL	COUNT	Last Acc	TOTAL	COUNT
	LOAD	+0	0								
	STORE	TOTAL	0	0							
	LOAD	+10	10	0							
NEXT	STORE	COUNT	10	0	10	9	6	9	1	56	1
	IN		6	0	10	9	6	9	4	56	1
	ADD	TOTAL	6	0	10	15	6	9	60	56	1
	STORE	TOTAL	6	6	10	15	15	9	60	60	1
	LOAD	COUNT	10	6	10	9	15	9	1	60	1
	SUBTRACT	+1	9	6	10	8	15	9	0	60	1
	JIZERO	END	9	6	10	8	15	9	0	60	1
	JUMP	NEXT	9	6	10	8	15	9			
END	LOAD	TOTAL							60	60	1
	OUT								**60**	60	1
	DIVIDE	+10							6	60	1
	OUT								**6**	60	1
	HALT								6	60	1

Data: 6 9 11 3 2 5 7 8 5 4

6

	Program		Dry run First Acc	X	Second Acc	X	Third Acc	X
START	IN		101		5	101	0	5
	JIZERO	END	101		5	101	0	5
	STORE	X	101	101	5	5		
	SUBTRACT	+100	1	101	−95	5		
	JINEG	START	1	101	−95	5		
	LOAD	X	101	101				
	OUT		**101**	101				
	JUMP	START	101	101				
END	HALT						0	5

Data: 101 5 0

*7 This program is dry run for the first, second, ninth and tenth numbers only.

	Program		Dry runs First Acc	INT	Second Acc	INT	Ninth Acc	INT	Tenth Acc	INT
	LOAD	+1	1							
NEXT	STORE	INT	1	1	2	2	9	9	10	10
	MULTIPLY	INT	1	1	4	2	81	9	100	10
	OUT		**1**	1	**4**	2	**81**	9	**100**	10
	LOAD	INT	1	1	2	2	9	9	10	10
	SUBTRACT	+10	−9	1	−8	2	−1	9	0	10
	JIZERO	END	−9	1	−8	2	−1	9	0	10
	LOAD	INT	1	1	2	2	9	9		
	ADD	+1	2	1	3	2	10	9		
	JUMP	NEXT	2	1	3	2	10	9		
END	HALT								0	10

Data: none

*8 Separate memory cells for length, breadth and area are not needed. One cell is needed for the loop counter, and one for the length. The program is dry run for the first, second and last repetitions of the loop only.

	Program		Dry runs First Acc	LEN	COUNT	Second Acc	LEN	COUNT	Last Acc	LEN	COUNT
	LOAD	+6	6								
NEXT	STORE	COUNT	6		6	5	7	5	1	2	1
	IN		7		6	6	7	5	8	2	1
	STORE	LEN	7	7	6	6	6	5	8	8	1
	IN		4	7	6	3	6	5	6	8	1
	MULTIPLY	LEN	28	7	6	18	6	5	48	8	1
	OUT		**28**	7	6	**18**	6	5	**48**	8	1
	LOAD	COUNT	6	7	6	5	6	5	1	8	1
	SUBTRACT	+1	5	7	6	4	6	5	0	8	1
	JIZERO	END	5	7	6	4	6	5	0	8	1
	JUMP	NEXT	5	7	6	4	6	5			
END	HALT								0	8	1

Data: 7 4 6 3 5 8 9 4 2 7 8 6

Notice that the data is in the order: length, breadth, length, breadth, etc.

Exercise 14a

1 See Glossary of Terms.

2 A high level language is problem oriented. It relates to the application of the computer, and not to the structure of the computer. High level language programs consist of a set of statements, using base ten numbers and, in most cases, English words.

3 Subprograms considerably reduce the length of a program by eliminating unnecessary repetition of statements.

4 The test data did not try out all the logical paths in the program.

5

High level language	*Low level language*
Programs consist of statements	Programs consist of instructions
Problem oriented	Machine oriented
Programs are shorter and easier to write	Programs are longer and harder to write
Programs are slower to run on a computer	Programs are faster to run on a computer.

Exercise 14b

1

BASIC	CESIL		Dry run Acc	A	B	C
5 READ A, B	IN		45			
	STORE	A	45	45		
	IN		9	45		
	STORE	B	9	45	9	
10 LET C = A/B	LOAD	A	45	45	9	
	DIVIDE	B	5	45	9	
	STORE	C	5	45	9	5
15 PRINT C	LOAD	C	5	45	9	5
	OUT		5	45	9	5
20 STOP	HALT		5	45	9	5
	%					
25 DATA 45, 9	45 9 *					
30 END						

2

BASIC	CESIL		Dry run Acc	L	B	H	V
5 READ L,B,H	IN		8				
	STORE	L	8	8			
	IN		3	8			
	STORE	B	3	8	3		
	IN		5	8	3		
	STORE	H	5	8	3	5	
10 LET V = L*B*H	LOAD	L	8	8	3	5	
	MULTIPLY	B	24	8	3	5	
	MULTIPLY	H	120	8	3	5	
	STORE	V	120	8	3	5	120
15 PRINT V	LOAD	V	120	8	3	5	120
	OUT		120	8	3	5	120
20 STOP	HALT		120	8	3	5	120
	%						
25 DATA 8, 3, 5	8 3 5 *						
30 END							

3

BASIC	CESIL		Dry run Acc	R	A
5 READ R	IN		14		
	STORE	R	14	14	
10 LET A = 22/7*R*R	LOAD	R	14	14	
	MULTIPLY	R	196	14	
	MULTIPLY	+22	4312	14	
	DIVIDE	+7	616	14	
	STORE	A	616	14	616
15 PRINT	LOAD	A	616	14	616
	OUT		616	14	616
20 STOP	HALT		616	14	616
	%				
25 DATA 14	14 *				
30 END					

BASIC	CESIL			Dry run First loop Acc	F	I	Third loop Acc	F	I
5 READ F	START	IN		4			0	9	108
		STORE	F	4	4		0	0	108
10 IF F = 0 THEN 30		JIZERO	FINISH	4	4		0	0	108
15 LET I = 12*F		MULTIPLY	+12	48	4				
		STORE	I	48	4	48			
20 PRINT F, I		LOAD	F	4	4	48			
		OUT		4	4	48			
		LOAD	I	48	4	48			
		OUT		48	4	48			
25 GO TO 5		JUMP	START	48	4	48			
30 STOP	FINISH	HALT					0	0	108
	%								
35 DATA 4,9,0		4 9 0 *							
40 END									

Exercise 15

1 See Glossary of Terms

3 Some others are:

BOS/360: The Basic Operating System on IBM 360 series computers.

VME/B and VME/K: Used on ICL 2900 series computers, these operating systems may be adapted for multiprogramming, multi-access, batch processing or remote job entry.

MULTICS: Used by Honeywell 645 computers.

4 **(a)** Multiprogramming **(b)** Single program operation **(c)** Batch processing.

5 **(a)** Some parts of the meal can be cooking while others are being prepared.
(b) The first coat can be drying in some rooms while the second coat is being applied in others.
(c) One load can be washing while another is spinning.

Exercise 16

1 See Glossary of Terms

2 **(a)** Installation engineer **(b)** Computer salesman
(c) Computer architect **(d)** Programmer
(e) Commissioning engineer **(f)** Systems analyst
(g) Programmer **(h)** Systems analyst
(i) Data processing manager
(j) Data processing manager
(k) Data preparation staff **(l)** Research enginner
(m) Computer operator **(n)** Operations manager
(o) Software writer

Exercise 17

1 See Glossary of Terms

2 It is hoped that pupils will recognize that each data processing system described in this question is very similar to one of the examples. The answers to the data processing questions, and the layout of the systems flow diagram can follow those of the appropriate example fairly closely.
Specifically:
Parts **(a)** and **(b)** resemble example 3.
Part **(c)** resembles example 4.
Parts **(d)** and **(f)** resemble the first part (accessing the database) of example 4.
Part **(e)** resembles example 5.

***6** The computerized system closely resembles the airline booking system, example 4.

Exercise 18

1 See Glossary of Terms

2 **(a)** name, address, telephone number **(b)** name **(c)** sequential.

3 **(a)** account number, name, address, date, balance.
(b) account number, date, transaction type, amount.
(c) Two are mentioned. One is in order of account number, the other is not.
(d) account number.
(e) account number. An error in an account number would cause the entry to go into the wrong account.

4 **(a)** 3878.41, 4359.63 **(b)** The fourth card
(c) 813, 17 138.37 **(d)** 110.37
(e) The number 27.41 in the fourth card. (It should be 68.41)

5 **(a)** Range checks
(b) Second card: account number too large.
(c) Third card: date wrong (4th month has only 30 days).
(d) Fourth card: transaction type 3.
(e) Sixth card: transaction amount exceeds £250.000.

6 60623**3** 31695**0** 72693**9**

7 correct incorrect correct

8 **(a)** 416**2**, 2125**1**, 20060**8**
(b) 275**3** should be 275**5**

9 **(a)**
1 4 3 5 2 no interchange
1 4 3 5 2 interchange
1 3 4 5 2 no interchange
1 3 4 5 2 interchange
1 3 4 2 5 largest number now last.
etc.

***10** If an entire set of comparisons results in no interchanges, then the numbers are already in order.

11 1 2 3 6 7 9 10 11 12 17 18 19 23 24 29

12 **(a)**
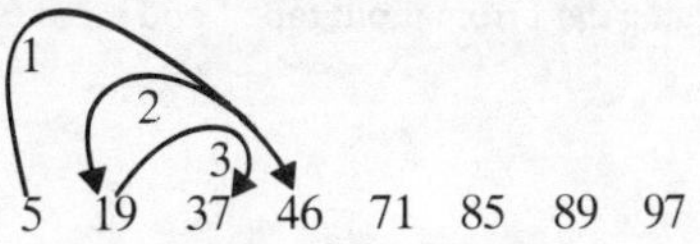

(b)
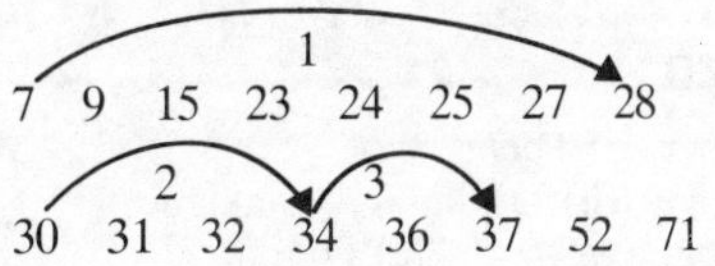

***13** Figure 18.6

Exercise 19

1 See Glossary of Terms and the text of the chapter.

2 Useful sources of information are the magazines *Computer Weekly* and *Computing* and publications from computer manufactuers.

3 The text singles out military uses and space research, but cases can be made for others.

4 Surgery monitoring in hospitals (with electrocardiographs). Traffic control (with television). Space research (with rockets and satellites). Ceefax/Oracle/Prestel with television). Weather forecasting (with satellites).

7

batch processing	*interactive processing*	*real time processing*
cheque clearing	electronic funds transfer	traffic control
	newspaper production	rocket guidance
	order processing	weather forecasting
	word processing	
	Prestel	

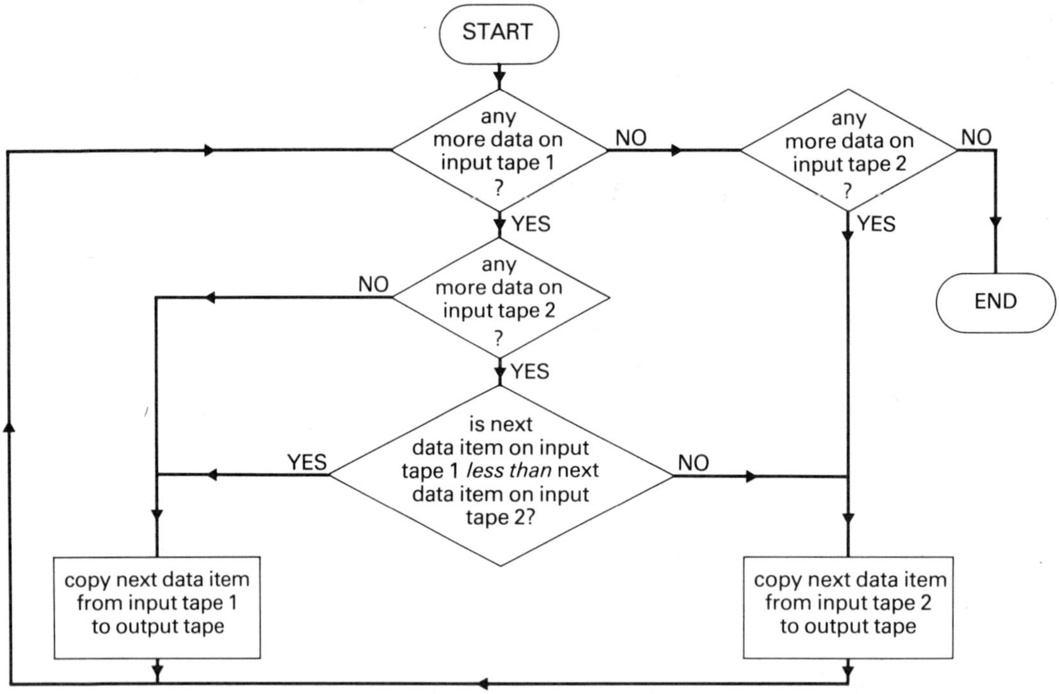

Fig. 18.6: Merging data from input tape 1 and input tape 2 to output tape

Exercise 20

1 See Glossary of Terms
2 **(a)** Analogue **(b)** Digital **(c)** Analogue **(d)** Analogue or digital **(e)** Digital
3 Analogue devices: gas or electricity meters (with dials), speedometers, thermometers, radio tuning dials, sundials.
Digital devices: gas or electricity meters (with figures), mileage meters in cars, tape position meters on tape recorders, floor indicators on lifts, traffic lights.
Hybrid devices: T.V. sets.
4 Commercial data is digital. Analogue computers have limited storage capacity.

Exercise 21

1 See Glossary of Terms and text of chapter.
2 **(a)** Lady Lovelace **(b)** M. V. Wilkes **(c)** George Boole **(d)** William Shockley **(e)** John von Neumann
3 **(a)** Alan Turing: (i) Proved that a small number of simple instructions can solve any problem capable of logical solution. (ii) Worked on COLOSSUS at Bletchley Park. (iii) Worked on ACE.
(b) Program, input – processor – output structure of computers.
(c) Both worked for the U.S. Census Bureau.
4 **(a)** ASCC, ENIAC **(b)** Analytical Engine **(c)** ASCC **(d)** TXO, IBM 7000, ATLAS **(e)** Hollerith's calculator.
5 Work of Jacquard, Babbage, Hollerith and later applications.
6 Work of Boole and Shannon, incorporated by Von Neumann.
7

ENIAC	*EDSAC*
base ten	base two
programmed by connecting wires	stored program

8 Some possibilities: Manchester University Mark 1: First computer using Von Neumann's principles.
Zuse computers: Probably similar to M. U. Mark 1, but constructed earlier.
ENIAC: First electronic computer.
Analytical Engine: First programmable computer with input – process – output layout.

Exercise 22

1 Name, address, age, whether married or not, number of children, occupation, wage, bank balance, value of house and household goods, endorsements to driving licence, amount of tax paid during current tax year.
5 One possibility is the storage of psychiatric records of patients. There is evidence of doctors and patients withholding information from these records, because they are not satisfied that their security is adequate.

Index